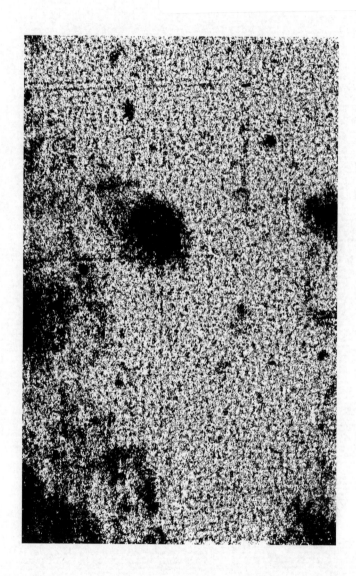

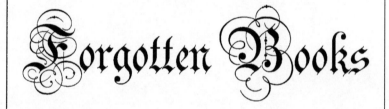

ISBN 978-0-260-23394-3
PIBN 11013492

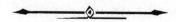

English
Français
Deutsche
Italiano
Español
Português

www.forgottenbooks.com

Mythology Photography **Fiction**
Fishing Christianity **Art** Cooking
Essays Buddhism Freemasonry
Medicine **Biology** Music **Ancient
Egypt** Evolution Carpentry Physics
Dance Geology **Mathematics** Fitness
Shakespeare **Folklore** Yoga Marketing
Confidence Immortality Biographies
Poetry **Psychology** Witchcraft
Electronics Chemistry History **Law**
Accounting **Philosophy** Anthropology
Alchemy Drama Quantum Mechanics
Atheism Sexual Health **Ancient History**
Entrepreneurship Languages Sport
Paleontology Needlework Islam
Metaphysics Investment Archaeology
Parenting Statistics Criminology
Motivational

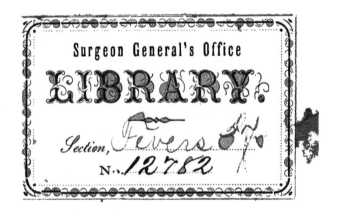

TREATISE

ON

FEBRILE DISEASES,

INCLUDING

INTERMITTING, REMITTING, AND CONTINUED FEVERS;
ERUPTIVE FEVERS; INFLAMMATIONS;
HEMORRHAGIES; AND THE
PROFLUVIA;

IN WHICH AN ATTEMPT IS MADE

TO PRESENT, AT ONE VIEW, WHATEVER, IN THE PRESENT
STATE OF MEDICINE, IT IS REQUISITE FOR THE
PHYSICIAN TO KNOW,

RESPECTING THE

SYMPTOMS, CAUSES, AND CURE

OF

THOSE DISEASES;

WITH

EXPERIMENTAL ESSAYS,

ON CERTAIN FEBRILE SYMPTOMS, ON THE NATURE OF INFLAMMA-
TION, AND ON THE MANNER ON WHICH OPIUM AND
TOBACCO ACT ON THE LIVING ANIMAL BODY.

BY

A. PHILIPS WILSON, M. D. F. R. S. Ed.

FELLOW OF THE ROYAL COLLEGE OF PHYSICIANS EDINBURGH, &c.

VOL. I.

FIRST AMERICAN FROM THE SECOND ENGLISH EDITION.

FIVE VOLUMES COMPRISED IN TWO.

HARTFORD:
PUBLISHED AND SOLD BY OLIVER D. COOKE.
SOLD ALSO BY JOHNSON AND WARNER, PHILADELPHIA; COLLINS
AND PERKINS, NEW-YORK; AND JAMES BURDETT
AND CO. BOSTON.

LINCOLN & GLEASON, PRINTERS.
1809.

CONTENTS.

CONTENTS.

CONTENTS.

CONTENTS.

PREFACE.

———◆———

WHEN I first turned my attention particularly to febrile diseases, I had no view of undertaking so laborious a work as that in which I am now engaged. For several years I devoted the whole of my time to the study of these complaints, in order to qualify myself for reading lectures on them, which I did in the summer of 1796, at Edinburgh.

My reasons for making choice of febrile diseases for the subject of my lectures, were that they form the most important branch of medicine, and that which is least generally understood. The practice in most other diseases is simple. In dropsy, for instance, we give a diuretic; if one fails we prescribe another; there is no nicety required in their exhibition; there are no minute circumstances to be considered in order to determine the propriety of prescribing the remedy; we have only to ascertain what the disease is, and what the proper dose of the medicine.

In febrile complaints the symptoms are infinitely varied; minute circumstances often point out essential differences in their nature, and consequently in the plan of treatment. A physician cannot spend too much time in the study of fevers, nor will any man find a little sufficient for acquiring a competent knowledge of them.

A very infirm state of health has obliged me to abandon the plan of continuing to give lectures; and I am inclined to think that I may render the result of my studies useful to others in another form.

Entering on the study of medicine, the student, anxious to abridge his labour, looks for some book where he may find nearly the sum of what is known on the subject; for the work of some author who had been at the trouble to collect together the valuable facts relating to the symptoms, causes, and cure of diseases, from the various sources through which they are scattered, and in which they are generally blended with many useless and ill founded observations. For such a work, however, he looks in vain.

The systematic medical writers of this country, intending their publications to serve as text-books to lectures, or mere introductions to the study of medicine, have given little more than the outline. This cannot be said indeed of those of other countries. But their arrangements of the symptoms of diseases, as well as their modes of practice, are in general so exceptionable, compared with those which have for some time been taught in Britain, that their works can only be recommended to those who have already studied medicine, and are capable of guarding against their errors, while they acquire a knowledge of the many useful facts they contain.*

The student then cannot acquire even a moderate knowledge of diseases from books without having recourse to the original writers and comparing them together, and for this, few students, I believe few practitioners, find leisure. It is to preclude the necessity of this labour, as far as relates to febrile diseases, that I have undertaken the following work.

It will be proper here to make a few observations on the plan I shall pursue, in considering the symptoms, causes, and cure of the diseases I am to treat of.

A physician about to prescribe must, in the first place, determine what the disease, and how great the danger, is. If he fails in determining these points, he acts in the dark. In treating of diseases then, we are led in the first place to attend to their symptoms.

It is customary in giving a regular view of the symptoms of any complaint, first to give a detailed account of all its symptoms; then, a separate view of such as form its *diagnosis*, that is, distinguish it from other complaints; and lastly, of such as give the *prognosis*, or those symptoms from which we prognosticate the event of the disease. This, it is evident, occasions much repetition. The symptoms which assist in forming the *diagnosis* and *prognosis* are the greater number of the symptoms of every complaint; but according to this plan, after detailing the whole symptoms, we must recapitulate them.

Notwithstanding this, in some cases, where the symptoms are very complicated, it is necessary to recapitulate those which chiefly serve to distinguish the disease from others, and prognosticate its event. In general, however, all this repetition may be avoided

---

* Foreign medical writers, although certainly much inferior in general to those of this country in their arrangement both of the symptoms and treatment of diseases, and in their modes of practice, yet greatly excel us (particularly the German writers) in a point of the greatest importance, in the number of facts which their writings contain. This proceeds from two causes, their field of observation being more extensive, owing to the communication between different parts of the Continent being much freer than between any part of it and this country; and to the writers being in general more laborious in their search after facts, than those of Britain. I have therefore, in the following work, availed myself of the writings of foreigners more than the authors of this country have generally done.

In most instances it will be as distinct a plan to notice, as we proceed in considering the detail of symptoms, those which assist in forming the *diagnosis* and *prognosis*.*

Why do we not pursue a plan still more concise, it may be asked, and confine ourselves merely to a view of the *diagnostic* and *prognostic* symptoms? Of what use can a knowledge of the other symptoms be to the physician? To this it may be answered, that the symptoms of diseases which have no share in forming the diagnosis or prognosis, may throw light on some of the functions of the system; they may assist in determining the nature of the complaint, and thus enable us to prescribe the proper remedies. But granting that they do neither, it is necessary for us to be acquainted with them, for two reasons, that their appearance may not disconcert us, and because we are not assured that as our knowledge extends, an acquaintance with these symptoms will not prove more useful.

Nothing, it is evident, would retard the progress of knowledge more, than only making such observations as at once lead to some useful inference. And the natural bias of the mind to neglect the observations which do not lead to such inferences, has in fact retarded the progress of medicine in all its departments. The physician has often marked only those symptoms of a disease which served to distinguish it from others with which he happened to be acquainted; so that, in a different part of the world, although the disease assumed the same appearance, his diagnostics have been found insufficient. The experimenter has often attended only to those appearances which affected a favourite hypothesis; so that when we repeat his experiments, we can hardly persuade ourselves that they are the same of which we have read so mutilated an account; and our hypothesis, or view in making the experiment, being different from his, the neglected circumstances may appear to us the circumstances of most importance.

Those whose observations have served most to advance the knowledge of diseases, have accurately observed and recorded every fact which presented itself, relating to the subject of which they treat; and, when they could make no useful application themselves of the facts they observed, left them for the consideration of their successors, who, in a more advanced state of science, have often derived from them important information. They have served to point out distinctions and analogies, which could not have suggested themselves to the first observer.

The symptoms of diseases then may be divided into three classes. Those which assist in forming the diagnosis; those which assist in forming the prognosis; and those which, in the present state of our knowledge, serve neither purpose. Of these

* This indeed is proper in all cases, even where we mean to recapitulate these symptoms, as it renders a shorter recapitulation necessary.

classes of symptoms, that which forms the diagnosis, that is, distinguishes each disease from every other, is unquestionably the
most important. The diagnostic symptoms of each disease have
been collected into one or more short sentences, and this collection has been termed its character or definition, by means of
which the learner is assisted in acquiring the power of distinguishing it from others. And for the purpose of farther aiding the
memory, the characters of diseases have been arranged in different
ways, or digested into systems.

The general principle on which such systems are constructed
is very simple.

From the symptoms common to the characters of those diseases
which resemble each other, a general character is formed, under
which the particular characters are arranged, and which is termed
the character of the order. And in like manner, from the characters of several orders having certain symptoms in common, the
character of a class including these orders is formed. Thus diseases are arranged under classes, orders, and genera. The genera
being occasionally divided into species, and these into varieties.*

We readily perceive the advantages of such a system to a
learner, but its advantages are not confined to learners. It is not
surely to be supposed that any man can construct a system of nosology from his own experience, equal in accuracy to that which
the combined experience of physicians for ages has constructed
with difficulty. The importance of a due attention to nosology,
therefore, I regard as unquestionable. It is of use to the experienced practitioner; it is absolutely necessary for those who
are only entering on the practice of medicine.

There are two things then aimed at by the nosologist; in the
first place he is to give an accurate character of each disease, by
which is meant (as appears from what has just been said) not an
account of all the symptoms of the disease, not a description of the
complaint as it really appears in practice, but merely an enumeration of a certain set of its symptoms; of those which either at
the same time, or in succession, are constantly observed to attend
it, and distinguish it from others. The second thing aimed at by
the nosologist is to arrange the characters of diseases in a methodical manner, that is, to adopt that mode of arrangement which best
assists the memory. In both we shall find there are difficulties
which appear to be insurmountable, so that a perfect system of
nosology is not to be looked for. But we have reason to believe,
there is still much room for improving our present systems.

* The plan I shall adopt in the following Treatise, not requiring so
many divisions, I have arranged diseases under classes, orders, and species.
A disease, according to the common acceptation of the term, being more
properly a species than a genus. The species are occasionally divided
into varieties.

. After the symptoms of diseases, we are led to consider their, causes, since these often assist both in distinguishing the complaint and prognosticating its event. Besides, as they tend to elucidate its nature, they are to be considered before the treatment.

The causes of diseases, like their symptoms, may be divided into three classes. The *predisposing* causes, comprehending those states of body which are favourable to the production of the disease, and the various causes which induce such states of body. The *occasional* or *exciting* causes, those which seem to excite the disease. These two sets of causes have been termed the remote causes. And the *proximate* cause, which has been defined, that which when present causes, when removed removes, and when changed changes, the disease. To this head (that of the proximate cause) belongs, what has been termed the *ratio symptomatum*.

. A division of the remote causes into predisposing and exciting, has been deemed necessary by almost every person who has attempted to give a methodical view of diseases. In many cases this division is proper, and if we aim at accuracy of arrangement, absolutely necessary. There are some diseases which have but few exciting causes; some, it has been ascertained, have but one, contagion. In such cases, any other circumstance which seems favourable to the production of the disease must be regarded as a predisposing cause, as a cause operating merely by bringing the body to that state which is favourable to the action of the exciting cause.

But there are many cases, where we cannot distinguish these two sets of causes, in which there is none of the causes which have been regarded as predisposing, that is, not itself capable of producing the disease. And so notorious is our want of precision in this particular, that they have almost become maxims in medicine, that a predisposing cause, applied in a greater degree, becomes an exciting cause; and, vice versa, that an exciting cause applied in a less degree, acts as a predisposing. Can we, in any case where these maxims hold good, admit of a division of the remote causes into predisposing and exciting ?

It is true, that in all cases, there are some causes which act more generally as exciting, others as predisposing ; and it is proper to adopt an arrangement which will point out this difference, which will shew the tendency of any particular cause to act in the one way or the other. But this difference cannot surely be regarded as a sufficient foundation for dividing them into predisposing and exciting. A division which implies that every cause acts only in the one way or the other. We constantly find the same circumstance placed by one author among the predisposing, and by another among the exciting causes of the same disease, according to the different opinions they entertained of the nature of the disease, and the modus operandi of its causes.

These considerations have induced me not to attempt such a division of the remote causes of diseases in every instance. In cases where it may be attempted with some degree of success, at the same time that I adopt the division, I shall point out those causes which belong properly to neither class, but act sometimes as predisposing, at other times as exciting.

With regard to the proximate cause of diseases, our knowledge is extremely deficient. There are few instances in which we can form even probable conjectures on this subject, and very few indeed in which we have any certain knowledge. In general therefore I shall employ little time in considering the proximate cause of diseases. It will be necessary now and then to point out the errors of prevalent opinions ; and we shall meet with a few instances in which observation has afforded some real knowledge respecting the proximate cause, which is not to be overlooked.

The common definition of the proximate cause is exceptionable ; since, in some instances, it applies to the remote causes, If we apply a considerable degree of pressure to the brain, by the finger for example, on the unossified bregma, apoplexy is the consequence. The degree of apoplexy is proportioned to the degree of pressure, and the pressure removed, the apoplexy ceases. The above definition of the proximate cause applies in this case then to the compressing force. It is not the compressing force, however, but the change it induces on the brain which is here the proximate cause of the apoplexy, the compressing force being evidently the exciting cause. It must surely be granted, that the proximate cause of diseases exists in the body ; but the compressing force, in this instance, is external.

A very slight alteration of this definition, however, removes the objection. The proximate cause may be defined, That state of the whole or any part of the system, which when present causes, removed removes, and changed changes, the disease. The proximate cause of dropsy, for instance, is in many cases a debilitated state of the vessels, in consequence of which the exhalation being increased, and the absorption diminished, watery collections are formed.

According to this definition of the proximate cause, every disease has several proximate causes. In the jaundice, for example, the definition applies to the accumulation of bile in the liver and gall ducts ; it also applies to the biliary calculus sticking in the duct ; if the presence of the stone in the duct is owing to a preturnatural constriction there, which is sometimes the case, the definition also applies to this. In cholera it applies to the increased action of the liver, and to the presence of an unusual quantity of bile in the alimentary canal, &c. ,—Some attempt to confine the term proximate cause to that which immediately, that is, without the intervention of other causes, produces the symptoms of the disease. But there is no common cause which immediately produces the symptoms of a disease. Each symptom has its own proximate cause, which has no share in producing any other symptom of the complaint. Thus in jaundice, the immediate cause of the pain is the irritation of the duct ; the immediate cause of the yellowness is the presence of bile in the circulating fluids ; and of costiveness, the want of it in the intestines. But is there not, it may be said, some cause, the last in the chain of proximate causes common to all the symptoms, which should be regarded as the immediate cause of the disease? When such a cause can be distinctly traced, it doubtless deserves exclusively the name of proximate cause ; this, however, can very rarely be done. And when we find any cause, to which it can be proved that the above definition applies, we are more fortunate than we are in nine cases out of ten.

With regard to the ratio symptomatum, that is, the application of the proximate cause of a disease to trace the proximate causes of its symptoms ; or when we are ignorant of the proximate cause of the disease, of our general knowledge of the animal œconomy to trace the proximate cause of some of its symptoms ; our knowledge is very defective. In most diseases indeed, the causes of some symptoms readily suggest themselves. If we meet with bilious vomiting, we are at no less to account for the nausea which preceded it ; if the internal fauces are swelled and inflamed, we readily explain, and could have foretold, the difficulty of deglutition which attends these symptoms. When the cause of any symptom is thus evident, it requires little comment ; when it is not, all that we can say of it is, in most cases, but conjecture. It is evident we can never give the ratio symptomatum of any disease fully, till we are acquainted with its proximate cause. This consideration alone is sufficient to convince us, how unsuccessful our attempts in this part of the subject must generally prove.

In attempting to trace the proximate cause of diseases, and still more in giving the ratio symptomatum, we are often assisted by observing the morbid appearances discovered by dissection after death. These are also frequently useful by tending more directly to point out the proper treatment of the disease. I say more directly, because every thing which tends to elucidate the proximate cause and ratio symptomatum, tends unquestionably to improve the treatment. It will often be necessary for us therefore to attend to the morbid appearances discovered by dissection after death.

In giving an account of these, there are three things which particularly demand attention. We must endeavour to distingulsh those changes which have been the cause of death, from those which were the cause of the disease; such as were the cause or consequence of the disease, from such as take place after death, and which are different in different circumstances; and such as were the cause or consequence of the particular complaint of which the patient died, from such as were connected with other disorders under which he had laboured. In these respects authors have been extremely negligent, often not even attempting to point out such distinctions. So that in giving a detail of the morbid appearances connected with particular diseases, (except when the change of structure observed is evidently such as must have produced the symptoms preceding death) much accuracy in these particulars cannot always be expected. But it is only in proportion as these points are ascertained, that we can make any use of the knowledge we acquire by opening bodies. In those cases, where no such distinctions can be made, our observations may prove useful to our successors, who will be enabled to make these distinctions in proportion as medical science becomes more perfect. To ourselves they are quite useless.

All the knowledge we derive from attending to the symptoms and causes of diseases, may be regarded as useful to the physician, only as far as it conduces to improve their treatment. It is not long since it was common with physicians to pretend, in most instances, to a knowledge of the proximate cause, and to boast of establishing on this foundation alone their rules of practice. But a juster mode of reasoning has convinced their successors, that they are able, in very few instances indeed, to determine the proximate cause of diseases; and that even in these instances, from the want of an accurate knowledge of the operation of remedies, they cannot with any degree of certainty determine, a priori, the modes of practice which will prove most successful.

Had we a perfect knowledge of medicine, such a work as that I am engaged in would be superfluous. There would then be no need for what is termed a system of the practice of medicine. A knowledge of another branch of the science, of the theory of medicine, of that branch which teaches the nature of the different functions of the body, the changes induced on them by disease, and the operation of the different means found capable of restoring their healthy state, would enable us to make the best use of every remedy we possess. But so deficient is our knowledge of the theory of medicine, that it often proves but of little use in practice. In many cases we have little else to conduct us in the treatment of diseases but the knowledge of what has formerly proved beneficial or hurtful. This is the most valuable information which the physician can acquire. It is the deficiency of our knowledge which renders a system of practice necessary; but this deficiency is so great, that such a system must at present be regarded as the most important branch of medicine.

Although we are unable to deduce the proper treatment of diseases from our knowledge of the different functions of the body, of their condition in the various complaints we are subject to, and the modus operandi of remedies, yet there are certain principles which regulate the treatment of many diseases, or even sets of diseases. With these it is of great consequence to be acquainted. They not only assist the memory, but in some measure serve, instead of a more perfect knowledge, to direct our practice in those diseases which have only lately made their appearance, or been distinguished from others, and of the treatment of which consequently our experience is but imperfect. These principles I shall take pains to trace as we proceed in considering the different orders of febrile diseases.

The best way of assisting the memory in recollecting the different means employed for the cure of diseases, is dividing these means into different heads ; pointing out the different ends we have in view in prescribing our remedies ; and arranging together the means which have been found to answer each of these ends.

This is what in medical language has been termed forming and fulfilling indications of cure. It is common to subdivide the means of fulfilling each indication ; and some have carried their divisions much farther, by which they have involved themselves in several difficulties. Their divisions and subdivisions have sometimes become so numerous, that so far from assisting the memory, it is easier to remember the treatment of a disease, without any arrangement at all, than their mode of dividing it. Besides, our knowledge is too imperfect in almost every instance to admit of such minute division, so that wherever it is attempted it is founded more or less on hypothesis.

It is evident, that before we can lay down any indications of cure, (except such as are so general that they hardly deserve the name and are quite useless) we must know something, both of the nature of the complaint, and of the operation of the remedies we are about to employ. If both the nature of the complaint, and the operation of the remedies that relieve it, be wholly unknown ; if our practice, as we shall find it in many instances, be wholly empirical, we cannot with any propriety lay down indications of cure, because they must then rest merely on the supposed nature of the disease, and the supposed operation of the remedies. Even in these cases indeed it has been customary to lay down indications, but they have always misled, and often been the source of much mischief.

In considering the treatment of diseases then I shall avoid numerous divisions. When our knowledge admits of it, I shall lay down indications of cure, and consider the means of fulfilling them; when it does not, I shall attempt some other mode of arrangement, which may equally assist the memory, and tend less to mislead. I shall not spend much time in considering remedies which have proved unsuccessful, or old modes of practice which are now abandoned. It will sometimes be proper to take notice of some of these, in order to warn against popular errors, and it will sometimes be of use to compare former modes of practice with those which have superseded them. But for the most part we shall find, that time may be better spent than in discussions of this nature. It is not only the most concise and simple, but in general the most useful way of laying down the mode of treatment in any diease, to give only the result of our experience in it; merely to point out that mode of practice which has proved most successful, together with the rational attempts which have been made to render it more so.

The modus operandi of remedies is the only head relating to the knowledge of diseases that remains to be mentioned. As we proceed I shall occasionally lay before the reader what appears to be ascertained in this part of the subject.

Such is the plan I shall follow in considering the symptoms, causes, and cure of the diseases I mean to treat of. A few general observations on my plan still remain to be made.

It is common with those who write, as well as those who deliver lectures, for the instruction of medical students, to speak as if all they say were the result of their own observation alone ; and this they do, not from any inclination to deceive, because they cannot for a moment hope that every thing they say will be regarded as having been unknown till ascertained by their observations, or that they themselves should be supposed to have seen all the varieties of diseases which they have occasion to mention. Provided they advance nothing but what has been thoroughly ascertained, they think it in general unnecessary to point out, or perhaps have forgotten, the sources from which they derived the information.

This is attended with more than one inconvenience to the student. His knowledge becomes confused and inaccurate, which it must always do when he is at a loss to discover the sources of it, by having recourse to which he may refresh the memory. This confused and inaccurate state of his knowledge prevents his advancing any thing with confidence, and at length even himself trusting with confidence to what he believes ascertained, but can neither point how, nor by whom. This mode of writing not only tends to render the student's knowledge inaccurate, but deprives him of an opportunity of becoming acquainted with medical authors, so that when he comes to be engaged in practice, he finds himself unacquainted with the merits, often even with the names of authors, which are the only source whence he can derive assistance. These considerations have induced me to make frequent reference to the best authors, and never to advance any thing which contradicts generally received opinions, or is not generally known, without a reference in support of it to the work of some author whose accuracy may be depended on.

I once intended to subjoin to each disease a short account of the best authors on it, to be met with in this country. It will answer every purpose to make frequent references to the authors of most importance, at the same time referring to those of less note, when I have occasion to quote from them any fact or observation of consequence.

Certain subjects will now and then present themselves, which (as they are less generally useful than most others) it will be proper to pass over without entering into a particular consideration of them. When this is done I shall refer to works, from which those who wish for a more accurate knowledge of such subjects may acquire it. By these means an opportunity will be offered of making out a list of writers on the different complaints I shall have occasion to consider, and likewise of becoming in some measure acquainted with their works.

I shall endeavour by attention to method, and adopting in every instance the simplest mode of arrangement which the subject seems to admit of, to adapt the following work to beginners ; and by comprising into a small compass a number of useful observations, to render it not unworthy the attention of the more advanced student, and an useful compendium to be occasionally consulted by the practitioner. I shall on this account avoid the narration of cases, and as much as possible the discussion of opinions, which consume much time.

I shall endeavour on the other hand, however, to avoid a great degree of conciseness, which is improper where it is of consequence to use every means of assisting the memory. The most effectual way of assisting the memory perhaps is endeavouring in every instance to account for phenomena of diseases, and explain the operation of the means which relieve them ; for even ill founded hypotheses may be useful in this way. The injury done by them, however, more than compensates for any advantage of this kind. We must therefore look for other means of assisting the memory. This will be done in some measure by a simple mode of arrangement. I shall also, with the same view, arrange together those diseases whose symptoms and treatment are similar ; compare the diseases which most resemble each other, point out analogies, and endeavour to trace certain principles, which I have already had occasion to observe regulate the treatment of many diseases, or even sets of diseases.

In the present volume I have endeavoured to free the different parts of the subject from hypothesis, which has been the bane of medicine, and at the same time to retain and enforce the maxims on which the treatment of idiopathic fevers is conducted.

These are simple deductions from facts, and must be admitted independently of all hypothesis. Dr. Cullen has severely criticised Lieutaud for attempting a system of practice independent of
hypothesis, and has justly observed, that he treats of diseases in
so unconnected a manner, and speaks with so little precision,
that his laborious synopsis may be regarded as nearly useless.
But this is not owing (as Dr. Cullen, anxious to find an apology
for introducing his favourite opinions, alleges) to the want of a
general system, but chiefly to Lieutaud's having overlooked
those maxims, which are nothing more than expressions for gener-
alized facts, that greatly assist us in acquiring a knowledge of medicine, and the knowledge of which forms the distinction between
the rational practitioner and the mere empiric. I have also endeavoured to give the different parts of the subject a more methodical arrangement than we find in the works of those who have
treated fully of fevers ; and attempted to simplify some of them,
particularly the treatment of continued fever, more than has formerly been done.

But if in none of these respects I have done any thing deserving
of notice, it will still be admitted, that if the following volume
enable another, by moderate application, to acquire in a few
weeks that knowledge which he could not otherwise acquire without much study, and for the acquisition of which, (prepared as
I was by having previously studied the subject) I found a twelvemonth's laborious application scarcely sufficient ; it cannot be regarded as an useless publication : and this is my apology for
offering it to the public.

A

TREATISE

ON

FEBRILE DISEASES, &c.

INTRODUCTION.

SOME observations on the nosological arrangement of febrile diseases form a proper, and indeed a necessary introduction to the following work. I have in the preface explained what is meant by a system of nosology, and for what purposes it is intended.

. Dr. Cullen* divides all diseases into four classes. The diseases arranged under the first class, are those I am to treat of. This class he terms Pyrexiæ. It comprehends all febrile diseases. These he subdivides into five orders, Febres, Phlegmasiæ, Exanthemata, Hæmorrhagiæ, and Profluvia.

The class Pyrexiæ he defines, " Post horrorem pulsus frequens, " calor major, plures functiones læsæ, viribus præsertim artuum " imminutis."†—The first order arranged under this class (the Febres) he defines, " Prægressis languore, lassitudine et aliis " debilitatis signis, pyrexia sine morbo locali primario."—The second order (the Phlegmasiæ) is defined, " Febris synocha; " phlogosis; vel dolor topicus, simul læsa partis internæ func- " tione; sanguis missus, et jam concretus, superficiem coriaceam " albam ostendens."—The third order of the Pyrexiæ (the Exanthemata) Dr. Cullen defines, " Morbi contagiosi, semel tantum " in decursu vitæ aliquem afficientes; cum febre incipientes;

---

* Dr. Cullen's System of Nosology, in every respect so greatly excels those which preceded it, that it will not be necessary to take notice of any other.—See a short view of the nosological systems of Sauvages, Linnæus, Vogelius, Sagare, and M'Bride, in the first volume of Dr. Cullen's Synopsis Nosologiæ Methodicæ.

† Characters of diseases are generally expressed in Latin, because it is difficult to remember accurately what is expressed in the language employed for the common purposes of life: we are apt to change the mode of expression, and consequently often the meaning.

" definito tempore apparent phlogoses, sæpe plures, exiguæ per
" cutem sparsæ."—His definition of the fourth order of the Pyrexiæ (the Hæmorrhagiæ) is, " Pyrexia cum profusione sanguinis
" absque vi externa ; sanguis missus ut in phlegmasiis apparet."
—The last order of the Pyrexiæ (the Profluvia) is defined, " Py-
" rexia cum excretione aueta, naturaliter non sanguinea."

Such is Dr. Cullen's mode of arranging febrile diseases. It is
far from unexceptionable. I shall here point out in what I mean
to deviate from this mode of arrangement, and my reasons for
doing so; which will make the reader further acquainted with
the plan to be pursued in the following work.

The orders arranged under Dr. Cullen's class of Pyrexiæ materially differ from each other in the following circumstance.

The fever in two of these orders (the Febres and Exanthemata)
is strictly idiopathic, that is, exists independently of any local
affection. It is true indeed that local affections accompany many
of the idiopathic fevers. The Exanthemata are attended with
eruptions on the skin ; but these appear a considerable time after
the commencement of the fever, and cannot therefore be regarded
as the cause of it. Besides, its degree is not at all proportioned
to that of the local affection in these complaints ; in some of them
so much the contrary, that the more violent the local affection,
the milder in general is the fever. This is the case in the plague
and the scarlet fever ; nay where certain causes conspire to prevent the fever, the local affection of the Exanthemata is often
present, and that to a considerable degree, without fever. This
frequently happens in the plague, and sometimes in the small-
pox, though not so strikingly, for there the local affection is inconsiderable when unattended by fever.

We shall find also, that in the Exanthemata, the fever, with all
its peculiar symptoms, has often appeared without any eruption ;
this is true of the plague, small-pox, and measles, and probably
of all the other Exanthemata. So far indeed is the local affection
in these complaints from occasioning the fever, that the latter
generally suffers an abatement, and is sometimes wholly removed,
on the appearance of the eruption. In the Exanthemata then,
the fever is as truly an idiopathic affection as in fevers properly
so called; and in laying down the practice in those complaints
we shall find it treated as such. The first and third orders of
Dr. Cullen's Pyrexiæ therefore agree in the most essential point
—in that which, we shall find, more than any other, influences
our practice in febrile diseases.

On the contrary, in the three remaining orders, (the Phlegmasiæ, Hæmorrhagiæ, and Profluvia) we shall find, that the fever
always accompanies some local affection ; being not only proportioned to it, but varying in kind as the local affection varies ; and
that the principles on which the practice in these orders of dis-

eases is conducted, are so modified by this circumstance, as to differ widely from those which regulate the treatment of the Febres and Exanthemata.

In the one set of diseases, the fever is the primary complaint; in the other, merely the consequence of some local affection. It cannot therefore appear surprising, that the principles which direct our practice in these two sets of diseases should essentially differ. In the former, our whole attention is directed towards removing the febrile symptoms; in the latter, the local affection demands our chief attention; and experience has taught us that if we succeed in removing this, we at the same time remove the fever which attends it.

These circumstances considered, does it not appear a proper, and, if we aim at any degree of nosological accuracy, a necessary alteration of Dr. Cullen's mode of arranging febrile diseases, to divide his Pyrexiæ into two classes, the idiopathic, and the symptomatic, fevers?

To arrange the Phlegmasiæ after the Febres, and before the Exanthemata, (diseases so much allied to the Febres) and after considering the Exanthemata, to return to the Hæmorrhagiæ and Profluvia, (diseases in their nature so nearly resembling the Phlegmasiæ) tends to perplex our ideas of the different orders of the Pyrexia. Why first consider the idiopathic, then the symptomatic, then return to idiopathic fevers, and then again to such as are merely symptomatic?

What induced Dr. Cullen and other systematic writers to adopt this mode of arrangement, seems either to have been, that they regarded the Exanthemata as complaints compounded of Fevers and Phlegmasiæ, and consequently considered it proper to treat of both the latter sets of diseases before the former; or they thought that their account of the inflammatory affection which appears in the Exanthemata, would be more readily understood after treating of the Phlegmasiæ; and thus repetition be prevented, which it cannot be if we first describe the eruptions of the Exanthemata, and afterwards the different species of inflammation.

The idea on which the former of these arguments is founded, is false, if by Phlegmasiæ we mean any thing more than a local affection, (as will presently more plainly appear) and may lead to errors in practice.

The latter seems a better argument; for almost every thing we say, when we describe the Phlegmon in the small-pox, for instance, must be repeated in describing Dr. Cullen's first genus of the Phlegmasiæ, the Phlogosis. This objection to the mode of arrangement which I propose is considerable, but it is less so in a system of practice, than in a nosological system. In the former, for the sake of perspicuity, nearly the same description of the eruption in the Exanthemata is necessary, whether the Phlegmasiæ have been previously considered or not. But however objectionable this mode of arrangement may be, it is certainly less objectionable than that of Dr. Cullen, who confounds together idiopathic and symptomatic fevers, diseases so different in their nature, and requiring very different modes of practice.

ι Here then, turn which way we will, we find a barrier opposed to our advancement in nosological accuracy : A probable inference from which is, that we are not proceeding on a proper plan. The error seems to be, that we are considering the more complicated, before we have treated of the more simple, diseases.

Not only the Pyrexiæ, but the Neuroses and Cachexiæ, ought to be placed after the affections which are merely local, by far the majority of which are constantly occurring in the general and more-complicated diseases.

In this class of local diseases, there should be an order for simple inflammations, for such inflammations as are not attended by fever, as pimples, and that habitual and superficial redness of the face and hands which never produces fever. These affections are trifling, and on that account have often been overlooked, at least not treated of separately from other inflammations ; but however trifling the complaints themselves may be, properly arranged they would prove useful in a system of nosology, by enabling us to give a methodical arrangement of more important diseases. Besides, such an order of simple inflammations would include some diseases of importance, certain species of Ophthalmia for instance, and the Aphthæ Infantum. With what propriety are these, in which no kind of fever ever appears, ranked in the class of Pyrexiæ?

Not one symptom of these complaints is mentioned in Dr. Cullen's definition of Pyrexiæ. They might as well be arranged under any other definition in the whole nosology.

The Phlegmasiæ, as defined by Dr. Cullen, are diseases compounded of simple inflammation and fever. There are the same reasons, therefore, for treating of simple inflammation before the Phlegmasiæ, which have induced nosologists to arrange the inflammations before the Exanthemata. But the latter also are compounded of simple inflammation and fever, not of Phlegmasiæ and fever. When a Phlegmasia supervenes on an Exanthema, the combination is of quite a different nature from that of the primary fever of the Exanthema and the simple inflammation which succeeds it.

There is no better reason then (resulting merely from a view of the complaints themselves) for arranging the Phlegmasiæ before the Exanthemata, than for arranging the Exanthemata before the Phlegmasiæ. But since both are complaints in which two more simple affections are combined, these should be considered before either. ▼ And since in the Exanthemata the fever is idiopathic, they should be arranged with other idiopathic fevers, and consequently before the Phlegmasiæ.

Dr. Cullen is led into several difficulties, by treating of the Phlegmasiæ without having previously considered simple inflammations. In the definition of the Phlegmasiæ, Phlogosis is mentioned; but Phlogosis is a genus of this order, so that this disease is arranged under an order, of whose definition it forms a part; just as if we were to define the Exanthemata, fever attended with eruption, and then arrange eruption as a genus of the order. Besides, Phlogosis is the name of a disease, and is here used before the disease has been defined.

Dr. Cullen perceived the difficulty; it is one indeed which it was impossible for him not to perceive, and he seems in this instance to have had recourse to a common subterfuge, a degree of obscurity. In the definition of the Phlegmasiæ he says, " Febris synocha, phlogosis," &c. evidently implying by Phlogosis, nothing more than an external inflammation unaccompanied by fever, and immediately after he informs us, that it is a febrile disease.

If Phlogosis is made a genus of the Phlegmasiæ, it must be a febrile disease; if not, there is no place for it in Dr. Cullen's system. It would have been easy for him in the definition of the Phlegmasiæ, instead of the term Phlogosis, to have used some other, expressive of simple inflammation; but he must then have mentioned a complaint not to be found in his nosology.

The same circumstance forces him into an error of no less consequence, in his definition of the Exanthemata. There again the want of a term expressive of simple inflammation recurs, and he is again obliged to employ Phlogosis, which he has defined to be a febrile disease. Phlogosis is an external inflammation occasioning fever; the eruption in the Exanthemata, instead of occasioning, usually even relieves, fever.

Had Dr. Cullen treated of simple inflammations, as well as simple fevers, before the more complicated diseases, he would have avoided all the foregoing difficulties. There would have been no reason for interrupting the consideration of idiopathic fevers, to introduce the order of Phlegmasiæ, which, as it stands in Dr. Cullen's system, can only be regarded as the sixth or seventh part of the whole nosology in a parenthesis.

He would not have been obliged to confound in one class, diseases so different as idiopathic and symptomatic fevers. This he certainly would have avoided, had not his mode of arrangement rendered it necessary to place the Phlegmasiæ before the Exanthemata, which he could not do without making one class of all kinds of fever.

He would not have been obliged either to exclude from his system the simple inflammations, or to arrange the genera of this order among febrile diseases.* He would not have found it necessary to employ the name of a disease before he had defined it, nor run into the inaccuracy (to use no stronger term) of arranging as a genus under an order, a complaint the name of which he finds it necessary to use in the definition of that order. In short, febrile diseases (the most essential part of a system of nosology) would have admitted of a more systematic arrangement.

Such are the circumstances, which have induced me to divide Dr. Cullen's Pyrexiæ into two classes, the idiopathic, and symptomatic, fevers. I am now to make a few nosological observations on each of these classes.

The former, I have already had occasion to observe, comprehends only two of the orders of Dr. Cullen's Pyrexiæ, the first and third, the Febres and Exanthemata. In every febrile complaint, which cannot be referred to one of these orders, the fever, we shall find, must be regarded as symptomatic.

However different the symptoms are which distinguish the different genera of idiopathic fevers, there are certain symptoms common to all of them, and which may therefore be allowed to constitute fever, or in other words to form the definition of this class of diseases. Let us endeavour to determine what these symptoms are.

We are informed by Van Swieten, that Boerhaave, with much labour, collected from a great variety of authors, all the symptoms which they had observed in fevers. From these he threw out such as did not appear in all fevers, and was much surprised to find the catalogue of symptoms common to all kinds of fever, so short. It reduced itself to the three following, shivering, or as it has been termed rigors, a frequent pulse, and heat.

But it may be observed that no one even of these symptoms constantly attends fever. The shivering is almost always confined to the commencement of the fever, or to that of its exacerbations, and sometimes is not observed at all. Both Boerhaave and his commentator allow, that although the shivering is present at the commencement of fever, when arising from an internal cause, such as the pestilential contagion, the contagion of small-pox, &c.; yet when it arises from what they call an external cause, such as rage, violent exercise, &c. it often comes on without any sense of cold.

* Dr. Cullen might have formed an order in the Locales for simple inflammations; but introducing them into any part of his system after the Phlegmasiæ, would have only rendered the difficulty of forming an accurate definition of the Phlegmasiæ the more apparent. The only means of avoiding the difficulties which have been mentioned, seems to be making the Locales the first class of diseases.

Many of the ancients, although they did not wholly overlook the state of the pulse, as appears from several passages in the works of Hippocrates, seem to have regarded the last of the three symptoms just mentioned (the increase of temperature) as that which constitutes fever.

It is well known, however, that in certain kinds of fever the temperature of the body often falls below the natural standard. In the commencement of the cold stage it generally does so, and very often in the progress of that species of fever which has been termed the low nervous fever. The shivering, or sense of cold, then, and increase of temperature, are symptoms, not only not present at every period of these complaints, but not even at any period essential to fever.

Thus one symptom only remains to constitute the disease, a frequent pulse, and to this conclusion Boerhaave was led. But we must go a step farther, and observe, that although a frequent pulse is the most constant of all the symptoms of fever, it is not universally present in these complaints ; in malignant fevers the frequency of the pulse is often observed to be no greater, and sometimes considerably less, than natural. In these fevers the pulse has been found to beat only 40, sometimes only 30, times in a minute. Besides, by considering fever as present wherever the frequency of the pulse is increased, we class together the most dissimilar affections. With fever, for instance, we must class palpitation of the heart.

The inference from these observations is plain, that no one symptom can be regarded as characteristic of fever. We ascertain its presence, not by attending to any one, but several of its symptoms. In selecting however the train of symptoms which characterise it, there is much difficulty.* The following is the selection made by Dr. Cullen : Languor, lassitude, and other signs of debility, followed by Pyrexia, (that is, by rigors, frequent pulse, increased heat, and derangement of the functions, particularly a want of vigour in the limbs) without any primary local affection.

Although I quote this, as the best definition of fevers which has been given, even its author confesses its faults, but pleads justly the difficulty of the subject. The most exceptionable part is the definition of Pyrexia contained in it.

' Fever, it has just been observed, is not always attended by rigors ; even increased heat is not uniformly present during its progress. Increased heat, however, it is necessary to retain as

---

* It is certainly impossible, by any enumeration of the symptoms of fever, to give a short definition of this complaint that will apply to all periods of every kind of fever ; and a long one would not answer the purposes of a definition. In a subsequent part of this volume I shall attempt a definition of idiopathic fevers, constructed on a different principle.

a part of the definition of fever, since it is very generally present, and the frequent pulse, without increased heat, often attends complaints of a very different na$_t$u$_r$e. The derangement
of the functions, particularly the debility of the limbs, does not
very properly enter into the definition; since the derangement of
some of the functions is observable in almost all diseases, and
the derangement particularly specified (the debility of the limbs)
is frequently absent in fever, in which indeed the vigour of the
whole system is often preternaturally increased.

Having arranged under the term Pyrexia so many diseases, Dr.
Cullen found it necessary so to define this word as to express
the striking characteristic features of a great variety of complaints. If we lay aside the term Pyrexia, (not attempting to
class together so many diseases) we shall considerably lessen the
difficulty of giving such a definition of idiopathic fevers, as shall
apply to all cases. Dr. Cullen's mode of arrangement obliges
him to introduce into his definition that of Pyrexia. By arranging separately the idiopathic and symptomatic fevers, we get rid
of this embarrassment. Idiopathic fevers, as far as I can judge,
may be defined pretty accurately as follows :—Prægressis languore, lassitudine, et aliis debilitatis signis; pulsus frequens, calor
auctus, sine morbo locali primario. This is the definition of
Dr. Cullen's first order of the Pyrexiæ, with this change, that
pulsus frequens, calor auctus is inserted, instead of Pyrexia. He
uses the definition as the character of an order, only comprehending fevers properly so called. I shall use it, with this alteration, as the character of a class comprehending both fevers properly so called, and the Exanthemata.

Under this class may be arranged three orders ; Intermitting
and Remitting Fevers ; Continued Fevers ; and the Eanthema-
ta. It will be proper to make a few observations on each of
these orders.

Dr. Cullen gives the following definition of intermitting and
remitting fevers :—"Febres miasmate paludum ortæ, paroxysmis
" pluribus, apyrexia, saltem remissione evidente, interposita: cum
" exacerbatione notabili, plerumque cum horrore, redeuntibus, con-
" stantes; paroxysmo quovis die unico tantum." In this definition
Dr. Cullen, very properly I think, includes both intermitting and remitting fevers ; because (as he observes) these fevers arise from the
same cause, are cured by the same means, and in the same person
the fever often changes from the one form to the other. " Miasmate
paludum ortæ" should be rejected from the definition. It is far from
being fully ascertained, (as will appear hereafter) that intermitting
and remitting fevers always arise from marsh miasma, even in
those who have not formerly laboured under them ; while it is
certain, that these complaints are often renewed by other causes,
in those who have lately been afflicted by them. Besides, we
should confine nosological definitions as much as possible to what

the practitioner can himself observe. The knowledge he derives from the information of the patient, or others, is always liable to error.

" Paroxysmo quovis die unico tantum" ought also to be omitted, since both in intermitting and remitting fevers, there are often two paroxysms in the same day. Dr. Cullen seems to have introduced this part of the definition to assist in forming a diagnosis between this set of fevers, and those termed continued. We shall presently see more clearly that it affords no mark of distinction between these complaints, and that such a diagnosis is not so necessary, as at first sight it may appear.

With these exceptions, Dr. Cullen's definition of intermitting and remitting fevers is extremely good, and sufficient we shall find after the objectionable parts are rejected, for distinguishing the fevers arranged under it. It is simple and short, and at once directs the attention to the leading features of the complaint. The species and varieties of this order I shall presently have occasion to consider at some length.

The second order of idiopathic fevers, that is, the second section of Dr. Cullen's first order of the Pyrexiæ, (continued fever) he defines, " Febres sine intermissione, nec miasmate paludum " ortæ, sed cum remissionibus et exacerbationibus, parum licet " notabilibus, perstantes, paroxysmis quovis die binis." As " mi- " asmate paludum ortæ" was rejected from the last definition, " nec miasmate paludum ortæ" should be omitted in this. The latter part of it, " paroxysmis quovis die binis," is also exceptionable, as this circumstance is seldom distinctly observed in continued fevers.

Dr. Cullen observes, that since continued fevers consist of repeated paroxysms, it may sometimes be difficult to distinguish them from remitting fevers; and this difficulty may seem increased by the changes I have proposed in his definitions. The truth is, that these two kinds of fever run into each other. The only difference, which can be specified between remitting and continued fever, is, that of the degree and length of their remissions. There is no symptom of the one, which does not occasionally attend the other. In this, however, and similar difficulties, we shall find, that when the symptoms of two diseases imperceptibly run into each other, the same is true of the modes of practice suited to them; so that a perfect diagnosis between them is unnecessary, for nosology derives all its importance from its being subservient to practice.

The ancients (Dr. Cullen remarks) mention fevers, in which there was not the least appearance of remissions throughout their whole course. Such however are seldom if ever observed. In all fevers we generally perceive some degree of remission, at least once, sometimes twice, in the day. It is therefore to fevers with slight remissions, that we apply the term continued.

Continued fevers have long been divided into acute and chronic; and many disputes have arisen concerning this division. In acute fevers the symptoms are generally more violent than in chronic, and the disease is sooner terminated. Some have confined the term acute, to those fevers which terminate before or on the twentieth day. Others extend this period to sixty days; and Galen divides the acute fevers into acute, which extend to between the seventh and the twentieth day; and peracute, those which terminate before or on the seventh. The peracute he subdivides into exactly peracute, those which are not protracted beyond the fourth day; and not exactly peracute those which extend to the seventh. The acute he in like manner subdivides into exactly acute, those which terminate on the fourteenth day; and not exactly acute, those which are protracted to the twentieth. All these days, we shall find, were regarded by the ancients as chief critical days.* These divisions are altogether arbitrary, and of little or no use in practice.

The division of continued fever into Inflammatory and Nervous, or, as they have been termed, Synocha and Typhus, is one of more consequence, and at present more generally adopted by physicians. It points out the only species of continued fever, which can be well defined; and greatly assists us in laying down the mode of treatment in this varied disease.

The following is Dr. Cullen's definition of Synocha, " Calor " plurimum auctus, pulsus frequens, validus, et durus, urina ru_ " bra, sensorii functiones parum turbatæ." Many objections might be started to this definition, but it would be difficult to give a better. In forming it, Dr. Cullen chiefly kept in view the cir_ cumstances which distinguish this species of fever from the Ty_ phus; and he rather gives the symptoms of the more strongly marked cases of Synocha, than of Synocha in general.

The same observation applies to the definition of Typhus. He rather gives the diagnostic symptoms of strongly marked Typhus, than such as characterise the generality of fevers referred to this head: " Morbus contagiosus, calor parum auctus, pulsus parvus, " debilis, plerumque frequens, urina parum mutata, sensorii func_ " tiones plurimum turbatæ, vires multum imminutæ." Nor does it seem possible to avoid this inaccuracy, since as Synocha and Typhus insensibly run into each other, it is only in the more strongly marked cases, that they can well be distinguished. Between the mildest cases of Synocha and Typhus, there is no line of distinction.

A simple Synocha or Typhus are fevers which we rarely, if ever, meet with. For however high the inflammatory symptoms at first run, however well marked the Synocha may be at the commencement of the complaint, the symptoms of Typhus always, at least in this country, shew themselves towards its termi-

* Days on which the great changes of fevers most frequently happen.

mation; and however well marked the symptoms of Typhus may be in the progress of fever, in almost every case the first symptoms are more or less inflammatory.

On this account Dr. Cullen makes a third species of continued fever, which he terms Synochus; and defines, " Morbus conta- " giosus, febris ex Synocha et Typho composita; initio Syno- " cha, progressu, et versus finem, Typhus."

The fevers mentioned by authors, under the names Synocha and Typhus, are in fact no other than varieties of the Synochus. When the symptoms of Typhus predominate, the fever has been termed Typhus; when the inflammatory symptoms are most remarkable, and present through the greater part of the complaint, it has been named Synocha. These varieties of continued fever so run into each other, the difference seeming often to depend on adventitious circumstances, that they are properly considered as one complaint; wonderfully varied indeed, but between the varieties of which no well marked line can be drawn.

There are other varieties of continued fever, however, which in some respects are better marked. Although continued fever is not in general attended with any eruption, yet eruptions of different kinds often appear in this complaint; and as they seem to modify its symptoms, or at least, as each particular eruption is apt to shew itself when a certain train of symptoms is present, they may serve to distinguish some varieties of continued fever.

After physicians became acquainted with the Exanthemata; after they had observed that a certain train of febrile symptoms are always followed by an eruption of a particular kind, and that every one infected by a person labouring under such a fever is seized with the same train of febrile symptoms, followed by the same eruption: I say after physicians became acquainted with these complaints, they seem to have inferred, that wherever an eruption occurs in continued fever, preceded by, or attended with, a particular train of febrile or other symptoms, the complaint is an Exanthema; that it is of a nature different from that of a common continued fever; and that when communicated from one person to another, it would always be attended with its peculiar symptoms and eruption, as happens in the small-pox and meazles. Thus they regarded the Petechial fever, thus they still regard the Miliary, the Aphthous, and several other varieties of fever, as Exanthemata.

A more particular attention to these complaints has long ago (at least in this country) convinced physicians of their error, with respect to the Petechial fever; and they begin to suspect it with respect to several others, which nosologists at present class with the Exanthemata. Let us consider the pretensions of each of those to the place it holds in our systems of nosology.

Although Dr. Cullen gives the Miliary fever a place among the Exanthemata, he expresses his doubts whether it properly be-

longs to this order, or may I rather say, he adduces sufficient arguments to prove that it does not. " There has lately been a
" warm dispute (he observes) concerning the nature of this fever,
" particularly among the German physicians ; the one party
" looking upon it as merely a symptomatic affection ; the other
" asserting that it is as completely idiopathic as the small-pox or
" meazles.

" For my own part (he continues) although I cannot in the face
" of very respectable authorities, positively assert that it never is
" an idiopathic fever, yet since experience in such cases is often
" fallacious, and physicians are too apt to adopt the opinions of
" their predecessors, I cannot help expressing my doubts on this
" point, and the more so, as I have in many years practice found
" this complaint for the most part symptomatic. I have never
" found it (he observes) contagious or manifestly epidemic ; al-
" though at certain periods, I confess, I have known it more fre-
" quent than at others. The miliary eruption appears in putrid
" as well as inflammatory fevers, and at no time in any, except
" when forced out by external warmth or sweats. Besides, in fe-
" vers where from various circumstances the miliary eruption
" was expected, I have known its appearance prevented by the cool-
" ing regimen, and by avoiding sweats. In some parts of the body
" I have even seen it induced as if by art. Lastly, the matter ex-
" citing the military fever, if there be any such matter, differs
" widely from other exanthematic contagions, both in not causing
" the eruption to appear about the same day of the complaint in
" different cases, and in attacking the same person more than
" once.* De hujus igitur materiæ natura specifica, (he adds)
" vel ad morbum quemvis idiopathicum gignendum apta, valde
" dubito. In hac re mecum sentientem experientissimum
" et peritissimum Carol. White habere mihi gratulor. Vide
" White on the Management of Lying-in Women."†

Dr. Cullen, to overcome the difficulty as far as possible, con-
sistently with the place it holds in his nosology, divides the miliary
fever into two varieties, the idiopathic and symptomatic. The
former, he confesses, he mentions, not from his own observations,
but those of foreign writers. All the cases of miliary fever which
he himself saw, he refers to the latter variety.‡

* Some authors even assert that the miliary fever is most apt to attack
those who have formerly laboured under it. See Vogel de Cog. et Cur.
Morh.—I know a woman who is subject to this eruption in almost every
indisposition under which she labours.

† See Cullen's Synop. Nos. Meth. genus 32.

‡ It is when the miliary eruption is of that kind which has been called
the White miliary eruption, that the complaint is supposed to have the
best claim to be considered an Exanthema ; but its claim seems no better
founded than that in which the red miliary eruption (the rash as it is called in England) appears ; both kinds of eruption frequently appear on the
same patient at the same time.

But I have found no facts in the writings of any foreign author
I have met with, who treats of the miliary fever, capable of war-
ranting this division, or of setting aside ,Dr. Cullen's mode of
reasoning with respect to any of the cases of which they give an
account.*

The miliary eruption has doubtless now and then attended the
raging fever; but so have Petechiæ. A variety of circumstances,
improper treatment for instance, (and we have reason to believe
that this is the circumstance which has most frequently operated)
may render the inhabitants of any particular neighbourhood sub-
jcet to the miliary eruption, while labouring under fever. Can
we suppose any thing peculiar in the fever produced by a fractured
limb? Yet Burserius mentions a case of this kind attended by the
miliary eruption. In what fever does it appear so frequently as
in the Puerperal, between which and the Exanthemata there is
surely very little analogy? This eruption in short appears in all
febrile diseases, when its peculiar causes happen to have been
applied. It appears in the Exanthemata, the Phlegmasiæ, the
Hæmorrhagiæ, and Profluvia, as well as in fevers properly so
called; nay, its appearance we shall find is not even confined to
febrile diseases. It seems to be nothing more than an accidental
symptom, which is most apt to occur in fever, but may appear in
any disease whatever. And, like Petechiæ, it also sometimes
appears unaccompanied by any other complaint.†

* The principal foreign authors I allude to are Hoffman in his Opera
Physico-Medica, Van Swieten in his Comment. in Aph. Boerhavii, Lieu-
taud in his Synopsis Praxeos Medicinæ, de Haen in his Ratio Medendi,
Burserius in his Institutiones Medicinæ Practicæ, Vogel in his work de
Cog. et Cur. Morb., Quarin in his excellent work de Febribus, Allionius
in his treatise de Miliarium Origine, and Planchon in his work de la Fievre Miliaire. The following works also, Welsch de Novo Pueper. Morbo,
Fantonus de Febre Miliare, Fischer de Febre Miliare, Gastallier sur la
Fievre Miliare des Femmes en Couche, have found their way to this
country, but I have not been able to meet with them. I was the less anxious to procure these treatises, as I found, after perusing what is said of
the miliary fever by a few of the authors just mentioned, there was little
to be met with in the works of others but a repetition of the same observations. It must always happen that after six or eight authors, who have
been conversant with a disease, have given a copious account of it, many
important facts relating to it will not remain to be mentioned by others.
If instead of facts, we are in quest of opinions, every publication indeed
presents us with novelty enough. But of all knowledge, that of medical
hypotheses is the most useless, not to say hurtful. No man, although he
could without pains procure this knowledge, would have his memory bur-
dened with it. With the hypotheses of some eminent writers indeed we
find it necessary to be acquainted; not that they are in general better
founded than more obscure opinions, but because the authority of a great
name has infused them extensively into the writings of succeeding authors.
It will therefore be necessary, in the present work, to take an opportunity of giving a short account of the hypothesis of a Boerhaave, a Cullen,
or a Brown.

. † For cases of the miliary eruption unattended by any other complaint,
see Huxham on Fevers, White on the Diseases of Lying-in Women,

There are nearly the same reasons for rejecting the Aphthous, as the miliary fever, from the number of the Exanthemata. " I " doubt, (says Dr. Cullen) whether or not the Aphthæ ought to " be arranged under the Exanthemata. Most cases of Aphthæ " which I have seen (he observes) appeared without fever; and " if at any time a fever did attend the Aphthæ infantum, the for- " mer generally supervened upon the latter. A fever indeed (he " continues) does accompany the Aphthæ of adults, but this fever " is of no particular kind, and the Aphthæ generally appear to- " wards its termination; nor as far as I know is there any fever " well defined, or even mentioned by medical writers, which con- " stantly attends Aphthæ."

The Aphthæ infantum is an idiopathic affection, and this form of the complaint has sometimes appeared in adults.* But a dis- ease unattended by fever does not certainly belong to the order of Exanthemata. We have to consider how far those cases in which Aphthæ appear in fever deserve a place in this order.

I have just quoted Dr. Cullen's observation, that Aphthæ do not appear in a fever distinguished by any particular symptoms, as the eruptions in the Exanthemata are observed to do.† They appear in all kinds of fevers, in the symptomatic, as well as the idiopathic. In many of the former indeed they are more com- mon than in the latter. Sydenham declares, that there is no complaint in which he found Aphthæ so common as in dysentery, and in those fevers on which dysentery had supervened. We know that this affection is one of the most common forerunners of death in Phthisis, &c. With what propriety then are Aphthæ ranked among the Exanthemata? We shall even find, when we come to consider them more particularly, that Aphthæ, when at- tended by common continued fever, (the only case in which there can be a shadow of reason for regarding them as an Exanthema) can generally be traced to causes different from those which pro- duce the fever in which they occur; very frequently to affections of the primæ viæ, or suppressed sweats.

Burserius's Institutiones Medicinæ Practicæ. Even Hoffman observes, that the red miliary eruption is often chronic, continuing a considerable time without fever, and often returning at certain seasons of the year. The white is more rarely unaccompanied with fever.

* Cases of this kind are mentioned by Boerhaave, by Ketelaer in his Treatise de Aphthis nostratibus, Arneman in his Commentatio de Aph- this, and others. Such cases however are extremely rare. Van Swieten lived for many years in a country where Aphthæ were very common, yet he never saw a case of Aphthæ in an adult not labouring under fever; and Dr. Cullen makes the same observation with respect to his own ex- perience.

† Certain symptoms indeed generally precede all eruptions; but in the cases we are at present considering, the attending symptoms appear oc- casionally in all kinds of fevers, and at all periods of them. Whereas in the true Exanthemata, the fever from its commencement is of a peculiar kind, at least attended with peculiar symptoms.

- Dr. Cullen has also expressed his doubts respecting the propriety of ranking the Erysipelas among the Exanthemata ; and regards the species which have been termed Erysipelas pestilens and Erysipelas contagiosum, as nothing more than Typhus attended by an Erythematic inflammation. ,

All the arguments urged for the exclusion of the miliary fever from the Exanthemata, are equally strong when applied to the Erysipelas : it is not a contagious disease ; the eruption often appears indeed, like those just mentioned, in contagious fevers, but it is not necessarily communicated along with such fevers. Like the miliary eruption, it appears in various kinds of fevers, in the symptomatic as well as idiopathic. External warmth and irritation are capable of producing the Erysipelas in the predisposed, as well as the miliary eruption. There is no particular period of the fever at which the Erysipelas shews itself ; and with regard to its recurrence, it is even most apt to attack those who have formerly laboured under it.

We shall afterwards find, that there is another complaint, in which the same kind of inflammation appears as in the Erysipelas, termed by Sauvages and Cullen (for other authors have used the word in a very indefinite sense) Erythema. The difference between the Erysipelas and Erythema is, that in the former, the inflammation supervenes on a fever ; in the latter, the inflammation is the primary affection, and the fever merely its consequence. The Erysipelas seems to be nothing more than an Erythema, supervening on any kind of continued fever ; and as such I shall consider it along with the other eruptions which appear in these fevers.*

* I have arranged the Erysipelatous fever among the varieties of Synochus, because, like those just mentioned, it has been arranged among the Exanthemata ; but if the view I have here taken of it be just, and that it is so will I think more fully appear when we come to speak of its treatment, it should have no place in a system of nosology, since it is a combination of a Phlegmasia and continued fever ; and it is of the combinations of symptoms, not of diseases, that nosology treats. It may be said indeed, that as all the eruptions we have been considering, occasionally appear unaccompanied by any other complaint, the same objection holds against admitting the other varieties of Synochus into a nosological system. And this cannot be denied. But most of these eruptions appear so rarely as a distinct complaint, and their appearance in continued fever, or rather the causes which produce them, so modify many of its symptoms without altering the nature of the fever, as we shall find the appearance of the Erythematic inflammation generally does, that it is useful in practice to regard those combinations as single diseases. The most methodical arrangement in a system of nosology is not always the most useful : for another proof of which I may refer to what was said of the definitions of Synocha and Typhus, in which we introduce symptoms not essential to these complaints, in order to draw a line of distinction which nature has not made, because the division is useful in the practice in fevers, and still more so in teaching the principles of that practice. This is one of the circumstances I alluded to, when it was observed in the preface that a perfect system of nosology is not to be looked for. Although for the reasons just given, I have arranged the Erysipelatous

The complaint I am now speaking of is Dr. Cullen's first species of Erysipelas, (the Erysipelas vesiculosum); the complaint which he arranges as a second species of this disease, differs from it considerably. This species he terms the Erysipelas Phlyctænodes. It is the same which is termed by Pliny, Zoster; by Hoffman, Zona ignea; in English, the Shingles:[*] it is certainly not very properly regarded as a species of Erysipelas; nor does its place in a system of nosology seem well ascertained.

Sydenham also ranks as a species of Erysipelas, the complaint termed Urticaria, (Dr. Cullen's 53d genus). This however we shall find differs essentially from Erysipelas, and seems to have a better claim to be regarded as an Exanthema.

Another complaint, to be regarded in nearly the same light with the foregoing, is the Pemphigus, or vesicular fever. There is no particular kind of fever in which the eruption appears; there is no particular period of the fever at which it shews itself. Dr. Cullen says it appears on the first, second, or third day; Sauvages observes that it sometimes appears on the fourth; and Dr. Dickson,[†] who seems to be better acquainted with this complaint than either of these authors, declares it may appear on any day.

The cases related by Salabert, in his observations des Fievres Inflammatoires, are evidently cases of common continued fever, in which the vesicular eruption proved critical.[‡]

Dr. Cullen was but little acquainted with the Pemphigus, as appears both from what he says in a note, and from the definition which he gives of it; the most exceptionable perhaps in his nosology. The more accurate observations upon this complaint indeed, have appeared since the publication of his system, so

fever as a variety of the Synochus, yet we shall find, on considering it more particularly, that it will be necessary to defer entering fully into its treatment till I come to speak of the Erythema; because it partakes so much of the nature of a Phlegmasia, that the principles, on which the practice in idiopathic fevers is conducted, will not apply to the treatment of Erysipelas.

[*] See an account of this complaint in the 2d vol. of Burserius's Inst. Med. Prac., in Schroeder de Feb. Erysip. in his Opusc. Med., in Vogel's Prælect Acad. de Cog. et Cur. Morh., and Smith's Essay on the different Species of Inflammation, in the 2d vol. of the Med. Communications; see also Kussel de Tabe Gland. p. 124.

[†] See Observations on Pemphigus, by Dr. Dickson, Prof. of Medicine in the University of Dublin, in the Transactions of the Royal Irish Academy for 1787.

[‡] The celebrated Morton, the contemporary and rival of Sydenham, takes notice of this complaint, but without particularly describing it. The name by which he calls it however seems to imply that he regarded it merely as a symptomatic affection, "Febris Synocha cum vesiculis per pectus et collum sparsis."

that he could not be acquainted with them ; yet the knowledge
he had of it led him to doubt of the Pemphigus being an idiopathic affection.) , And all that Burserius says in favour of its being
eo is, that we must at least allow those cases to be idiopathic, in
which the eruption is not attended by fever.*

This eruption, like the foregoing, also appears in other complaints, as well as in continued fever. We have a remarkable
instance in which it accompanied a Phlegmasia² (the Cynanche
Maligna) in the Pemphigus Helveticus, of which there is an
account in the Acta Helvetica by Dr. Langhans. Much difference of opinion has arisen among physicians respecting the nature of the complaint described by Dr. Langhans, from their not
admitting the vesicular eruption to be merely symptomatic ; for,
this granted, the difficulty is removed; we know that symptomatic eruptions appear in all kinds of fever, whether idiopathic
or not.

I may also add, that the vesicular, like some of the other symptomatic eruptions, (the Aphtha for instance) is not confined to
the skin, but often attacks the œsophagus, stomach, and intestines ;
a circumstance which has not been observed of any of the eruptions in the true Exanthemata.† There is every reason to believe
indeed, that all the symptomatic eruptions, as well as the Aphthous and Vesicular, occasionally attack the stomach and intestines. That the Erysipelatous does, appears from what Dr.
Cullen says of the Gastritis and Enteritis. I have myself seen
this eruption spread from the mouth and fauces to the stomach
and prove fatal. Of the miliary fever, Vogel observes, that the
peculiar pricking felt in the skin when the miliary eruption is
coming out, is also frequently felt at the same time in the intestines. And with respect to the petechial eruption, from what we
know of its nature, there is every reason to believe that it is apt
to appear wherever there is a lining of cuticle.

The complaints we have been considering then, the Petechial,
Miliary, Aphthous, Erysipelatous, and Vesicular fevers, are to be
regarded merely as varieties of continued fever. After treating
of continued fever in general, I shall consider each of these varieties separately ; that is, I shall point out the forms of continued
fever in which these different eruptions are most apt to appear,
the peculiar symptoms which generally attend their appearance,
the causes which produce them, and the change which their appearance renders necessary in the treatment of the fevers in
which they occur.

* This, he observes, frequently happens. See a case of this kind related by Dr. Winterbottom, in the 3d vol. of Medical Facts and Observations, p. 10. I have seen a similar case.

† It was once supposed that the small-pox was apt to attack the intestines; but since the publication of Cotunnius's Treatise, de Sede Variolarum, this is generally admitted to have been a mistake.

Petechiæ, it may be said, are improperly classed among these eruptions; as they are to be regarded merely as a symptom of debility, as the consequence of morbid tenuity of the blood, and relaxation of the vessels. This however does not seem to be precisely the case; other circumstances than the presence of debility are requisite for the appearance of Petechiæ. It often happens in Typhus, even where the debility is extreme, that no Petechiæ make their appearance; this was the case, for instance, in the jail fever of Winchester, described by Dr. C. Smith; it is very frequently the case in the plague. Besides, Petechiæ are often observed where there are no signs of debility whatever. Grant in his Treatise on the Fevers most common in London, Eller in his Obs. de Cog. et Cur. Morbis, and others, relate cases in which Petechiæ attended well-marked Synocha.

The second order of Idiopathic fevers then comprehends Synocha and Typhus, or the Synochus (for Synocha and Typhus are rather to be regarded as different stages of the Synochus, than distinct complaints) and its varieties, viz. the Synochus Petechialis, the Synochus Miliaris, the Synochus Aphthosus, the Synochus Erysipelatosus, and the Synochus Vesicularis; the definitions of which shall be considered when I come to speak of these varieties separately.

The third order of Idiopathic fevers comprehends the Exanthemata properly so called. The Exanthemata form the third order of Dr. Cullen's Pyrexiæ, and are defined by him, " Morbi " contagiosi semel tantum in decursu vitæ aliquem afficientes; " cum febre incipientes, definito tempore apparent phlogoses, " sæpe plures, exiguæ, per cutem sparsæ."

" Semel tantum in decursu vitæ aliquem afficientes," (as not strictly true of any of the Exanthemata, and certainly very far from being true of many of them) might with propriety be omitted in this definition;* which sufficiently distinguishes the diseases arranged under it without this addition. Dr. Cullen properly admits the contagious nature of the Exanthemata to form part of this definition. The true Exanthemata are always contagious.

I have already offered my reasons for rejecting from this definition the term Phlogosis; instead of which I shall use Papulæ, (pustules) which we must suppose to have been arranged, and consequently defined, among the Locales, which I have endeavoured to shew should form the first class of diseases in a system of nosology.

---

* The plague is generally admitted to attack the same person repeatedly; and there are many well authenticated instances on record of the small-pox and measles attacking the same person a second or third time, or oftener. See Burserius's Inst. Med. Prac., Rosen. in Haller's Disput. ad Morb. Hist. et Cur. Per. &c.

The following then may be adopted as the definition of the third order of Idiopathic fevers : Morbi contagiosi cum febre idiopathica incipientes, definito tempore apparent Papulæ, sæpe plures, exiguæ, per cutem sparsæ. Under this order are arranged the Variola, the Varicella, the Rubeola, the Scarlatina, the Pestis, and the Urticaria.

Such is the mode of arrangement I shall adopt in treating of idiopathic fevers; on the arrangement of the symptomatic, a very few words will be sufficient. This class of diseases comprehends the three remaining orders of Dr. Cullen's Pyrexiæ, viz. the second, fourth, and fifth, the Phlegmasiæ, Hæmorrhagiæ, and Profluvia; and may be defined, Morbus localis, calore aucto, pulsu frequente.

Dr. Cullen's definition of the first order of this class, the Phlegmasiæ, (the second order of his Pyrexiæ) is, " Febris synocha, " phlogosis, vel dolor topicus simul læsa partis internæ functione, " sanguis missus et jam concretus superficiem coriaccam albam " ostendens."

This definition requires considerable alterations. I have already given my reasons for rejecting the term Phlogosis. According to the arrangement I have adopted, this definition must also be made to include that of the class of which it is an order; and I think there are several reasons for rejecting the latter part of it, namely, " Sanguis missus et jam concretus superficiem co- "riaccam albam ostendens." The appearance of the buffy coat on the blood does not, we shall find, uniformly indicate the presence of inflammation; nor does it always attend inflammation. Besides, although its appearance did lead to a perfect knowledge of the nature of the disease, it should not enter into a nosological character, because we can only determine the presence of the complaint in this way after we have prescribed the remedies.

But as the other parts of the character are not always, though generally, sufficient for distinguishing the complaints arranged under it, I would propose, instead of sanguis missus, &c. to insert pulsus durus, which at least as constantly attends the Phlegmasiæ, as the buffy coat of the blood. Febris Synocha is also perhaps exceptionable, as we shall find that in certain species of Phlegmasiæ, the fever is a Typhus ; as, for example, in the Pneumonia Putrida of foreign authors, and the Cynanche Maligna. In the Gastritis and Enteritis too, notwithstanding a degree of hardness in the pulse, the fever is certainly more of the nature of Typhus than of Synocha. There is an evident inaccuracy in admitting Synocha into the definition of an order, when we find it necessary in several of the genera of that order to call the fever Pyrexia typhodes.* Dr. Cullen's reason for ma-

---

* See Dr. Cullen's definition of the Gastritis and Enteritis.

king Synocha a part of the definition of the Phlegmasiæ, is evident, namely, because in a great majority of the Phlegmasiæ, the fever is of this kind ; it may be thought therefore the alteration I here propose is not for the better. I have already more than once had occasion to observe that our view is to form an useful, not a perfect, system of nosology.* But as far as I can judge, the introduction of pulsus durus into the definition answers every purpose which that of Synocha can serve, and it seems proper for other reasons that pulsus durus should make a part of this definition.

For these reasons I would propose the following definition of the Phlegmasiæ : Febres symptomaticæ, pulso duru ; quibus est pro morbo locali, vel inflammatio externa, vel dolor topicus simul læsâ partis internæ funcione. Still supposing simple inflammation to have been defined in the class Locales.†

The Hæmorrhagiæ (the fourth order of Dr. Cullen's Pyrexiæ) form the second order of symptomatic fevers. They are defined by Dr. Cullen : " Pyrexia cum profusione sanguinis absque vi " externa ; sanguis missus ut in Phlegmasiis apparet."

" Sanguis missus ut in Phlegmasiis apparet," cannot here be objected to, for the same reason that " Sanguis missus et jam," &c. was omitted in the last definition. But as the buffy coat is not always observed in Hemorrhagies, as its degree is regulated by a variety of accidental circumstances, and as the definition, without this addition, is sufficient to distinguish the diseases arranged under it, it is better I think to omit it. It is also necessary to alter the definition, in order to suit it to the general mode of arrangement I have adopted. It may be expressed in the following manner, Febres symptomaticæ, quibus est pro morbo locali, sanguinis profusio absque vi externa.

The Profluvia, the third and last order of symptomatic fevers, (which Dr. Cullen makes the last order of his Pyrexiæ) he defines, " Pyrexia cum excretione aucta naturaliter non san- " guinea."‡ This definition requires no farther alteration than the mode of arrangement I follow renders necessary ; Febres symptomaticæ, quibus est pro morbo locali, excretio aucta naturaliter non sanguinea.

Such is the mode of arrangement which I mean to adopt. It may be proper to present it to the reader at one view.

* See the notes in the 43d and 44th pages of Dr. Cullen's Syn. Nos. Meth.

† Before entering on the consideration of the Phlegmasiæ, it will be necessary to make some observations on the simple inflammations.

‡ Naturaliter non sanguinea, is introduced into this definition, in order to exclude from the diseases arranged under it the Menorrhagia. With what propriety this is ranked among the Hæmorrhagiæ it is difficult to say : it is still doubtful whether the menstrual discharge is a discharge of blood, or a secretion.

ARRANGEMENT

OF

FEBRILE DISEASES.

——•——

CLASSIS I.

FEBRES IDIOPATHICÆ.

, Prægressis languore, lassitudine, et aliis debilitatis signis, pulsus frequens, calor auctus, sine morbo locali primario.

ORDO I.

FEBRES INTERMITTENTES ET REMITTENTES.

·· Febres idiopathicæ, paroxysmis pluribus apyrexiâ, saltem remissione evidente, interposita, cum exacerbatione notabili, et
plerumque cum horrore redeuntibus, constantes.*

ORDO II.

FEBRES CONTINUÆ.

Febres idiopathicæ, sine intermissione, sed cum remissionibus
et exacerbationibus, parum licet notabilibus, perstantes.

SPECIES 1.

SYNOCHA.

Calor plurimum auctus, pulsus frequens, validus, et durus,
urina rubra, sensorii functiones parum turbatæ.

SPECIES 2.

TYPHUS.

' Morbus contagiosus, calor parum auctus, pulsus parvus, debilis,
plerumque frequens, urina parum mutata, sensorii functiones
plurimum turbatæ, vires multum imminutæ.

---

* The species and varieties of these fevers are very numerous. It will
be necessary to consider them in a separate chapter, I therefore say nothing of them here.

SPECIES 3.

SYNOCHUS.

Morbus contagiosus, febris ex synocha et typho composita ; initio synocha, progressu et versus finem, typhus.

Varietas 1ma.
 Synochus Simplex.
Varietas 2da.
 Synochus Petechialis.
Varietas 3tia.
 Synochus Miliaris.
Varietas 4ta.
 Synochus Aphthosus.
Varietas 5ta.
 Synochus Erysipelatosus.
Varietas 6ta.
 Synochus Vesicularis. *

ORDO III.

EXANTHEMATA.

Morbi contagiosi, cum febre idiopathica† incipientes ; definito tempore, apparent papulæ, sæpe plures, exiguæ, per cutem sparsæ.

SPECIES 1.
VARIOLA.
SPECIES 2.
VARICELLA.
SPECIES 3.
RUBEOLA.
SPECIES 4.
SCARLATINA.
SPECIES 5.
PESTIS.
SPECIES 6.
URTICARIA.

---

* The definitions of these varieties, and of the following species, shall be considered when I come to treat of them separately.

† A single word would be preferable to the circumlocutions Febris Idiopathica and Febris Symptomatica, but I wished to avoid the introduction of new terms.

CLASSIS II.

FEBRES SYMPTOMATICÆ.

Morbi locales, calore aucto, pulsu frequente.

ORDO I.

PHLEGMASIÆ.

Febres symptomaticæ, pulsu duro; quibus est pro morbo locaíli, vel inflammatio externa, vel dolor topicus simul læsâ partis internæ functione.

SPECIES 1.
　　PHLOGOSIS.
SPECIES 2.
　　OPHTHALMIA,
SPECIES 3.
　　PHRENITIS.
SPECIES 4.
　　CYNANCHE.
SPECIES 5.
　　PNEUMONIA,.
SPECIES 6.
　　CARDITIS.
SPECIES 7.
　　PERITONITIS.
SPECIES 8.
　　GASTRITIS,
SPECIES 9.
　　ENTERITIS.
SPECIES 10.
　　HEPATITIS.
SPECIES 11.
　　SPLENITIS,
SPECIES 12.
　　NEPHRITIS.
SPECIES 13.
　　CYSTITIS.
SPECIES 14.
　　HYSTERITIS.
SPECIES 15.
　　RHEUMATISMUS.
SPECIES 16.
　　ODONTALGIA.

SPECIES 17.
 PODAGRA.
SPECIES 18.
 ANTHROPUOSIS.

ORDO II.

HÆMORRHAGIÆ.

Febres symptomaticæ, quibus est pro morbo locali, sanguinis profusio absque vi externa.

SPECIES 1.
 EPISTAXIS.

SPECIES 2.
 HÆMOPTYSIS.

SPECIES 3.
 HÆMORRHOIS.

SPECIES 4.
 MENORRHAGIA.

SPECIES 5.
 HÆMATEMESIS.

SPECIES 6.
 HÆMATURIA.*

ORDO III.

PROFLUVIA.

Febres symptomaticæ, quibus est pro morbo locali, excretio aucta natúraliter non sanguinea.

SPECIES 1.
 CATARRHUS.

SPECIES 2.
 DYSENTERIA.†

---

* The Hæmatemesis and Hæmaturia, regarded by Dr. Cullen as always symptomatic, are sometimes, though rarely, idiopathic. I have seen the Hæmaturia idiopathic. The Cystirrhagia (his last species of Hemorrhagy) is perhaps never idiopathic.

† At the end of the work we shall be enabled to take a more detailed view of that part of a nosological system which relates to febrile diseases, when we shall have considered the definitions and varieties of these complaints.

PART I

OF IDIOPATHIC FEVERS.

IDIOPATHIC fevers, it has been observed in the introduction, are distinguished by the following symptoms: Languor, lassitude, and other signs of debility, followed by a frequent pulse and increased heat, without any primary local affection. This class comprehends three orders, Intermitting and Remitting Fevers, Continued Fevers, and the Exanthemata, or Eruptive Fevers.

BOOK I.

OF INTERMITTING AND REMITTING FEVERS.

ACCORDING to the definition given in the introduction, intermitting and remitting fevers consist of repeated paroxysms, returning with an evident exacerbation, and generally with shivering, complete apyrexia, or at least an evident remission being interposed. I am now to consider the phenomena of these complaints more fully.

CHAP. I.

Of the Species and Varieties of Intermitting and Remitting Fevers.

INTERMITTING and remitting fevers have long been divided into Quotidians, Tertians, and Quartans, that is, fevers returning every day, every second day, and every third day. To which are to be added, those whose paroxysms recur at a longer interval.*

The revolution, interval, or period, as it is called, is divided into two parts, that during which the fever prevails, and that during which it is absent or nearly so. The former, is termed the paroxysm; the latter, the intermission or apyrexia, if the fever ceases altogether; it is termed the remission, if the symptoms only suffer an abatement.

* The interval, it must be remembered, is the space of time occupied by what is called a complete revolution or period of the fever, that is, the time from the accession of one fit to that of the next. And when physicians talk of a Tertian, Quartan, &c. they count from the beginning of a revolution. Thus, in a Tertian, the day on which the fever appears is the first day; the next, the second; and the next, on which the fever again takes place, the third; this fever therefore is termed a Tertian. Some confusion of names has arisen among the vulgar, from not attending to this mode of reckoning.

Hippocrates mentions intermittents which returned on the fifth, seventh, or eighth days. Boerhaave says he saw a Septenary, that is, a fever returning every seventh day; and Van Swieten saw a Quartan change to a Quintan. Many similar observations have been made. Burserius enumerates no less than twelve authors who saw a Quintan distinctly marked, nine who met with Septenaries, sixteen who met with Octans, several who met with fevers returning on the ninth, the tenth, and even the fourteenth or fifteenth day. We also read of fevers which are said to have returned once a month, once in two months, &c. These have been termed Menstruæ, Bimenstruæ, &c. and some authors even speak of fevers which returned yearly, termed Annuæ.

How far the observations of those who mention fevers with such intervals are accurate, it is difficult to say; on comparing them with the observations of others, we cannot help suspecting their accuracy. Galen, whose practice was more extensive perhaps than that of any other physician, never saw a fever with a longer interval than a Quintan, and very rarely this.† The particular state of the weather at certain times of the year, by producing fever in the predisposed, often gives rise to the appearance of an annual intermittent. But the fever in such cases is always of the continued kind, and never assumes the appearance of the paroxysm of an Ague.

Besides the Quotidian, Tertian, Quartan, and the fevers of more protracted periods, there are other intermittents and remittents,‡ in which the return of the paroxysm is irregular, that is, whose revolutions are not performed in equal times. These are considered by Dr. Cullen, as varieties of the Tertian and Quartan. They have been termed Erratica, Quintana, Septana, Octana, Nonana, Lunatica.||

Each intermittent has also been divided into Benigna, Maligna or Corruptiva, Primaria, Secondaria or Symptomatica, Periodica; Partialis, that is, affecting the body partially; Sporadica, appearing at the same time with other diseases; Endemica, appearing in a place which from its natural situation is peculiarly apt to produce the disease; and Epidemica, prevailing generally at any particular season. Such divisions (as may be inferred from the meaning of the terms) are quite useless.

† Even the Quintan has been suspected by later writers to be a variety of the Tertian.

‡ In the following pages what is said of intermittents (in order to shorten the expression) is implied of remittents, except where the meaning evidently points out the contrary.

|| There are many fevers of this kind mentioned in the works of Etmuller, Van Swieten, De Haen, by different authors in Haller's Disp. ad Morb. Hist. et Cur. Pert. &c.

Intermittents have also been regarded as varying according as they are accompanied by certain symptoms, by coma for instance, syncope, convulsions, an efflorescence on the skin, much sweating, great inquietude, nausea, vomiting, delirium, &c. hence the names Elodes, Assodes, Syncopalis, &c. This division also is quite useless.

The same may be said of that division which regards intermittents, as varying according as they are accompanied with other complaints; Scurvy, Syphilis, Worms, Dysentery, Epilepsy, Gout, &c. and of that which makes them vary according to the nature of the remote cause. We shall find, in considering the remote causes of intermittents, that there is very little room for any division of this kind.

Of all the species of intermittents, it will be necessary to consider particularly only three. The others have not been accurately observed, very rarely occur, and are suspected by many, and not without reason, to be only varieties of these.

The intermittents which deserve a particular consideration are the Quotidian, Tertian, and Quartan. Of these, the most noted is the Tertian. It occurs most frequently; so much so indeed, that Dr. Fordyce* and others are of opinion, that all fevers, whether continued or intermitting, are varieties of this: an opinion not to be admitted however, as will be sufficiently evident, I think, after we shall have considered the symptoms and varieties of these complaints.

SECT. I.

Of the Varieties of the Tertian.†

THE Tertian is defined by Dr. Cullen, " Paroxysmi similes " intervallo quadraginta octo circiter horarum, accessionibus me- " ridianis."

The Tertian, whose paroxysm does not exceed twelve hours, is called the true simple Tertian; that whose paroxysm exceeds twelve hours, is called the spurious simple Tertian. The former, Dr. Cleghorn‡ remarks, frequently comes on about the middle

* See Dr. Fordyce's first Dissertation on Simple Fever.

† In considering the varieties of intermittents, it is proper to begin with the Tertian, because its varieties have been better marked, and are more numerous than those of the Quotidian and Quartan. However uninteresting this part of the subject is, the practitioner must be acquainted with it, since the varieties about to be pointed out are constantly occurring in practice; and it is necessary to know the meaning of terms employed by the authors who treat of these fevers.

‡ See Cleghorn's Treatise on the Diseases of Minorca.

of the day, and goes off the same evening; the other comes off much earlier, and often lasts for eighteen hours.*

The Tertian varies in the frequency of the recurrence, as well as the length of its paroxysms; instead of every second day, it sometimes returns every day; it is then distinguished from the Quotidian by its alternate paroxysms being similar, that is, by the paroxysms of the odd days being similar, but more or less severe, in all, or some of their stages, making their attack at an earlier or later time of the day, &c. than the paroxysms of the even days. When the paroxysms recur in this way, the fever is termed Tertiana duplex; and there might be a division of the Tertiana duplex into that in which the most severe paroxysm happens on the even, and that in which it happens on the odd, day, counting from the beginning of the complaint. And this division is not so useless as at first sight it may appear; it assists, we shall find, in forming the prognosis, particularly in double Tertian remittents.† It has been observed that the most severe fit is followed by the most complete apyrexia. Double Tertians, if the fit does not exceed twelve hours, are termed true double Tertians; when it exceeds twelve hours, spurious double Tertians.

When the fits are so protracted that one begins almost as soon as the preceding fit ends, this as well as other remittents have been termed subintrant, or sub-continued. Subintrant fevers are almost always remittents, complete apyrexia rarely taking place in them.

The Tertian sometimes returns twice every second day, the intermediate day having no paroxysm; it is then termed Tertiana duplicata.

It sometimes returns twice every second day, while one paroxysm takes place on the intermediate day; the fever is then termed Tertiana triplex. And Tulpius relates a case of the Tertiana quadruplex, which has escaped the observation of most authors, in which two paroxysms take place every day.‡ It is still to be remembered that the Tertian type is discovered by the paroxysms being similar on alternate days. When we come to consider the manner in which intermittents suffer a reduplication of their paroxysms, we shall find, that as often as an additional paroxysm takes place in any of these fevers, both the new and the

* Hippocrates observes, and the observation is confirmed by Vogel (see Vogel de Cog. et Cur. Morb.) and others, that the paroxysms of Tertian, as well as other intermittents, are less frequently protracted when the patient is young, his general health good, and particularly when he is not troubled with visceral obstructions.

† See Cleghorn on the Tertian, in his Treatise on the Diseases of Minorca.

‡ The case mentioned by Tulpius supervened on a double Tertian. See his Observationes Medicæ, l. iv. c. 46.

original paroxysms are more protracted than the latter, were before the accession of the former. Considering this circumstance, and the frequency of the paroxysms in a quadruple Tertian, the remissions must be extremely slight, and the complaint consequently must assume entirely, or in a great measure, the appearance of a continued fever, according to the foregoing definition of this complaint.

When a single paroxysm takes place every day, but the remission between the first and second paroxysm is more considerable than that between the second and third, the remission between the third and fourth more considerable than between the fourth and fifth, and so on;* the Tertian has been called Hæmitritæus or Semitertiana. Different authors however do not always employ these terms in the same sense.†

The interval of the Tertian, it was observed, is forty-eight hours, but sometimes it is rather less, the fit coming on at an earlier time of the day; and sometimes it is more, the fit coming on at a later time of the day than that which preceded. When the former happens, the fever is called an anticipating Tertian (Tertiana prævertens); when the latter happens, a postponing Tertian (Tertiana tardans). And Dr. Cleghorn has observed of the double Tertian, that the more severe fit often comes on a little earlier in each period, while the slight fit returns at the same hour of the day, or perhaps later.

It is remarkable, that postponing agues, after the accession of the paroxysm is postponed to eight o'clock in the evening, frequently have their next accession early in the morning of the day following that on which the fever should have returned; and in like manner, after an anticipating paroxysm has occurred at eight o'clock in the morning, the next accession is often on the evening

* This indeed is generally the case in double Tertians; but when it is more remarkable than usual, it has given rise to a particular division of this fever.

† The following account of the Hæmitritæus by Celsus, does not correspond to this definition. There are two kinds of Tertians, he observes, the one coming on and terminating like the Quartan, with this only difference, that between the paroxysms the patient remains well for only one day, the fever returning on the third, (this is the common simple Tertian); the other, he continues, is much more pernicious; this indeed, like the former, returns every third day, but of the forty-eight hours almost six and thirty are occupied by the fever, and during the remainder the fever never wholly disappears, but only suffers an abatement of its symptoms. "Id genus (he adds) plerique medici Hæmitritæen appellant." In this account of the Hæmitritæus, Celsus wholly overlooks the remission which takes place, according to the above definition, between the unequal and equal days, the first and second, third and fourth, &c.
The sense in which others use the term Hæmitritæus differs still more widely from the above definition, and approaches very nearly to that given of the Tertiana triplex. It is used in this sense by Lommius in his Observ. Medic. libri tres, p. 22, and Eller in his Observ. de Cog. et Cur. Morb. sect. 4, p. 83.

of the day preceding that on which it should happen.* A post-poning intermittent is a safer fever than an anticipating one.

SECT. II.

Of the Varieties of the Quartan and Quotidian.

HAVING considered the varieties of the Tertian at some length, it will not be necessary to spend much time in consider-ing those of the Quartan and Quotidian. The former (the Quar-tan) is defined by Dr. Cullen, " Paroxysmi similes intervallo sep-" tuaginta duarum circiter horarum, accessionibus pomeridi-" anis."

This, like the Tertian, varies in the length of its paroxysms, and the manner and frequency of their recurrence. There are sometimes two paroxysms every fourth day ; the fever is then called Quartiana duplicata. At other times there are three par-oxysms every fourth day ; it is then called Quartiana triplicata. Sometimes, of the four days, the third only is without a parox-ysm ; a single paroxysm taking place on the first, second, and fourth days ; each paroxysm being similar to that which occurs on the fourth day before it ; the fever is then called Quartana duplex. The paroxysm returns sometimes every day ; the par-oxysms happening on every fourth day being similar ; it is then called Quartana triplex.

The following is Dr. Cullen's definition of the Quotidian, " Paroxysmi similes intervallo viginti quatuor circiter horarum, " paroxysmis matutinis."

This fever varies chiefly in the length of its paroxysms, and the degree of remission. Some Quotidians, Celsus observes, suffer so complete a remission, that the patient is free from the fever between the paroxysms. In others, though an abatement of the symptoms takes place, yet more or less of the fever re-mains throughout the paroxysm. This is the only way in which Celsus regards the Quotidian as varying. According to Burse-rius, however, it varies also in having one, two, and even three paroxysms in the day, and these varieties he terms the simple, double, and triple Quotidian. But a Quotidian with the appear-ance of two or three paroxysms in the day, (for they are never very distinctly marked) is not to be distinguished from a continued

---

* Thus, if the paroxysm of an anticipating Tertian comes on at nine o'clock on Monday morning, the next paroxysm at eight o'clock on Wed-nesday morning, the third paroxysm will probably not occur at seven o'clock on Friday morning, but some time on Thursday evening. In like manner, if a postponing Tertian make its attack at seven o'clock on Mon-day evening, and the next paroxysm appear at eight o'clock on Wednes-day evening, the third paroxysm will probably take place, not at nine o'clock on Friday evening, but some time on Saturday morning.

fever. The terms anticipating, postponing, subintrant, &c. applied to the Quartan and Quotidian, are employed in the same sense as when applied to the Tertian.

All these fevers, it may be observed, are said in the definitions to make their attack in the day time. The Quotidian in the morning, the Tertian at noon, and the Quartan in the afternoon. It is remarkable of all fevers, that nine perhaps out of ten make their attack between eight o'clock in the morning and eight in the evening The cause of this may be, that a state of natural sleep is opposite to that of fever.

Such are the different species and varieties of intermitting fevers. Before we leave this part of the subject, it may seem proper to consider the manner in which the different types* assume more or less of the continued form; but it will be better to defer this till we shall have considered the symptoms of these fevers.

CHAP. II.

Of the Symptoms of Intermitting and Remitting Fevers.

IN treating of the symptoms of intermitting and remitting fevers, I shall in the first section give a detail of the symptoms which more properly belong to these fevers. In the second, I shall give the reader a view of what may be termed the anomalous symptoms of intermittents. In the third section, I shall point out the diseases with which these fevers are most frequently complicated. In the fourth, we shall consider more particularly the prognosis in intermittents. In the fifth, take a view of the symptoms which characterise the different types. And in the last, consider the manner in which these assume more or less of the continued form.

These heads, with what has been said, comprehend all that relates to the symptoms of intermittents, except what may be said of their crises. The term crisis has not been used in a very definite sense; I shall generally employ it to express certain symptoms which are often observed to attend the change from fever to health. As it will be proper to throw together the observations which it is necessary to make on the crises of fevers; and as the crisis which in intermittents is almost always the same, is, in continued fevers, very various, I shall defer the consideration of this part of the subject till I come to speak of the latter set of complaints. I am in the first place then to lay before the reader the symptoms of intermittents in general.

* By type is meant the species of the intermittent. All Quotidians are of the same type; Quotidians and Tertians are of different types.

SECT. I.

Of the Symptoms of Intermitting and Remitting Fevers.

A short account of intermitting and remitting fevers has already been given. We are told, in the definition of those diseases, that they are fevers consisting of repeated paroxysms, complete apyrexia, or at least an evident remission, being interposed. It is necessary however to take a more particular view of their symptoms.

A regular fit or paroxysm of an intermittent is divided into three stages. The most striking symptoms of the first stage are, a sense of cold and shaking; this is therefore termed the cold stage. The second is characterised by an increase of temperature; it is therefore called the hot stage; and the chief symptom of the last, which is termed the sweating stage, is a copious secretion by the skin.

1. *Of the Symptoms of the Cold Stage of Intermittents.**

At the commencement of the fit the patient is more indolent than usual, frequently yawning and stretching himself. The aversion to motion increases till it arrives at an uneasy weariness over the whole body; and sometimes the weakness is such, that he is scarcely able to support himself. He is restless, soon tired of the same posture, yet feels an uneasy exertion in changing it. His thoughts succeed each other more rapidly than usual, and he feels it irksome to bend his attention for a considerable time to one object. The pulse is now weaker and sometimes slower an natural.

At the commencement of these symptoms the patient does not always complain of cold, but his skin, especially in the extremities, often feels cold to another person. The nails soon begin to grow pale, the same gradually happens to the fingers, toes, lips, &c. and the skin becomes rough as when exposed to cold, and less sensible than usual.

The patient now complains of a sense of cold, which indeed sometimes from the first attends the foregoing symptoms. After this, which on its first coming on is generally referred to the

* That the following account of the symptoms of intermittents may be less complicated, I have omitted many which will be mentioned under the head Prognosis, and shall here give those which may be regarded as more properly constituting the disease. It is necessary to have recourse to this, or some other such means when the symptoms of diseases are very numerous, in order to avoid confusion; which is not to be done, when the reader is at once presented with a great variety of symptoms. We have sufficient proof of this in the manner in which the symptoms of diseases are generally laid down by foreign systematic writers, Lieutaud, Burserius, Frank, &c.

back, has continued for a short time, a trembling begins in the lower jaw, and gradually spreads over the whole body.*

In some cases the sense of cold is partial, being confined to one or more of the limbs; while at the same time the rest of the body perhaps glows with heat; and while the cold is severe on the surface, a burning heat is sometimes felt internally.

For a short time after the shaking begins, the skin continues cold to the feeling of another person, and measured by the thermometer is found considerably below the natural temperature. Its temperature has been observed as low as 74°. After the shaking has lasted for some time, however, the patient still complaining of cold, the warmth of his skin to the feeling of another person, or measured by the thermometer, gradually increases.

The pulse during the cold stage, is small, frequent, sometimes irregular, and often hardly to be felt; the respiration is also considerably affected. It is frequent and anxious, accompanied with a cough, or interrupted by sighing; there is a sense of weight and often tightness and oppression about the præcordia, and that dejection of spirits which constantly attends these symptoms.

This is not the only change which takes place in the mind. The remembrance of things at other times desirable now disgusts; and the hurry of thought which attended from the beginning of the paroxysm increasing, a degree of confusion takes place. If these symptoms continue to increase, they rise to delirium; or more frequently the patient becomes stupid and a considerable degree of coma, or what has been termed the febrile apoplexy, supervenes. Delirium is a more frequent attendant on the hot stage, and coma on the cold; the latter often appearing almost at the very commencement of the paroxysm.

Although neither delirium nor coma attend the cold fit, it is not uncommon at this period of the disease for some of the senses to be considerably impaired; the patient often complains of numbness in the limbs; and in some instances both sight and hearing have been almost lost. When this happens, the stomach is generally loaded with bile.†

* The teeth strike against each other, often with such force, that instances are on record of the teeth of old people being knocked out by the cold fit of a Quartan. The trembling over the whole body indeed is sometimes so severe, that after the cold fit the patient has hardly strength to move his limbs. Even syncope is apt to occur during this stage when the strength has been much reduced; and it seldom occurs repeatedly without endangering life. In very severe and long continued cold fits, particularly in old people, the body has been known to become stiff almost like that of a dead person.

† We know that the stomach is oppressed, when there is a bitter taste in the mouth, when the breath is fœtid, the tongue yellowish and covered with thick mucus, when the patient is troubled with eructations, anxiety,

Pains of the back, limbs, and loins, generally attend the cold stage, or the patient complains of a sensation as if the body had been bruised.

There is, especially soon after the beginning of this stage, a shrinking of the extemities, so that a ring at other times tight, drops off the finger. Ulcers often dry up, during the cold stage of agues; and tumors subside.*

The natural functions are much deranged. At the beginning of the paroxysm the appetite ceases, and as the cold stage advances nausea frequently occurs, often succeeded by a vomiting of bile, which, in the intermittents, and still more in the remittents of sultry climates, and even of the warmer seasons of temperate climates, is sometimes poured into the stomach and intestines in prodigious quantity. Less frequently the matter rejected by vomiting, is a ropy, transparent fluid, nearly insipid ; often secreted in no less quantity in various kinds, or rather, in many cases of all kinds of fevers.

When the quantity of bile in the stomach and intestines is very great, it is frequently (particularly towards the beginning of the hot fit) passed by stool as well as vomiting ; bile indeed often predominates so much in these fevers, that the patient looks like a person in the jaundice, and the serum of the blood and the urine are tinged with yellow.

With these symptoms the thirst is constant, the mouth and fauces dry and clammy. The urine, if not tinged with bile, is in the cold stage almost colourless and without cloud or sediment ; and, if there be no bile in the primæ viæ, stools are uncommon at this period.

Such are the symptoms of the cold stage of an intermittent. It must be recollected, however, that in different cases there is great variety ; we are not to expect that these symptoms will be equally remarkable in every patient, or that all of them will, be observed in any one. Even the leading symptoms, the sense of cold, shaking, &c. are sometimes absent, so that we can hardly say there is any cold stage at all.† This however rarely happens.

and a sense of oppression, pain or heat about the stomach, nausea, vomiting, heaviness or pain of the head, vertigo, thirst, and spontaneous diarrhœa. When these, or part of these, symptoms are present to a considerable degree, they form one of those useless divisions of intermitting fever above alluded to, termed Intermittens Gastrica. See a copious account of this species of intermittent, in the first volume of Frank's excellent work, entitled Epitome de Cur. Morb.

* During the hot stage, or after the paroxysm is over, tumors generally regain their former size, and ulcers again discharge matter as before the paroxysm.

† See the section of the anomalous symptoms of intermittents.

The duration of the cold fit varies much ; sometimes it contin-ues four or five hours, or more, particularly in the intermittents of long periods; at other times it does not last above half an hour, or even a shorter time, particularly in remittents, and especially those approaching to the continued form. Its mean duration per-haps is between one and two hours.*

During the first paroxysms, the cold stage is often longer than at a later period, becoming shorter as the disease increases in vi-olence, and particularly, as it suffers a prolongation and redupli-cation of its paroxysms ; till, at length, when the paroxysms have been so protracted as almost to run into each other, the cold fit is sometimes hardly perceivable. This part of the subject will be considered more particularly when speaking of the man-ner in which the different types assume more or less of the con-tinued form.

2. Of the Symptoms of the Hot and Sweating Stages.

The hot stage succeeds the cold. It is sometimes ushered in by the vomiting which follows the nausea in the first stage ; or the cold and shivering, after alternating for some time with short fits of heat, gradually abate, and more permanent heat is at length diffused over every part of the body. The paleness and shrinking, together with the peculiar constriction of the skin which attend the cold stage, now disappear, and are succeeded by a general redness and fulness, which however give the appear-ance rather of turgescence than relaxation, the skin still remain-ing parched.

The heat in this stage often raises Farenheit's thermometer five, six, or more degrees above the natural temperature. Dr. Fordyce states 105° as the greatest degree of febrile heat which he has observed. Other writers mention higher degrees.

As the hot stage advances, other changes take place in the state of the vital functions. The pulse from being small, weak, and often irregular, becomes regular, strong, and full. And this state of the pulse generally increases till the sweat breaks out. The breathing, from being hurried, interrupted, and anxious, becomes more full and free, while the sense of tightness across the breast is in some measure relieved. In most cases, however, the breathing still continues more frequent and anxious than in health.

With regard to the animal functions; the sensibility which is impaired in the cold stage, is morbidly increased in the hot. The patient cannot endure the least noise ; and the light is offen-sive. The pains of the limbs continue during the hot stage ; and the pain of the head, which is often wholly absent in the cold fit, now comes on or increases, frequently accompanied with a throb-

* See M'Bride's Introduction to the Theory and Practice of Medicine.

bing of the temporal arteries and tinnitus aurium. The confusion of thought is upon the whole greater in this than in the former stage, and more frequently rises to delirium.*

The state of the natural functions suffers but little change. As the hot stage advances the nausea and vomiting abate, but the thirst still remains or increases. The urine, from being limpid, often becomes high coloured, but is still without sediment ; in other respects the state of these functions is nearly the same as in the cold fit. Except when a diarrhœa accompanies the complaint, stools seldom occur till the end of the paroxysm, and then a general relaxation of the excretories taking place, there is usually a loose stool.

It is in the hot stage that hemorrhagies most frequently occur, at least those hemorrhagies which relieve the symptoms. They happen from various parts of the body ; from the uterus ; from the rectum, if the patient happens to labour under the hæmorrhoids ; sometimes from the lungs ; from the ears ; but most generally from the nose. If the hemorrhagy from the nose be free, it is almost always a favourable symptom, and sometimes brings immediate relief ; but a few drops of blood falling from it, Cleghorn says, he generally found to portend danger, and others have made the same observation.

The hemorrhagies which appear about the commencement of the hot stage, however, it may be observed, are generally the consequence of too rapid a circulation ; and if not favourable, are seldom to be regarded as affording a bad prognosis. When we come to consider the symptoms of typhus I shall have occasion to take notice of another species of hemorrhagies, which seldom attend the fevers I am speaking of, till, in consequence of a debilitated state of the system, they have nearly assumed the continued form, and which almost always afford a bad prognosis.

It is to be observed, that the appearance of hemorrhagies only assists us in judging of the event, when we attend to the symptoms which accompany them, and the parts of the body from which the blood flows. They may afford the most favourable or the most fatal prognosis. They will be considered more particularly among the crises of fever. It may be remarked at present, that when the excitement is considerable, they frequently prove favourable, and seldom do harm ; when the excitement is too low, they are rarely beneficial, and often followed by the worst consequences.

* It is not uncommon at this period for the patient to complain of pain, heat, and tension, accompanied also with a sense of pulsation in the stomach and bowels; this, however, is a less frequent symptom, and seems generally to depend on the presence of some irritating matter, and sometimes indicates inflammation, in the primæ viæ.

' When the fever has lasted for a considerable time, and the re-missions have become less complete, especially when the epidemic is of a malignant nature ; a variety of symptoms denoting great debility, and affording a very unfavourable prognosis, shew themselves. But these, like the worst species of hemorrhagics, belong rather to continued, than intermitting, fevers. I shall have occasion to speak of them at large, when we come to consider the symptoms of typhus, the fever in which they most generally make their appearance. It is sufficient here to have observed, that the symptoms alluded to sometimes, though rarely, occur, while the remissions are still very evident.

The violence of the hot stage is not, at all times, proportioned to that of the preceding cold fit. Dr. Cleghorn informs us, that the most violent fevers he ever saw came on without any cold stage. It is often observed, however, that the longer the cold stage is, the more violent is the succeeding hot fit, the type of the fever being the same. We shall find that, with respect to intermittents of different types, this is by no means the case, but rather the contrary.

The hot stage is at length terminated by a profuse sweat, which forms the last stage of the paroxysm ; and soon relieves the patient. The sweating generally begins about the head and breast, extending gradually to the back and extremities. The strength and frequency of the pulse are now diminished, and the breathing becomes free. The urine deposits a sediment like brickdust, which has been termed lateritious ; or a copious reddish or white sediment, which writers have confounded with the other ;* and the patient generally falls into a sleep, while the symptoms of the fever abate, leaving him weak and wearied. If the fever be an intermittent, complete apyrexia succeeds. If a remittent, the symptoms of the hot stage, but with an evident abatement, continue till the recurrence of the paroxysm, which is regulated by the type of the fever, as has been shewn.

Although the patient, between the paroxysms of an intermittent, is free from fever, yet he seldom finds himself in perfect health, especially if the paroxysms have been severe. He is easily fatigued, complains of want of appetite, the skin is parched, or he is more liable to sweat than in health. Sometimes he is subject to vomiting or purging, and is often dejected and drowsy. The more the patient is harrassed by such symptoms during the apyrexia, the more reason there is to dread that the ensuing paroxysm will be severe.

Such are the phenomena of intermitting fevers in general; they vary much in the violence and duration of the paroxysm, and in the proportional violence and duration of the different

* It will be necessary to make some observations on these depositions from the urine, when I speak of the crises of fevers.

stages constituting the paroxysm, as well as in the degree and
length of the remissions, and the general health of the patient
during them.

All intermittents are apt to change to a more or less continued
form, the tendency to become continued is always unfavourable ;
the prognosis is good when they change from a less to a more
intermitting form.

SECT. II.

Of the Anomalous Symptoms of Intermittents.

THERE is another class of symptoms belonging to intermittents in general. These may be termed anomalous, a great
variety of which have been observed.

The anomalous appearances belonging to intermittents, may
be divided into four classes. The first, comprehending those
cases in which the order of the different stages constituting a
paroxysm is deranged, or in which some of these stages are
wholly wanting. The second comprehending those cases, in
which the whole paroxysm or some of its stages are confined to
particular parts of the body. The third, those in which certain
symptoms prevail so much as to alter considerably the appearance of the disease. And the last, those in which other diseases
or particular symptoms assume the form of an intermittent.

Without giving a particular account of such cases, I shall refer
to different works where the reader will find a variety of them,
falling under each of these heads.

In the first place, of those in which the order of the stages is
deranged or some of them wholly wanting.

It is observed, by Cleghorn,* Senac,† and others, that the
cold stage is sometimes wanting. Sometimes it accompanies only some of the paroxysms : intermittents have been
observed to recur without the shivering for several of the first
paroxysms. Frank‡ remarks, that even the hot stage itself
is sometimes scarcely perceptible ; at other times, as in cases
mentioned by Senac,|| the hot and sweating stages occur together.
The hot fit does not always follow the cold ; Frank observes, that
the former sometimes precedes the latter : nor does the sweating
always follow the hot ; the skin sometimes remaining perfectly
dry during the whole paroxysm.§ " The tumult and uneasiness

* See Cleghorn on the Diseases of Minorca.
† See Senac de Febribus.
‡ See Frank's Epitome de Cur. Morb.
|| De Febribus.
§ See Senac de Febribus.

" (says Dr. Jackson,*) of intermittent fever, which terminate in
" most cases by sweat, went off in some by urine or stool, or per-
" haps declined in others without the appearance of any preter-
" natural evacuation." Dr. Cleghorn also observes, that tertians
sometimes terminate by urine or stool, rather than by sweat.
And there are cases mentioned in the works of Burserius† and
Schenkius,‡ in which the order of the stages was so far inverted,
that, in one instance, the cold stage was the last of the paroxysms,
and in another, the sweating stage was the first.

The second class of the anomalous cases of intermittents comprehends those in which the paroxysm, or some of its stages, is
confined to particular parts of the body. Vogel‖ observes, that
the cold sometimes seizes on one member only, for instance the
arm, and is sometimes confined to one half of the head. This
is a less uncommon occurence; but it is remarkable, that the
whole fit should sometimes be confined to a particular part of the
body, that a particular member should be seized with the symptoms of the cold, hot, and sweating stages, while the rest of the
body remains unaffected.§

The third class of anomalous cases of intermittents comprehends those in which certain symptoms prevail so much, as to alter considerably the appearance of the disease.

" Sometimes one or two symptoms of the fit (Dr. Cleghorn¶
" observes) predominate with such violence that the rest are ob-
" scured or altogether eclipsed. Hence we so frequently meet
" with hemicranias, choleras, dysenteries, and chincough, re-
" turning regularly at stated periods; and several fevers of
" this class, upon account of some predominant symptom, have
" had particular names bestowed on them." I formerly had occasion to mention these, which indeed are of no use; it is necessary however to be acquainted with them, since they are used by
authors. Tertians, Dr. Cleghorn observes in another place, are
sometimes so complicated with pains of the head, breast, belly,
back or limbs, as to appear like a pleurisy, phrenzy, hepatitis,
lumbago or rheumatism, particularly when the remissions are
obscure.

I have known patients, says Stork,** who along with fever were
every day, at a certain time, seized with palpitation of the heart,

* See Jackson on the Fevers of Jamaica.
† See Burserius Institut. Med. Pract.
‡ See Schenkius Observat. Med. Rariores.
‖ See Vogel's Prælect. Acad. de Cog. et Cur. Morb.
§ There is a striking instance of this kind related in the Nosologia Me-
thodica of Sauvages.
¶ Diseases of Minorca.
** See Stork's Anni Medici.

or great anxiety about the præcordia, with fruitless and violent coughing ; others were attacked with a violent pain of the whole, or part of the head. Sir John Pringle* observes, that among the intermittents which prevailed in the army in marshy countries, there were some which attacked the head so suddenly, and with such violence, that the men without any previous symptom of indisposition ran about in a wild manner, and were believed to be mad till the solution of the disease, and its periodical return, shewed its real nature.

Dr. Rush,† and many others, mention cases of intermittents coming on with delirium, particularly Mr. Clark in the fourth volume of the Medical Observations and Inquiries. Great swelling of the tongue, a strangury, dreadful horror, with a desire to die, and boils on the skin, mentioned as frequent symptoms in the bilious remittent fever of Bussarah, may also be regarded as anomalous.‡ In the sixth volume of the Edinburgh Medical Essays there is a case related by Mr. Bain, in which epilepsy attended the paroxysms of an intermittent ; and in the fifteenth volume of the Medical Commentaries, another related by Mr. Davidson in which the paroxysms were accompanied by amaurosis.

In short, the anomalous appearances of intermittents belonging to this class are very various. It is impossible to enumerate all that have been observed ; those just mentioned are sufficient to put the practitioner on his guard, and prevent embarrassment when such cases occur. It appears from the observations of a variety of authors, that when we succeed in removing the fever by the ordinary means, such anomalous symptoms yield along with it. This even happened in the two cases just alluded to, in which epilepsy and amaurosis were complicated with the intermittent.

It is to be observed, that when such violent symptoms occur, they often derange the fever, so that it is impossible to say of what type it is. But when the symptoms become more moderate, it generally assumes the same type which it had before the accession of such symptoms. And what tends still farther to perplex intermittents, and render them irregular, though indeed it rarely happens, is, that in one paroxysm certain symptoms shall predominate, and in another, symptoms of quite a different nature.

The last class of anomalous cases, which may be regarded as belonging to the fevers we are speaking of, comprehends those in

* See Sir John Pringle's Observations on the Diseases of the army.

† See Rush's Medical Obs. and Inq.

‡ There is a good account of this dreadful fever in a work entitled the Transactions of a Society for the Improvement of Medical and Surgical Knowledge, for 1793.

which other diseases, or particular symptoms assume the form of
an intermittent.

Certain symptoms, such as pain in some part of the head, coma, delirium, even hiccup, recurring for several paroxysms,
with intermitting fever, at length take place, at stated intervals,
after every symptom of fever is removed. Cases of this kind
are related by Senac and a variety of other authors. But it does
not always happen that the symptoms which thus recur periodically have accompanied an intermittent, They sometimes appear from the first without fever, and continue to recur at the
quotidian, tertian, or quartan interval.

Stork* relates a case of amaurosis which recurred in this way.
Rheumatic pains have often been observed to do so. Dr.
Rush† relates several cases of this kind. There is a very curious
account of pulmonary complaints assuming the form of an intermittent, by Dr. Chapman, in the first volume of the Medical
Commentaries. Dr. Strack‡ enumerates many of the anomalous
symptoms belonging to this class. He relates one case which
never appeared in any other form but that of coma. He also met
with inflammation of the eyes appearing as an intermittent, and
enumerates pleuritis, cholera, cholic, gout, histeria, and convulsions, as apt to assume the same form.

Of all such cases it is remarkable, and deserves particular attention, that they almost always yield to the same means which
remove intermittents, however dissimilar to these fevers they
may be in all respects, except in their periodical recurrence.
This curious fact has been established by very extensive observation.

I shall only add, before I leave the anomalous symptoms of
intermittents, that they have sometimes left behind them irreg-,
ular shakings, which often prove very obstinate. There are cases of this kind related by Dr. Monro in the second volume of
the Edinb. Med. Ess. and Obs. and in the fourth volume of the
same work by Mr. Andrew Willison. The case related by the
latter yielded to the cold bath.

SECT. III.

*Of the Diseases with which Intermittents are most frequently com-
plicated.*

With regard to a variety of symptoms which often appear in
intermittents, arising from their being complicated with other
diseases, little can be said here, as I am not at present to treat of

* See his Anni. Medici.
† See his Med. Obs. and Inq.
‡ Strack de Feb. Intermit.

the different complaints to which they belong. The diseases
with which they are most frequently complicated are, diarrhœa,
cholera, dysentery, obstructions of the different viscera, dropsy,
jaundice, and different species of inflammation.

Inflammation of some of the viscera and remittent fever is one
of the most common of these combinations. ·De Haen* and
others relate many cases of remittents, in which the stomach
and bowels were found on dissection inflamed and sphacelated.
This combination has been observed to be remarkably frequent
in certain epidemics. Bartholine† in particular gives an account
of an irregular remittent that raged at Copenhagen, which was
always accompanied with inflammation of the stomach and duodenum ; and we have an account of a similar fever which raged
at Leyden, by Professor Silvius de la Boe.‡ The brain is also
frequently the seat of inflammation in remittents, as appears
from the account of dissections by Sir John Pringle‖ and others ;
and rheumatism, another inflammatory affection frequently accompanies the intermittents of cold climates.§

The vernal intermittents are most commonly accompanied
with inflammatory affections. In autumn these fevers are more
frequently combined with the disorders that have been termed
putrescent, particularly dysentery.

The frequent concurrence of some of the above-mentioned
complaints and intermittents is owing to something peculiar in
particular epidemics, or in the climates or constitutions in which
intermittents generally occur ; but some of them are the effects
of the fever itself: schirrous indurations of the viscera, for instance, and their consequences, jaundice and dropsy. The liver
and spleen are the viscera most frequently affected.

When we recollect the nature of the circulation in the liver,
and consider whence the greater part of its blood is supplied, we
are at no loss to account for the ascites that sometimes attends
its induration. Nor is it difficult to conceive in what manner an
induration and enlargement either of this viscous or the spleen
frequently produce an anasarca of the inferior extremities, gradually extending over the whole body, when we reflect that the
cava ascendens is exposed to the pressure of the enlarged viscera. That jaundice must frequently be the consequence of an
induration of the liver or pancreas, (for this viscus is also sometimes indurated in those who have suffered much from agues) is
also evident from considering the situation of the biliary ducts,

* See his Ratio Medendi.
† Barthol. Hist. Anatom. Rar. hist. 56.
‡ Prax. Med. Append. tract x.
‖ See his observations on the diseases of the army.
§ See the epidemics described by Sir John Pringle, in his Observ. on
the Dis. of the Army.

which may be pressed upon by enlarged portions of either of these organs.

'To these consequences of intermittent fever may be added cachexy and atrophy, a bad habit of body, and wasting from obstructions of the mesenteric, pancreatic, and other glands of the abdomen. Agues also sometimes check habitual discharges, the menstrual and hemorrhoidal flux, and sometimes interrupt the secretion of milk in nurses. They also now and then occasion excessive discharges by sweat or stool, of the menses, lochia, &c.*

If intermittents sometimes induce, they also now and then remove, other complaints. It has long been the opinion of physicians, that intermittent fevers, if not accompanied with any uncommonly bad symptoms, pre-dispose to good health and long life. Unless these fevers, says Boerhaave,† are malignant, they dispose the body to longevity, and purge it from inveterate disorders. Nor do I believe, his commentator Van Swieten observes, that any physician who has considered this disorder will deny that after quartan fevers, disturbed by no powerful remedy, but gradually resolved by a good diet, in the spring time, the body has been found more firm, and much less subject to diseases than before.‡ These opinions however are far from being well founded, and have often done harm by preventing the endeavours of the practitioner to stop the fever at an early period, which we shall find in at least ninety cases of a hundred ought to be done.

But it is not to be denied that agues supervening on other diseases, sometimes relieve them. Habitual rheumatisms, inflammations, cutaneous eruptions, indigestions, epilepsy, histeria, &c. Dr. Fordyce|| observes, are relieved by a regular tertian. The quartan, says Vogel,§ has often prevented gout, asthma, convulsions, and hypochondriacal affections; and even Hippocrates says that the quartan is a safe fever and prevents others. Those affected with convulsions, he adds, are relieved from them by a quartan. Intermittents are also said to relieve or remove palsies and other complaints. Some are inclined to doubt of many effects of this kind which have been ascribed to them.¶

When an intermittent relieves a worse disease, it should not be stopped without caution; and we shall find that in certain

* See observations on these effects of intermittents, in Strack de Febribus Intermittentibus, Brocklesby on the Diseases of the Army, Jackson on the Fevers of Jamaica, &c.

† Aph. Boerhaavii.

‡ Comment. in Aph. Boerhaavii.

|| First Dissert. on Simple Fever.

§ Prælect. Acad. de Cog. Cur. Morh.

¶ See some observations on this part of the subject, in a Treatise on Malignant Intermittents by Aurivilius, in Baldinger's Sylloge Opusculorum.

cases, even where this does not happen, attempting to stop the fever early, is attended with bad consequences. In by far the greater number of agues, however, more is to be apprehended from too late than too early an use of medicine.

SECT. IV.

Of the Prognosis in Intermittents.

ALTHOUGH the prognosis in intermittents might be gathered from what has been said, the danger being upon the whole in proportion to the violence of the paroxysm, and the shortness and incompleteness of the apyrexia, or remissions; yet, on account of the number and variety of the symptoms of those fevers, a few observations on it here will be proper; notwithstanding such observations must partly consist of a repetition of what has already been said. This, however, I shall endeavour to avoid as much as possible.

As the prognosis in intermitting fever is collected from the symptoms of the paroxysm, and the state of the patient between the paroxysms, it may be divided into two parts. I shall, in the first place, take a short view of the state of the different functions, which during the paroxysms chiefly indicates danger.

The weakness and irregularity of the voluntary motions become more and more remarkable, as the state of the patient becomes more dangerous. He is troubled with involuntary twitchings of the muscles, (subsultus tendinum) and startings, which often terminate in general convulsions, in which he expires.

For some time before this happens a degree of coma generally comes on, and as death approaches it is often impossible to rouse the patient by any irritation whatever. Nor is delirium a more favourable symptom. In intermittents, indeed, it is to be regarded as denoting even more danger than coma. The danger is very great when delirium is among the first symptoms of the complaint, as happened in several epidemics above alluded to, and that of Bengal, described by Dr. Lind, in which the patient generally died in the third paroxysm.

To this head belongs the depravation of particular senses, especially false vision, which in all fevers is among the most fatal symptoms.

Such are the principal changes in the state of the animal functions which indicate much danger. With regard to the vital functions, palpitation of the heart and much anxiety are unfavourable symptoms. The pulse before death generally becomes very frequent, weak, and irregular, except when a considerable degree of coma is present; it is then often slow and regular: but, while the coma continues, this state of the pulse by no means indicates that the patient is not in immediate danger; it frequently portends a fatal apoplexy. In this, as in most other diseases, death often approaches with a paleness, shrinking, and coldness of the extremities; the pulse then for the most part cannot be felt at any considerable distance from the heart. Nor, on the other hand, is the complaint to be regarded as free from danger, when the pulse is remarkably strong and full; this state of it however we have it more in our power to correct

The respiration is also much affected as the patient draws towards his end; it becomes anxious and quick, though often at the same time less frequent than natural, interrupted with sighs and groans, and a little before death sometimes suffers considerable intermissions.* Under the head of respiration, it may be observed, that hiccup is a dangerous symptom, if it occurs while the others are alarming, especially if accompanied with vomiting.†

Every change in the voice from its natural tone indicates danger, and the total loss of speech is often the forerunner of death.

Of the state of the natural functions indicating danger. Much nausea, the abdomen swelled, hard and painful to the touch, with obstinate costiveness, are dangerous symptoms; a hard belly, and a swelling of the tonsils, are regarded by Sydenham as fatal symptoms in autumnal agues. It often happens that for some time before death the patient is unable to swallow, the tongue, mouth, and fauces generally becoming very foul. " The danger " (says Dr. Jackson) is very great when the tongue is immode- " rately dry or black, or covered with a white slimy gelatinous

* This intermission of the respiration is seldom very remarkable except when the patient dies much exhausted, and affected with coma. It is frequently more considerable in other complaints where the brain is more particularly the seat of the disease. Dr. Whytt takes notice of its being a common symptom in the hydrocephalus internus. I happened to meet with a case in which it was more remarkable than in any I have read of; the patient (a boy suspected to labour under an affection of the head) had been long complaining and was much reduced. Before his death a considerable degree of coma came on, and his breathing for about the last half hour was so much interrupted that there were not less than six or eight minutes between each inspiration, so that his friends thinking him dead, repeatedly closed his eyes, and were astonished a short time after to hear him make a very sonorous inspiration.

† When this is the case, although the patient does not complain of much pain, there is reason to suspect inflammation of the stomach or duodenum, especially if he complains of pain on pressure about the region of the stomach. It must also be kept in view, in the treatment of agues, that whenever much difficulty of breathing occurs, especially if attended with a degree of hardness in the pulse, we have reason to suspect inflammation of the lungs or its membranes. In speaking of the phlegmasiæ we shall have occasion to consider at length the symptoms denoting the presence of inflammation in the different viscera, and the circumstances in which it is most apt to occur. I make these observations respecting it here, because in the treatment of intermittents we must always be prepared for its appearance.

u termittents, Vogel* observes, are often removed by cutaneous eruptions, particularly the miliary eruption, and small pox, by the hæmorrhois, by a salivation, or by an ulcer of the lips. A variety of quotations from different authors might be given to the same purpose. My reason for not entering at present into a particular consideration of this set of symptoms, which have been termed critical, I have already given.

It is to be observed, that the most obstinate intermittents are not always the most dangerous. Of all intermittents, tertians upon the whole are removed with most case, and quartans with most difficulty. Hippocrates has pronounced a quartan the long-est and safest of fevers. This observation applies only to the simple quartan; when the quartan has suffered a reduplication of its paroxysms, the prognosis in it is no better than in other intermittents. The quartan is a safe fever (Celsus observes) and is never fatal; but if it become a quotidian, the patient is in great danger.

Upon the whole, intermitting fever, though often a very obsti-nate, is not generally a very dangerous, complaint. The symptoms enumerated as affording an unfavourable prognosis, seldom make their appearance, unless it has suffered a reduplication and pro-traction of its paroxysms, or is complicated with other disorders, and then the danger cannot be ascertained without being ac-quainted with the prognosis in those disorders. Epidemics in-deed occur, which form an exception to this observation, as that of Bengal, described by Dr. Lind.

Death may happen in any of the stages of intermittents. It most frequently happens in the hot stage. In the quartan in-deed, Sydenham observes, death in most cases happens in the cold fit; we shall presently find that the cold fit is more severe in the quartan than in other intermittents. The patient rare-ly dies in the sweating stage; if he is much reduced however, and the sweating profuse, death may happen at this period also; and now and then he is carried off during the remission, often in consequence of the violence of the preceding paroxysm.

If the first paroxysms of an intermittent are mild, the progno-sis is good; if from being severe they become mild, it is still better. But we must not form a decided prognosis from the mild-ness of one or two paroxysms, and the health of the patient du-ring their intermissions. It often happens that the first appear-ance of intermittents is very deceitful.

It may upon the whole be remarked, that the danger is rath-er to be estimated from the severity of the paroxysms, than from the length and completeness of the apryexia.† It has been ob-

* Præ. Acad. de Cog. et Cur. Morh.

† There are some good observations on this part of the subject, in the first chapter of the third book of Torti's Therapeutice Specialis.

" substance. To the above we may add, a sodden or parboiled-
" appearance of the tongue, which indicates much danger." A
spontaneous, or what has been termed colliquative, diarrhœa frequently precedes death. And the uncommon fetidness of the
stools sometimes gives reason to suspect that some part of the
intestines is sphacelated, which is always a fatal accident.* A
black matter like coffee grounds, discharged either upwards or
downwards, denotes much danger; this symptom is generally
the consequence of hemorrhagy from the stomach or bowels.
In the remittents of warm climates the vitiated bile sometimes
produces a similar appearance, and sometimes in the stools it
assumes that of tar or molasses. Whatever be the matter evacuated, vomiting, although not attended with hiccup, is dangerous,
if it does not abate towards the end of the paroxysm, especially
if attended with much anxiety, and if the discharge does not bring
relief.†

The urine or sweat being offensive, the former of a dark colour,
and depositing a brown or blackish sediment; the latter, which is
a more rare occurrence, tinging the patient's linen with a brown
colour; both of which appearances proceed from an admixture
of blood; and the eyes being suffused with blood; are among
the most alarming symptoms.‡ The sphincters are relaxed before death, so that the urine and fæces are frequently passed
involuntarily.

It may be observed upon the whole, that much danger is indicated by the various symptoms denoting great debility in the
natural functions. These will be enumerated more at length
when we consider the symptoms of typhus, to which fever they
properly belong.

In the last stage of the paroxysm, a free and thin sweat universally diffused, not occasioning much loss of strength, tends to
form a favourable, the opposite of these, an unfavourable, prognosis.

I shall conclude this part of the prognosis with the following
observations from Dr. Rollo's account of the diseases of St. Lucia.
" A comatose disposition, (he observes) remarkable dejection,
" coldness of the skin, partial cold. sweats, hiccup, involuntary
" stools, subsultus tendinum, loss of speech, &c. were certain
" signs of danger. When flies become numerous about the
" patient's bed in any period of the disease (he adds) and adhere
" to his lips and eyes without his being sensible of their attach-

---

* If there is much bile in the primæ viæ, the stools may be unusually
fetid without indicating sphacelus.

† In this case also we have reason to dread inflammation of the stomach
or duodenum.

‡ These are the most fatal of the hemorrhagies above alluded to, which
almost always afford a bad prognosis.

" ment, it is a certain mark of danger. Indeed these insects ne-
" ver made their appearance in any number until danger, by
" other signs, was too apparent.

With respect to the prognosis during the remission, or apyrexia, in proportion as these are shorter, and less complete, the
danger is greater. A simple quartan is a safer fever than a
tertian; a simple tertian is safer than a quotidian; and this becomes the more dangerous, the more its paroxysms run into
each other. These observations by no means apply universally,
but they should be kept in view.

If the patient, during the apyrexia, even although this be complete, feels himself weak and oppressed, especially if there be a
tendency to œdema in his feet and legs, he is not free from danger, We should inquire, Burserius observes, if on the days of
intermission the tongue be dry and rough; if the patient be un-
quiet, listless, and apt to sigh; if he be subject to vomiting or
purging; if he be drowsy; or, in short, disordered in any other
way; for then we may suspect some lurking mischief. If these
symptoms proceed from no evident cause, he adds, we dread in
the ensuing paroxysm cardialgia, cholic, lethargy, or some such
alarming symptom.*

All combinations of other complaints with intermittents, are
to be regarded as dangerous. Visceral obstructions are apt to
render the fever more obstinate, as well as to give rise, (as has
been observed) to other complaints.

THE state of the symptoms affording a favourable prognosis,
may be readily collected from what has been said of those affording an unfavourable one. The symptoms of the paroxysm being
moderate, the patient bearing them without much loss of strength,
and enjoying good health during a long apyrexia, are the best
signs. In fevers in general, as well as in those I am speaking of,
the failure of the sight above alluded to is an unfavourable symptom, while deafness on the other hand is generally, though not
universally, a favourable one.

There is a particular set of symptoms which occur now and then
in all kinds of fever, and have generally been observed to attend,
and generally supposed to occasion, a favourable change in the
state of the complaint, and often perfect recovery. " An erup-
" tion about the mouth and ears, (says Dr. Rollo†) with a swelling
" of the upper lip, either in this fever, or in the intermittent,
" happening when the paroxysm was going off, was a certain
" sign of recovery, except when the other symptoms were dan-
" gerous; these then assisted the unfavourable prognosis." In-

* Frank gives a good account of the symptoms which afford a bad
prognosis during the apyrexia. See his Epit. de Cur. Hominum Morb.
vol. 1, p. 59.

† See his Obs. on the Dis. of St. Lucia.

served of complicated intermittents, that those are most to be dreaded whose paroxysms are most severe on the even days.

Some attempt to foretel the period at which the fever will terminate favourably, by attending to that at which it comes to its height ; that is, the time at which the paroxysms from becoming more violent, begin to become less so ; for it is common in these fevers for every paroxysm, during the first intervals, to be more violent than that which preceded it. " The tertian inter- " mittents, or remittents, which come to their height in the " fourth period, (Cleghorn observes) terminate in the fifth or " sixth ; those which come to their height in the fifth, termi- " nate about the sixth or seventh." Cleghorn speaks of the tertians of Minorca. No general rules of this kind can be laid down. Every one must make such observations for himself in the particular climate, and even epidemic, in which he practises. It is sufficient to be warned, that by making such observations he will be enabled with more accuracy to foresee the event of the disease.

When a paroxysm occurs, which, without any evident cause, is considerably more severe than those which preceded it, it has often been observed to be the last paroxysm of the fever, the patient after it remaining well.*

TO the head of prognosis, belongs the doctrine of critical days.

This doctrine the reader will find noticed in the writings of physicians ever since the days of Hippocrates, who paid particular attention to it.

Some regard the doctrine of critical days as wholly unfounded, This opinion, however, appears to be the result of a careless view of the subject. In this country indeed the facts brought in support of it are seldom to be observed. But the complaints of different climates vary much, and the observations on which the doctrine of critical days is founded, have been too frequently repeated to permit us to doubt that there is a tendency to certain periodic changes in the fevers of warmer latitudes.

Physicians were soon led to observe the crises of fevers, viz. changes, often sudden, either for the better or the worse, which take place in them, and to mark the days on which these, particularly the favourable, changes were observed to happen. Having observed a crisis take place in more than one patient on the same day of the fever, they were led to pay attention to this day in other cases, and when they found a day, as the 2d, 3d, 4th, &c. of the disease on which a crisis happened more frequently than on most other days, this day they termed a critical or judicial day.

* Fordyce's second Dissertation on Simple Fever.

⋅⋅Thus the days, during which a fever lasts, came to be divided into those which are, and those which are not, critical. It is to be observed, however, that there is no day on which a crisis never happens ; but there are some on which it is observed to happen more rarely than on most others. Thus, the 7th is a critical day, since crises happen frequently upon it ; whereas the 12th or 16th are not critical days, since crises very rarely take place on them.

Those numbers which are made up by adding alternately four and three (with an exception I shall presently point out) denote the chief critical days, the 4th, 7th, 11th, 14th, &c. that is, the 4th and last day of each week, counting from the beginning of the complaint.*

The other days on which crises frequently happen are termed, by Galen, coincidental; and are esteemed an inferior class of critical days, on which crises do not happen so often as on the true critical days. When crises happen on the coincidental critical days, Galen taught that the natural course of the disease is disturbed by some irritation of the system, or by a new attack of the complaint; thus he calls the 7th a good critical day, but the 5th a bad one ; for he supposed that a favourable crisis happening on a coincidental, was less to be depended upon than that happening on a true critical, day.†

In the first septenary, that is, the first week, there are many coincidental critical days, because, according to the Ancients, the violence of fevers which run their course in so short a time as one week, often disturbs the crisis which ought only to happen on the 4th or 7th day. In the second septenary, the ninth is esteemed almost the only coincidental critical day ; thus it is, that after the 14th day, the coincidental critical days are of little consequence, the crises generally happening on the true critical days.

* Dr. Cullen considers all the uneven days, the 3d, 5th, &c. to the 11th, as critical days. After the 11th he regards every third day as critical, the 14th, 17th, and 20th. He marks no critical day beyond the 20th. " Because (he observes) though fevers are sometimes protracted beyond " this period, it is however more rarely, so that there are not a sufficient " number of observations to ascertain the course of them ; and further, " because it is probable that in fevers long protracted, the movements " become less exact and regular, and therefore less easily observed." See Dr. Cullen's First Lines, vol. i.

† The opinion that the course of the fever is disturbed when the termination happens on any other but a critical day, seemed farther confirmed by the observations of Hippocrates ; from which it appears, that although the fatal, like the favourable, terminations generally happen on critical days, yet a much larger proportion of the former, than of the latter, happen on the non-critical days.* Thus, Dr. Cullen remarks, all the terminations of fevers mentioned in the writings of Hippocrates, which happened on the 6th day, were either fatal, or not finally salutary.

. Hippocrates observed, that the crises happened very often on the 4th day of the first and second week, that is, on the 4th and 11th days of the disease. These days he therefore esteemed of much importance in fevers. But as he observed the crisis to happen very frequently on the 17th day, he considers this the 4th day of the third week, so that he makes the third week begin on the same day on which the second ends. Then the 20th day, not the 21st, is the last day of the third week, and this also he thought a chief critical day; of all these days crises are said to happen most frequently on the 17th.

The critical days which follow the 20th are the 24th, 27th, 34th, 40th, not the 41st, which is the 7th day from the 34th, for the same thing takes place in the 6th week, which happens in the 3d, namely, as the 3d begins on the same day on which the 2d ends, so the 6th begins on the same day on which the 5th ends; thus we count but six days for each of these weeks. The same happens in the 9th, 12th, 15th, and every succeeding 3d week, therefore the 60th, 80th, 100th, 120th days, are critical days.

Notwithstanding what is here said, Hippocrates remarks, that fevers, unless they leave the patient on uneven days, usually return; the most favourable termination therefore generally takes place on uneven days. In some places he calls the 21st a critical day; these passages are by many believed to be spurious. This, says Van Swieten, is very probable, since there is no mention of the 21st day in the histories of the cases given in his book of epidemics.*

Certain terminations, according to the Ancients, are more apt to take place on certain critical days than on others; thus Galen says a fever seldom terminates by sweat on the 4th day, and Hippocrates omits this day in enumerating the days on which fevers are generally terminated by sweat. It was supposed indeed that fevers seldom terminate by sweat on an even day; and in the aphorism just alluded to, Hippocrates calls the 21st, not the 20th, a critical day. Sweats, he observes, in febrile patients are good, if they begin on the 3d, 5th, 7th, 9th, 11th, 14th, 17th,

---

* In the doctrine of critical days, as delivered by Hippocrates, however, there certainly are contradictions; this Dr. Jackson attributes to his having related some cases from memory, and others only in part given him by different persons; he observes also, that when the fever begun in the evening, or during the night, Hippocrates generally reckoned the following the first day of the disease. Dr. Jackson adds, that the 21st is too frequently mentioned in the writings of Hippocrates as a critical day, to be considered, as Van Swieten and Dr. Cullen suppose it to be, an error in the original manuscript. Dr. Cullen ascribes many of the contradictions in the doctrine of critical days, as delivered by Hippocrates, to his opinion respecting the supposed power of numbers, to which he attributes his doctrine of the quartenary and septenary periods, and his opinion respecting odd days.

21st,* 27th, 31st, or 34th days, for the sweats which happen not on these days denote length of the disease, difficulty, and return of it.

It was also taught by the Ancients, that each critical day serves for indicating what may be expected on the next; and in this way the doctrine assists to form the prognosis.

If on a critical day the patient finds himself better, although on the next day he relapses into his former state, the physician may expect a more remarkable remission on the following critical day. On the contrary, if the patient finds himself worse on a critical day, a still more unfavourable change is to be looked for on that which follows, although during the intermediate days the symptoms become milder. From critical days being serviceable in this way, they have been termed indicating or judicial days; the physician forming his judgment respecting the future changes of the disease from what happens on these days. Thus every critical day is an indicating day to that which succeeds it.

Admitting this, it follows that by carefully attending to the severity of the symptoms on these days, or the degree of relief obtained, we may not only form a conjecture respecting the termination of the fever, but also concerning the distance of that termination. If on the critical days the violence of the symptoms be much increased, we dread a fatal termination, and we judge this nearer or more distant according to the degree of exacerbation which takes place; on the other hand, if a remission of the symptoms happens on the critical days, we expect a favourable termination, and judge of its distance from the degree of the remission.

In proportion as the disease is slower in its progress, the critical days are more distant from each other: thus in fevers which do not exceed three weeks, the 4th, 7th, 11th, &c. are critical days; but if the disease extend itself beyond three weeks, then only one critical day in the week is to be looked for; lastly, when the disease continues above forty days, Hippocrates esteems only every 20th day critical, to wit, the 60th, 80th, and 100th, &c. It is also to be remembered, that in lingering fevers the crisis does not happen precisely on the day called critical, but about that day.

Such is the doctrine of critical days delivered by the Ancients,

---

* It has already been observed that Dr. Cullen supposes the 21st day by mistake put for the 20th. He alleges that in continued fevers the tertian type prevails on the 11th day, and from this day to the 20th the quartan type. But, admitting what he says of the 21st day to be just, he attempts in vain to reconcile his view of the doctrine of critical days with what is said of the 4th day in the writings of Hippocrates, unless we admit what he alleges, and what in part is probable, that the writings attributed to Hippocrates are in fact the works of different people, and that the most genuine of them have suffered corruptions.

and we do not find in modern authors any addition of consequence to their observations on it, if we except what is said of the application of this doctrine to intermittents of complicated types by Dr. Jackson, in his account of the diseases of Jamaica.

The reduplication of paroxysms, which often takes place in intermittents, occasions some difficulty in applying the doctrine of critical days to them. Dr Jackson, in making this application, considers a double intermittent as two fevers, the one consisting of the original, the other of the new, paroxysms.

" Thus if the fever (he observes of tertians) which began on
" the odd day was critical, that is, if the paroxysm of the odd day
" terminated the disease, the crisis was necessarily on an odd
" day ; but if that fever, (namely that consisting of the paroxysms
" which supervened upon the original ones) the first attack of
" which was upon the even day, consisted of an equal number of
" paroxysms with the other, or continued after that had ceased,
" the crisis was then on an even day, reckoning from the begin-
" ning of the illness, though still on an odd day dating from the
" commencement of the second fever. It was the observation of
" this fact which first gave me the idea of calculating the critical
" days by the periods of the disease."*

By simplifying intermittents in this way, Dr. Jackson observes that their crises will be found to happen as regularly on the critical days as those of continued fever. Of 60 cases which under his care terminated favourably, ten terminated on the 3d day, ten on the 5th, twenty on the 7th, ten on the 9th, five on the 11th, three on the 13th, and two on the 17th. This nearly coincides with what Hippocrates says of the days on which fevers are terminated by sweats, which has just been quoted.

" Of nine cases which terminated fatally, (Dr. Jackson con-
" tinues) one terminated on the 6th, one on the 7th, six on the
" 8th, and one on the 10th." The even days, he observes, were fatal in the proportion of three to one, which he accounts for in the following manner. The paroxysm which destroyed life, like most other changes, took place on the odd day ; this paroxysm seemed to decline after the usual duration. It left the body in some measure free from disease, but so completely deranged the vital functions, that life, although it went on for a little could not be long continued, so that death generally happened on the next, that is, the even day ; but it was the consequence of a violent paroxysm which had taken place on the odd day.

It also sometimes happened that the patient was tolerably well

* Dr. Jackson always reckoned the period of the tertian 48 hours, allowing that time for every revolution, although it was sometimes completed in less. As for quotidians, he observes, their crises were generally on an odd day. How shall we reconcile the crises of quartans with the foregoing observations?

after this severe paroxysm, but a new one recurring after a
short interval, speedily terminated his existence on the even day.
" Hence we may see, he observes, why the patient sometimes
" died on the odd day when the fever was very violent, for then
" he died in the height of a severe paroxysm, often carried off
" by convulsions, apoplexy, or some other accident."

Dr. Cleghorn has observed, indeed, of complicated intermittents, that the great changes of the fever are always most apt to
happen on that day on which the most severe paroxysm takes
place, whether this be the odd or the even day.   This observation
is readily reconciled with Dr. Jackson's, as Dr. Cleghorn reckons
in the usual way without simplifying the complicated types.*

Many of the first physicians of antiquity endeavour to assign
the cause of these periodic movements in fevers.   Most of their
opinions, however, are now justly regarded as without foundation,
and many of them indeed are quite whimsical.   The most ancient was founded, on the Pythagorean doctrine of the power of
numbers.   Hippocrates seems to have been of this opinion ; Galen disclaims a doctrine so absurd, and conceives that the crises
of fevers are caused by the changes of the moon.   This opinion
long met with the general assent of medical authors, and we shall
find that an opinion very similar to this, and claiming the authority of extensive observation, has been maintained by some late
writers.†

SECT. V.

Of the Symptoms peculiar to the different Types.

We have now considered the symptoms essential to, or attendant upon, intermitting fevers in general.   It is proper, however,
before we leave this part of the subject to say something of the
symptoms peculiar to each of the three species, the varieties of
which have been considered.   In the first place, of those peculiar
to the quotidian.

The quotidian is comparatively a rare fever ; we often indeed
meet with intermittents whose paroxysms return every day ; but
most of these are double tertians, in which the fits do not return

---

* It is remarkable, that we still find something in the severity of the
paroxysm which disposes to health.   It was formerly observed of double
tertians, that the most severe paroxysm is generally followed by the most
complete apyrexia, and that in intermittents in general an usually severe
paroxysm often proves the last of the disease ; the patient remaining well
after it.

† These are the most celebrated opinions on the subject ; it would be
equally mispending time to trouble the reader with any more, or to enter
on any refutation of these.   The more modern opinion alluded to in the
text, which is not wholly unfounded, I shall presently have occasion to
consider.

every day at the same hour, or if they do, are dissimilar, that is, not of the same duration or degree of violence, or not having the violence and duration of their different stages in the same proportion.*

It is observed by Dr. Cullen, in his definition of the quotidian, which has been quoted, that its paroxysms occur in the morning. This is generally, but not always, the case.

In the quotidian the cold stage is shorter, less severe, and more frequently wanting than in the tertian or quartan. But the whole paroxysm is generally longer than in either of these fevers ; and the quotidian is more apt than any other to assume the continued form. Any of the others, about to become continued, in the first place so far assume the appearance of the quotidian, as to have a paroxysm every day.

Galen says, every physician ought to know, from the appearance of the first fit, of what type an intermittent will be. He gives the following diagnosis for distinguishing the paroxysm of a quotidian. The heat is more moist than in other intermittents, and joined with a kind of acrimony,† which is not immediately perceived on applying the hand ; the thirst is less, and there is a discharge of phlegmatic humours, by vomiting and stool ; the body abounds with crude humours ; the patient's age or habit is too moist, and the season of the year, or state of the weather, is damp. In a quotidian, he adds, there is never so great heat as in the paroxysm of a tertian.

We cannot, however, trust to this diagnosis in predicting the type of the fever, although it is not to be altogether overlooked. The most prudent plan, in all cases, is to watch the return of the paroxysm before we give a name to the disease. Whatever the extensive practice of Galen may have enabled him to do, it is now generally admitted that we can seldom determine the type of an intermittent from the symptoms of one paroxysm.

Upon the whole, however, a mild paroxysm coming on in the morning, particularly in the spring, often proves a fit of the quotidian.

The simple tertian, for the most part, comes on about mid-day, and returns every second day at the same time. The cold stage is generally longer and more severe than that of the quotidian,

* The quotidian, Eller observes, is a more uncommon fever than either the tertian or quartan, and some writers have regarded all quotidians as double tertians, altogether denying the existence of a simple quotidian. But we thus distinguish the quotidian and double tertian ; all the fits of the former are similar and come on at the same time of the day ; this can only be said of the alternate fits of the latter. See Eller de Cog. et Cur. Morb.

† See Observations on the Heat in Typhus, in b. ii, c. i. of this vol.

but the whole fit is shorter, in most cases not exceeding ten or twelve hours, and often terminating in five or six.

The cold stage in the tertian is upon the whole less severe than in the quartan, and of shorter duration ; but the whole paroxysm of the former is generally longer.

Galen observes, that at the commencement of the paroxysm of a tertian, there is often a painful sensation like pricking ; the thirst (he remarks) is always urgent, the heat very great, and universally diffused over the body ; that this heat strongly affects the hand of the physician on first touching the patient, but soon after seems to be less than that of his own hand. Such observations on the heat in fevers seem at first view whimsical ; we shall find, however, when we come to consider certain kinds of continued fever, that they are not altogether unfounded.*

Eller maintains that the cold is more considerable in the tertian, and confirms Galen's observation that the heat is greater (calor magis urens) than in other intermittents ; Hoffman, Huxham, and others, have also endeavoured to point out some circumstances which characterise a paroxysm of the tertian, but there is no diagnosis which enables us with any certainty to distinguish it from the paroxysms of other agues. Nor are we enabled to do so by the time of the day at which this fever appears. It is observed indeed, in the definition, that its accession is about midday, and it frequently is so, but it also often makes its attack at other times. In double tertians the fits are sometimes alternately before and after mid-day ; in these cases it has been observed, that the paroxysms which occur towards evening are generally more severe than the morning fits.

The tertian is sometimes, but rarely, protracted for several months ; in autumn it now and then becomes a quartan, and is protracted for a much longer time. The tertian, as observed above, is upon the whole less obstinate than other intermittents. But Frank† has justly remarked, that of all intermittents it is the most apt to become malignant, and appears most frequently as an epidemic. If any exception may be made to the former of these observations, it is with respect to the quotidian when it appears in autumn, which it rarely does.

The vernal intermittents are almost always either quotidians or tertians. Vernal intermittents, Sydenham‡ considered as not

* It is almost unnecessary to observe, that it is not here meant that there are two kinds of heat, but the peculiar secretion from the skin in certain fevers, affecting the hand at the same time, modifies the sensation produced by the increase of temperature. See the observations of Sir John Pringle, Huxham in his work on Fevers, Moore in his Medical Sketches, and others on this subject. I shall have occasion to quote part of their observations, when speaking of continued fever.

† Epitome de Cur. Hom. Morh.

‡ Sydenhami Opera Sect. de Feb. Intermit.

only safe but salutary, and if protracted till the autumn, he observes, which season is unfavourable to these species of intermittents, they generally cease spontaneously. It may be observed, however, on the other hand, that if autumnal tertians are protracted to the following spring, it also generally puts a period to them.

The vernal intermittents are less liable to become continued, to be accompanied by dangerous symptoms, or by bilious complaints, or followed by dangerous consequences, than the autumnal; they are also less disposed to return. I speak exclusively of the quotidian and tertian; the two first observations do not apply to the quartan, which generally appears in autumn. It has already been observed, that it is less apt to become continued, or to be accompanied by alarming symptoms, than either of the other species.

In the vernal intermittents, a considerable degree of excitement generally prevails; in the autumnal, a deficiency of excitement, debility. We shall afterwards find the following observation fully illustrated; that we always have it in our power to diminish excitement as much as we please, but in general we find it difficult and often impossible sufficiently to increase it, when it has fallen much below the healthy standard. It is chiefly owing to this circumstance that autumnal agues are more dangerous than vernal; and it will appear, as we proceed in considering febrile diseases, that this circumstance also, more than any other, influences our practice in all idiopathic fevers.

The regular quartan is an autumnal ague. Dr. Brocklesby[*] informs us, that he never saw an instance of a quartan which made its attack in the spring, and his experience was very extensive.[†]

The quartan generally attacks in the afternoon; the cold stage upon the whole is more severe, and of longer duration, than that of either the quotidian or tertian; it generally lasts for about two hours, and sometimes longer. Dr. Grant[‡] says, he has seen a cold fit of the quartan last fifteen hours; but it is not always accompanied with much sickness or vomiting; and Eller and others observe, that the sensation of cold is not in general so great as in the cold fit of the tertian.

The whole fit of the quartan is generally shorter than that of either the quotidian or tertian.

[*] Dr. Brocklesby's Observations on the Diseases of the Army.

[†] We shall find, in speaking of the causes of intermittents, that in the climates where the changes of the seasons are remarkable, spring and autumn are those in which intermittents most frequently appear.

[‡] Dr. Grant's Observations on Fevers most frequent in London.

At the invasion of quartans, Galen observes, the pulse is as if it were bound up and drawn inwards, nor is there that sense of painful pricking which we meet with in the cold fit of the tertian, but the patient feels as if all the soft parts were bruised. The following short quotation from Eller's Observations, contains perhaps the best diagnosis that can be given of the paroxysm of a quartan: The cold, he observes, is not so violent as in the tertian, but of longer duration; the heat is more gentle and dry, and the sweating is scanty.*

The quartan is more apt to be followed by obstructions of the viscera than other intermittents, owing probably to its being more obstinate, for although its paroxysms are shorter than those of the quotidian or tertian, its duration is generally much longer. It is often the most obstinate of all fevers, and has like the gout been termed the Opprobrium Medicorum. Some authors assert that they have known a quartan last for twenty or thirty years.

It is a remark of Sydenham, however, (how far it is generally applicable it is difficult to say) that if a person be attacked by a quartan for the second time it generally goes off after a few fits. After a quartan, which has proved obstinate, and in which the fits have been attended with delirium, the patient has been known to remain in a state of fatuity for a long time, as happens more frequently after that species of continued fever, which is most apt to be attended by delirium.

The quartan is particularly severe on old people; young people generally get the better of it, if not improperly treated, on or before the succeeding spring. Sydenham says, he has been surprised to see infants labour under a quartan for six months, and stand it out well.

Upon the whole, the principal difference between the paroxysms of the different species of intermittents, consists in their duration, and the proportional duration of their different stages. In the quotidian the cold fit in general is shorter than in the other two species, but the whole paroxysm is longer. The cold fit of the tertian is longer than that of the quotidian, but shorter than that of the quartan, and the whole paroxysm is shorter than that of the quotidian, but longer than that of the quartan. The quartan in general has the longest cold fit, but the shortest paroxysm. The duration of the cold fit then in the different types is proportioned to that of the intermission. The contrary is true of the duration of the whole paroxysm, which is generally the longer, the shorter the intermission. We are now to consider the manner in which the different types assume more or less of the continued form. Many of the facts relating to this part of the subject indeed have already been mentioned; it may be useful to present them at one view.

* Eller de Cog. et Cur. Morb.

SECT. VI.

On the Manner in which the different Types assume more or less of the continued Form.

PHYSICIANS have long endeavoured to assign a cause for some fevers assuming the form of intermittents, while others appear continued, at least so much so that the slight remissions which take place in them can often hardly be perceived. But how fruitless their labours in this part of the subject have been, appears at the first view of their several opinions. Even Sydenham's speculations on this subject are but ill warranted by observation. It would be mispending time to enter on the merits of these hypotheses; let us take a short view of the facts which gave rise to them.

When the fits of a quotidian are lengthened, there is no time for any apyrexia, and thus the intermittent is changed into a remittent. As the paroxysms are protracted, the remissions appear less remarkable, and the fever at length completely assumes the continued form.

The tertian, we have seen, is apt to suffer a reduplication of its paroxysms, and then this fever also may readily assume the continued form : for it is an observation generally applicable, that when a reduplication of the paroxysms takes place, the new are not only more protracted than the original paroxysms, but these also become more protracted than they were before the accession of the former. Although the paroxysm upon the whole is protracted, the duration of the cold fit is diminished as that of the hot is increased, so that when the fever has assumed the continued form, the cold fit in general is scarcely to be perceived. It is also to be observed, that when an intermittent assumes the continued form, the symptoms of the hot stage in proportion as it is protracted generally become more severe, and those of the cold stage in proportion as it is shortened become milder.

The quartan rarely assumes the continued form. The quartana triplex, in which a paroxysm happens every day, sometimes though rarely appears. This form of the quartan if it suffers a reduplication of its paroxysms may readily become continued.

The new paroxysms added to a tertian or quartan, when they become double for instance, always resemble the paroxysms of the first fever in this, that they are of the same type. Thus in a double tertian, the paroxysms of every second day are similar, and this is as constantly the case with respect to the new as the original paroxysms. But the new are seldom similar to the old, or recur at the same time of the day. It is by this circumstance, we have seen, that we distinguish a quartan or tertian in which the fits return every day from a simple quotidian.

Van Swieten observes that, as far as he knows quintans and other intermittents of more protracted types are never changed into continued fevers.

It will afterwards appear, that the chief if not the only circum-stances which determine intermittents to assume more of the continued form, are the presence of much debility, or of what has been termed the phlogistic diathesis, which is that state of the system that prevails in synocha, and may be considered sy-nonimous with increased incitement. This is in fact saying nothing more than that the severity of the disease determines it to assume more of the continued form. For we shall find, that in all idiopathic fevers, the two circumstances here mentioned, debil-ity and increased incitement, are the only sources of danger. It is the latter we most frequently have to combat in intermitting fevers ; the means of removing this with safety therefore (that is, without running the risk of inducing the opposite and more dan-gerous state of debility) forms an essential part of their treat-ment.

Instead of becoming more continued, intermittents sometimes become less so ; if a reduplication of the paroxysms of a tertian or quartan has taken place, they again become simple, and in proportion as they do so, the remaining fits at the same time become shorter while the cold stage again occupies a greater share of the paroxysm. Intermittents sometimes assume a more in-termitting form in another way, that is, by changing their type. It is not uncommon for an autumnal quotidian or tertian to be changed into a quartan after the violence of the fever is to a cer-tain degree broken.

Continued fevers also change to a more or less intermitting form. When this happens, the continued fever, for the most part, has formerly been an intermittent, or has appeared with in-flammatory symptoms while intermittents were epidemic.; we shall afterwards find, however, that all kinds of continued fever, though rarely, now and then assume the intermitting form.

CHAP. III.

Of the Morbid Appearances discovered by Dissection, in those who die of Intermitting Fevers.

MANY diseases prove fatal, without leaving any trace to be discovered by dissection. This strictly speaking is true of inter-mitting as well as continued fever. A variety of morbid appear-anecs indeed has been observed in those who laboured under agues ; none of these however can be regarded as essentially con-nected with the fever ; none of them seem at all connected with its cause, nor are there any which can be regarded as its immedi-

ate consequence. It is true, intermittents sometimes prove the
cause of other complaints, indurations of the different viscera,
&c. and in this view may be regarded as the cause of the morbid
appearances belonging to such complaints. But we must be
careful not to confound these fevers with their consequences, as
some have done, which has given rise to the opinion of intermittents depending on certain states of the bile, and to other ill-founded hypotheses. I have had occasion to enumerate the diseases
most frequently complicated with agues ; the consequences of
these diseases in the different cavities of the body, are those
which we find mentioned by writers as the consequences of intermittents.

The stomach, intestines, omentum, and mesentery are frequently found inflamed, or of a dark colour, and sometimes quite
sphacelated. The omentum and mesentery sometimes appear
wasted ; in other cases have tumours formed on them ; the stomach and intestines are often enlarged, the consequence of having
been distended with air ; and in various parts of the latter, pre-
ternatural constrictions are frequently observed. The gall bladder is often turgid, and an unusual quantity of bile is found in
the stomach and intestines. The liver is frequently indurated
and enlarged, sometimes diminished and of a whitish colour,
and it has now and then been found, only six or eight hours after death, soft, and it is said putrid. In some cases it seems
gorged with blood, the venæ portarum being much enlarged ; in
others, it is tinged with bile. The pancreas is also found enlarged,
and sometimes ulcerated, more frequently indurated. The spleen
is particularly apt to be affected in intermittents ; it is often enlarged, frequently weighing many pounds. Its structure has
sometimes been so completely destroyed, that it presented the
appearance of congealed blood wrapt in a membrane. In a greater proportion of cases, however, it is indurated, as well as enlarged ; in this state it has got the name of ague cake, and is
felt by the patient himself through the integuments of the abdomen. This affection of the spleen is particularly apt to occur
in the bilious remittents of tropical climates. Strack thinks that
boys are more liable to it than adults. The mesenteric and other
smaller glands of the abdomen are also frequently found indurated.

The viscera of the thorax are sometimes considerably affected.
Traces of inflammation in the lungs and pleura frequently appear, and the former are sometimes found soft and gangrenous.
The heart too is often flaccid and enlarged, and the vessels of the
lungs turgid, with dark coloured blood.* When the skin is tinged with yellow, the serum in the thorax and other cavities is of
course of the same colour.

* This state of the heart and blood-vessels is the consequence of the
circulation in the lungs having been much impeded for some time before
death, so that it is most remarkable in those cases where the dyspnœa
has been most considerable.

Morbid appearances of the head in intermittents are less frequently observed. Polypi are sometimes found in the sinuses.
But these are frequently met with whatever be the complaint of
which the patient dies, and must be ranked among those changes
which take place after death or in articulo mortis. Traces of inflammation, and even abscesses, are now and then met with in
the brain ;* and the serum in the head, like that of the thorax, is
frequently found of a yellow colour.

If the patient die in the cold fit, an unusual accumulation of
blood, it is said, is observed in internal parts. This is the only
morbid appearance which has been mentioned, that can be regarded as essentially connected with the fever, and it is more than
probable it has been magnified for the purpose of serving certain
hypotheses.

CHAP. IV.

Of the Causes of Intermitting Fevers.

IT was observed in the preface, that in considering the remote
causes of complaints, I should not always treat separately of
what have been termed the predisposing and exciting causes, the
circumstances which render the body liable to the disease, and
those which excite it, since in many instances it is impossible to
say to which of these classes any particular cause belongs, as in
many complaints the same circumstances act sometimes as predisposing, at other times as exciting, causes.

In intermitting fevers, however, the remote causes may be
more properly divided into predisposing and exciting, than in
most other complaints ; since a variety of observations seem to
prove that these fevers can only be excited, at least are generally
excited, by one cause, namely, exposure to an atmosphere of a
particular kind ; so that the other circumstances observed to co-
operate with this in their production, can only be regarded as increasing the power of that cause or producing a state of body favourable to its operation.

SECT. I.

Of the predisposing Causes of Intermittents.

OF the various circumstances favourable to the action of the
exciting cause of intermittents, (the marsh maisma or putrid effluvia from marshy grounds) there are some which operate by ren-

---

* These various morbid appearances will be considered at greater
length when speaking of the diseases to which they belong.

dering the body more susceptible of its action ; others which seem to act by increasing the power of the cause itself ; and some which act in both ways : so that it will be the most distinct plan, and save repetition, to consider the whole, under the head of marsh miasma, as circumstances favourable to its action in producing intermittent fever.

SECT. II.

Of the Marsh Miasma.

THE effects of an atmosphere loaded with noxious vapours on the animal body, are often striking. White females born and constantly residing in the lower districts of the province of Georgia, we are informed, have seldom lived beyond the age of 40 ; males sometimes approach to 50. Similar observations have been made respecting some parts of Egypt near the banks of the Nile.* There are swampy situations in the Carolinas and Virginia which are destructive of life in a still more remarkable degree. " I am credibly informed (says Dr. Jackson†) that there " is not on record an instance of a person, born in Peterborough " in Virginia, and constantly residing in the same place, who has " lived to the age of 21." Dr. Jackson saw a native of this town who was in his 20th year, but he was said to be the first who in the same circumstances had lived to that time of life ; he was decrepid as if from the effects of age, and it did not appear that he could survive many months.

The influence of marsh miasma, that is, of the vapours arising from marshy grounds, in producing agues, was first observed by Lancisi, about the middle of the last century. The justness of the observation is now so generally admitted, that it is unnecessary to adduce many facts in support of it.

It is almost an universal observation indeed that intermittents prevail in low marshy countries ; we have ample proof of the fact in our own. Our climate on the whole cannot be regarded as favourable to the production of these complaints. In Lincolnshire, however, and the other fenny counties, there are few complaints more frequent. Near stagnant pools, especially when the weather is warm, they are often so frequent as to deserve the name of an epidemic.

In other countries we have still more remarkable proofs of the effects of marsh miasma in producing agues. In Egypt, after the Nile retires, leaving the wet ground covered with a variety of putrifying animal and vegetable substances, these fevers begin to rage. We are informed that the Arabs, when they wish to be revenged on the Turks of Bussarah, break down part of the banks

* Bruce's Travels to Abyssinia, &c.

† Dr. Jackson's Account of the Diseases of Jamaica.

of the Euphrates, by which the deserts in the neighbourhood of that city are laid under water. The stagnating water and dead fish soon become putrid, and the most dreadful fevers, generally of the remitting form, are the consequence. The fevers induced by a single inundation of these deserts have been known to destroy between twelve and fourteen thousand of the inhabitants of Bussarah.*

When the cause applied is so violent, as in this case, we seldom meet with intermittents. Intermittents and remittents arise from the same cause, but from different degrees of it. " In Ja-" maica (Dr. John Hunter observes) the fevers in the most heal-" thy seasons are generally intermittents ; in the rainy and other " unhealthy seasons, remittents." When the degree of, heat and moisture, is not considerable, the regular intermittents prevail, and are in general readily removed by the ordinary means. In proportion as the season becomes hotter and more moist, a reduplication and protraction of the paroxysms take place, till the disease comes at length to differ but little from a continued fever. And in the more temperate climates, even when the autumnal fevers are of the most continued kind, if they arise from marsh miasma, they begin to intermit as the cold weather sets in, and before the winter is far advanced, often terminate in simple tertians or quartans.

The true intermittent fever is a complaint neither of very warm nor very cold climates. Bontius,[†] Lysons,[‡] Clark,[||] and others remark, that it is seldom met with near the equator. The putrid remittent may be regarded as the endemic of sultry latitudes. It is also to be observed, that in the more temperate climates, where intermittents are more frequent, they prevail most at the most temperate seasons of the year, spring and autumn. Upon the whole however, of the climates which may be called temperate, the warmest are the most favourable to the production of these fevers. In such climates as our own they generally prevail most when the weather has been for some time unusually warm, particularly when the rains suddenly set in after a warm summer.

The dreadful remittent of Bussarah, just mentioned, is always most feared in the hottest seasons ; and the heat of a country where the thermometer often rises in the shade to about 115°, may well be supposed to increase the malignity of every epidemic,

---

* The overflowing of the Euphrates, says a person who resided at Bussarah, and its waters stagnating on the desert, have always been accounted the principal cause of the remitting fever of this place. See the Observations on the Fever of Bussarah above alluded to, in the Transactions of a Society for the Improvement, &c. for 1793.

† De Medicina Indorum.

‡ Essays on Fevers, &c.

|| On the Diseases in long Voyages to hot Climates,

although it acted in no other way than by the irritation it occasions. " When the heats come on soon," Sir John Pringle observes of Flanders, where from the low, damp situation of the
grounds intermitting fever is very frequent, " and continue-
" throughout autumn, not moderated by winds and rains, the
" season proves sickly, the distempers come on early, and are
" dangerous ; but when the summer is late, and tempered by
" frequent showers and winds, or if the autumnal colds begin
" early, the diseases are few, their symptoms mild, and their
" cure easy. For in marshy grounds, intense and continued
" heats, even without rain, occasion much moisture by the ex-
" halation which they raise and support in the atmosphere;
" whereas frequent showers during the hot season cool the air,
" check the rise of the vapours, dilute and refresh the corrupted
" water, and precipitate the noxious effluvia." Heat then may
be regarded as a principal circumstance favourable to the action
of marsh miasma.

Sudden changes of weather indeed, whether from hot to cold,
or the contrary, are favourable to the production of intermittents,
and may therefore be regarded as another circumstance favourable to the operation of marsh miasma. It is constantly found,
says Raymond* of the yearly intermittents of Mettleburgh, that
if the cold and wet weather of autumn suddenly succeed an unusually dry and warm summer, these fevers rage more generally,
and show a greater tendency to become malignant.

It is particularly observed also by army physicians, that agues
are frequent if the warm day is succeeded by a cold damp night.
This often happens in marshy countries: For the exhalations
which rise during the day being condensed when the influence
of the sun is withdrawn, the ground is covered for some hours
with a thick mist.

Another circumstance particularly favourable to the operation
of the marsh miasma, is damp. It is observed that those who
live on small eminences, though equally exposed to the marsh
miasma, are less liable to agues than others living in lower situations; and it has been remarked, that people inhabiting ground
floors are more liable to them than those in higher parts of the
same houses. Sir John Pringle even observes, that of two bat-
talions, quartered near each other, and on ground of the same
height, the one in a town, the other in the peasants' houses in the
country, the latter was more subject to such complaints than the
former, from the greater dampness of the cottages. " The
" lower and moister the camp or garrison, (says Dr. Donald
" Monro) and the more moist the season, the more subject an
" army is to agues." And Dr. Brocklesby informs us, that he

* See Raymond on the yearly Intermittents of Mettleburgh, in Baldinger's Sylloge Opusculorum.

found nothing conduce more to the production of agues among the soldiers than lying on the damp ground in camps.

It might be urged, that moisture cannot be supposed favourable to the action of marsh miasma, as agues are more frequent when there is but little water remaining on the surface, than when the whole country, or many parts of it, are converted into pools. The inhabitants of Egypt, for example, are but little troubled with intermittents while their country lies under water; it is after the Nile retires within its banks that they chiefly prevail. " It has generally been remarked (says Dr. Rollo) that the efflu- " via of marshes are most active when the water is drained off " and the earth appears, which was certainly the case in St. Lucia: " The greater part of the regular intermittents, that is, of the " milder fevers, we had, happened when the rains were most " frequent, and before the stagnating pools discovered their bot- " toms; but the most dangerous remittents appeared when the " marshes had no water, but a slimy matter on their surface."

But it is to be observed, that when the country is under water, there is less marsh miasma than when the moist ground is exposed to the action of the sun, and this alone is sufficient to account for agues being less frequent in the former situation, although we admit that a greater quantity of moisture is constantly applied to the body. But this is far from being the case. The rapidity of evaporation we know is proportioned to the extent of surface which the fluid exposes to the air, and the degree of heat applied to that surface. When the ground is wholly overflowed, it presents a smooth and consequently the least possible surface, while, from the water being nearly pellucid, the rays of the sun have but little effect in raising its temperature. It appears from the experiments of Mr. Melvil, in the Edinburgh Literary Essays, that light only communicates heat when it is obstructed, reflected, or refracted. As soon as the water is drained off, the surface is increased in proportion as it is rendered unequal, and the sun acting now, not on the pellucid water, but the moist ground, has a great effect in raising its temperature, which is farther increased by the putrefaction which in such circumstances proceeds rapidly; so that the evaporation upon the whole is much greater. We frequently observe a thick mist over damp ground, but seldom on the surface of water.

Moisture seems to have so great a share in the production of agues, that at first view we are inclined to attribute the whole tendency of marsh miasma in producing these fevers to the damp that accompanies it. Dr. Lind* observes, that a person may be seized with an ague in the most wholesome spot of ground in England. There is occasional dampness in all places, but in many no degree of marsh miasma; and Dr. Moseley† remarks,

* See the Appendix to his Essays.
† See Dr. Moseley on Tropical Diseases.

that agues are often frequent during the rainy season in warm climates where there are no marshes. It is not a fair objection to this opinion, that an atmosphere loaded with moisture is not found to produce agues at sea, since on ship-board every thing can be, and always is, kept much freer from damp than in damp situations on land.

There are some facts, however, which lead us to believe that intermittents arise not merely from moisture, but a particular effluvia disengaged from marshy grounds. Dr. Lind observes, that ships lying at a considerable distance from a swampy shore, escape intermittents; while others lying nearer, about the distance of a mile perhaps, are subject to them. We cannot in this case attribute them to the moisture of the land breeze, since the thickest fogs on ship-board are found incapable of producing agues. But the question still remains, (on the supposition that in general they arise from marsh miasma) whether or not they ever are to be attributed to damp alone.

Extensive woods deserve a place among the circumstances favourable to the action of marsh miasma. Nothing conduces more to damp. They shed a constant moisture on the ground, and prevent both the rays of the sun from falling upon it, and the wind from passing over it. Besides, they confine the moist air, so that those who inhabit woody places are constantly exposed to an atmosphere loaded with moisture.

Soldiers encamped in woods seldom escape agues. There is ample proof of the truth of this observation in the works of Sir John Pringle, Dr. Cleghorn, and others. It appears from other observations, however, particularly those of Dr. Jackson and Dr. Rush, that scattered woods are of service, and in particular tend to prevent agues among those who live in the open country. One very evident way in which they may have this effect, is by preventing the diffusion of marsh miasma. Army physicians therefore have recommended having a wood if possible between marshy grounds and an encampment.

If Dr. Rush's observations be just, however, this is not the only way in which they tend to prevent agues. It would lead into too tedious a discussion to consider this subject at length; the reader will find some observation on it in Dr. Rush's Observations on the Causes of the Increase of Intermitting Fevers in Pennsylvania.*

The banks of rivers, if not swampy, have been recommended for the encampment of troops, with a view to prevent agues; the motion of the water occasioning a constant circulation of air, and thus tending to carry off the noxious vapours.

* See the 2d vol. of Rush's Med. Inq. and Obs.

Whether damp alone be capable or not of occasioning the first attack of intermittents, there can be no doubt of its renewing these fevers in those who have lately laboured under them, as daily experience evinces. It is doubtful how far the baneful effects of the night air in warm climates are to be attributed to moisture.

There are few things found to promote the action of marsh miasma in producing agues more than exposure to night air. It appears from the observations of Mr. Badinock,* that this is a principal cause of the bilious remitting fever of sultry latitudes; and to the same cause Bontius wholly attributes the worst fevers of Batavia. Of the baneful effects of the night air at Batavia Dr. Lind relates a striking proof. " During the sickly season, " a boat, belonging to the Medway man of war, which attended " on shore every night to bring fresh provisions, was three times " successively manned, not one of her crew having survived that " service." It is well known indeed, both in the East and West-Indies, that people are often attacked with agues from passing a single night abroad, especially in the woods.†

Respecting the predisposing causes of agues in general, it may be observed, that whatever tends to weaken the body, predisposes to these fevers, whether it be excessive heat or a cold and damp atmosphere, a poor and scanty diet, or gluttony and an abuse of fermented liquors, too much exercise or habitual indolence, bad cloathing, strong passions, long watching, the habitual use of irritating medicines, particularly strong purges, and whatever else is received into the body and tends to disorder it, an improper use of the warm or cold bath, suppressed sweats or eruptions, or the ceasing or increase of any habitual discharge. In short, those who live well and at ease, who are not given to excess in eating or drinking, nor disturbed by strong passions, and who use moderate and regular exercise, are least subject to intermittents.

Some have thought that particular kinds of food predispose to these fevers. Aurivillius maintains that those who live on pork and fish, are more subject to them than others ; those at least are so who live on food of a bad quality and difficult digestion.

There is a curious circumstance, that seems to deserve a place among the predisposing causes of intermitting fever, but which, like the doctrine of critical days, has not gained general credit; although like that also, it seems to rest on extensive observation.

Dr. Lind, Dr. Jackson, and others, have made some observa-

* See the 4th vol. of the Medical Observations and Inquiries.

† Dr. Hales, in the 1st vol. of the Medical Museum, proposes wetting the body with salt water as a means of preventing the bad effects of exposure to the night dews of warm countries, and adduces some facts in support of the benefit derived from this practice.

tions relating to the influence which the changes of the moon are supposed to have in determining the accession or renewal of fevers, particularly those of warm climates.

After stating briefly what has been done by others on this subject, the latter observes, " In order to ascertain the truth of " this conjecture, which I considered a matter of some impor- " tance, I provided myself with the almanack of the year 1776, " and marked in the blank leaf of it the precise date of attack of " all those fevers which came under my care." On looking over those memoranda at the end of the year, he found he had set down 30 cases of proper remitting fever, 28 of which made their attack on one or other of the seven days immediately preceding new or full moon, that is, in the second or last quarter. He continued the same plan through the following year, the result of which was similar. Besides the cases of proper remitting fevers, there were also marked in the almanack many slight feverish disorders, the accession of which in like manner was for the most part on the second and last quarters of the moon. It is also to be observed, that the greatest number of these accessions were within three or four days of the new or full moon, for the nearer these periods, the more frequent were the attacks.

Dr. Jackson supports these observations by others, and from the manner in which they were made, there was little room for fallacy. Dr. Lind accounts for the frequency of fevers at the new and full moon by the greater height of the tides at these periods. This, however, Dr. Jackson thinks cannot be admitted, since the influence of the moon in fevers is as observable in inland situations as on the coast.* Concerning this subject, future and very extensive experience must decide.

* For further information on this subject, the reader may consult the work from which the above quotation is extracted. Dr. Jackson's Treatise on the Fevers of Jamaica; he may also consult Dr. Lind's Thesis, and Dr. Balfour on Putrid Fevers.

In some parts of the West Indies, Dr. Wilson, in a treatise entitled Observations on the Influence of Climate, remarks, the changes of the moon influencing the accession of fevers, is a general opinion among the vulgar ; a circumstance in favour of the opinion, as popular creeds are seldom without foundation, especially when they regard a subject on which every individual is capable, and has opportunities, of making observations for himself.

We know from the laws of gravitation, that at new and full moon every body in those parts of the earth where the sun at twelve o'clock of the day is a certain number of degrees above the horizon, has its attraction for the earth, that is, its weight twice in the 24 hours more diminished and more increased than it ever is when the moon is in its quarters, and the nearer the sun is to the zenith at twelve o'clock, the greater is the difference of weight. What effect this may have on the human body, we neither can nor probably ever shall be able to determine. It is in vain to say that the difference is too inconsiderable to produce any effect when we speak of a machine so complicated, in many of its parts so sensible, and of which it must be confessed we know so little. This is worthy of re-

It is a common opinion, that salt water, mixed with the fresh water of marshes, produces a more noxious exhalation than salt water alone. Sir John Pringle considers this fact as undoubted. The opinion has gained ground by its having been found that a small proportion of salt promotes fermentation. This at first view contradicts a fact generally known, that common salt is one of the best antiseptics we have. But although a large proportion of salt prevents, a small quantity certainly promotes, fermentation. The author just mentioned, who made experiments in order to determine this point, observes, " Nothing could be " more unexpected than to find sea salt a hastener of putrefaction ; " but the fact is thus—One dram of salt preserves two drams of " fresh beef in two ounces of water about 30 hours uncorrupted, " in a heat equal to that of the human body ; or what amounts to " the same, this quantity of salt keeps flesh sweet 20 hours lon- " ger than pure water ; but half a dram of salt does not preserve " it above two hours longer than pure water. Now I have since " found (he adds) that 25 grains have little or no antiseptic virtue, " and that 10 grains both hasten and heighten the putrefaction."[†]

By others, however, it is asserted, that whatever be the septic power of a small quantity of salt, the admixture of salt water with the water of marshes is not found to increase their tendency to produce intermitting fevers. " So far as I have observed, " (says Dr. Jackson) the usual epidemic was less frequent and " less formidable on the banks of rivers after their waters became " mixed with those of the sea, than before this happened, un- " less the circumstances were in other respects more favourable " for the production of the disease."

He also affirms, that although sea and river water are mixed together in various proportions in Savanna la Mar, in Jamaica, and in the numerous islands on the coast of the Carolinas, yet these parts are seldom more unhealthy than where the lakes and rivers are unmixed.

Such are the circumstances which deserve attention relative to marsh miasma considered as the exciting cause of agues. Concerning the manner in which marsh miasma acts in producing these fevers, notwithstanding all that has been said on it, we can say nothing with certainty. It would be a waste of time therefore to enter on this part of the subject. Nor has it even been ascertained indeed what the marsh miasma is. We know that it is the effluvia, together with the moisture perhaps, of marshy

mark, that it is in those parts of the world, where the difference of weight just alluded to is most considerable, namely, within the tropics, that the changes of the moon have been observed to influence the accession of fevers. It is a curious fact, mentioned by Lind, that several sailors and others were attacked with fevers during an eclipse of the moon ; that is, at the very time of full moon.

- [†] Appendix to Sir John Pringle's observations, &c.

grounds; and this is all that has been determined concerning it. Is it the particular gas disengaged in the process of putrefaction?

It is to be observed, that almost all the circumstances which have been mentioned as favourable to marsh miasma in producing, are capable of renewing, intermitting fever; independently of the cause which first produced it.

Intermitting fever seems in general to arise from repeated exposure to marsh miasma. In most cases we cannot observe that the patient at the time the fever makes its attack, is particularly exposed to its action. In the authors I have had occasion to mention, however, the reader will find instances in which its effects were more sudden. " In the month of August, 1765," Dr. Lind observes, " the thermometer often rose to 82° in the mid-" dle of the day, and the marines, who were exercised early in the " morning on the south sea-beech, from the effects of the stag" naut waters of an adjoining morass, suffered much, half a dozen " at a time were often taken ill in their ranks when under arms."

I have already had occasion to observe, that the marsh miasma is generally regarded as the only exciting cause of intermitting and remitting fevers. Contagion, however, seems to have a claim to be ranked as such. With regard to intermittents indeed, contagion is not the cause in perhaps one of a thousand cases. Truka, in his elaborate treatise, entitled, Historia Febrium Intermittentium, quotes a variety of authors, in order to prove that even intermittents are sometimes contagious. As to remittents, they are more frequently contagious, and in general the more so the more they assume the continued form. I shall have an opportunity of speaking of contagion at some length in treating of the second species of continued fever.

SECT. III.

Of the proximate Cause of Intermittents.

THE proximate cause of intermittent and continued fever has generally been supposed the same; so that I shall defer the observations which I have to make on this part of the subject, till I come to consider the latter complaint. It is one of the many opinions which have generally prevailed indeed respecting the proximate cause of intermittents, that they arise from an increased secretion, or vitiated state of the bile; and as continued fevers have not been attributed to this cause, it will be proper to make a few observations on it here. The particular state and frequent redundancy of the bile in the intermittents, and still more in the remittents, of warm climates, gave rise to this hypothesis. These Dr. Cullen justly ascribes to the heat of the climate or season in which such fevers chiefly prevail, and which frequently occasion bilious complaints in those whose bodies are weakened by any cause whatever. The same author remarks, that frequent vomiting, which often accompanies intermittents, emulges the biliary ducts, and generally throws out much bile.

" But after all (says Sir John Pringle) the bile seems to be
" more the effect than the cause of intermitting fever ; for where-
" ever these fevers come to fair intermissions, they give way
" to the bark, a medicine which, as far as we know, has no direct
" influence upon that humour. All therefore that can be said
" in favour of the ancient doctrine is, that though the bile is not
" the first cause, yet from its redundance and depravation, owing
" perhaps to the fever, it frequently becomes a secondary cause
" of irritation, and supports the disease."*

If the bile be the cause of intermittents, Senac observes, it must have acquired some particular properties ; for it is often discharged both upwards and downwards, without inducing any fever of this kind. Nor are those who labour under jaundice more subject to agues than others ; and in these circumstances, if ever, the bile should induce fever, since the whole fluids of the body are mixed with it.†

It would be superfluous to attempt any addition to what these and others have said respecting this hypothesis, which, unfounded as it is, is very generally blended with the writings of medical authors.

CHAP. V.

Of the Treatment of Intermitting Fever.

THE treatment of intermitting and remitting fever is properly divided into two parts, that during the paroxysm, and that during the remission or apyrexia. The former is to be regarded as palliative only ; it is on the treatment during the apyrexia or re- mission that we depend for the cure. As the physician gene- rally first sees his patient during the paroxysm, we are in the first place to consider the treatment at this period.

SECT. I.

Of the Treatment of an Intermittent during the Paroxysm.

OUR view in the treatment of the paroxysm of an intermittent, is constantly to put a period to the stage which is present, by in. ducing that which naturally succeeds it ; till a free flow of sweat takes place. The crisis we aim at is then obtained, and we dis- continue the use of our medicines.

* Observations on the Diseases of the Army.

† Senac de Febribus.

a There are two indications then in the paroxysm of an intermittent; the first, to endeavour during the cold stage to induce the hot; the second, while the patient labours under the hot stage, to promote a flow of moisture by the skin. The following observation, however, is always to be kept in sight; that although it is our view during the cold fit to induce the hot, we are not indiscriminately to employ every means which tends to this effect. Many are otherwise so hurtful, that their bad effects more than compensate for any advantage to be procured by shortening the cold fit. The same observation applies to the means employed in the hot stage ; all the means we employ at this period tend to promote sweat, but every thing which has this tendency is not proper in the hot fit of an intermittent. I am now to point out what the proper means of fulfilling each of the foregoing indications are.

1. *Of the Means to be employed during the Cold Fit.*

The patient's feelings generally point out to us the greater part of the treatment necessary in the cold fit. He should be put to bed and kept warm, and some have recommended the warm bath. We are informed by Dr. John Hunter,* that the Negroes and others in Jamaica derive considerable advantage in the cold stage of agues, from stretching themselves out in the sunshine.

During the cold fit the patient is generally allowed the use of warm diluting liquors, but not stimulating, for these are apt by their irritation to heighten the symptoms of the hot fit that succeeds ; all kinds of aromatics therefore, distilled liquors, and wines, should be used with caution at this period, and altogether forbidden when there is any tendency to an inflammatory diatbesis, that is, to the symptoms enumerated in the definition of Synocha. Many do not allow drink of any kind in the cold fit, except to promote vomiting, as much fluid in the stomach and bowels generally increases the oppression.†

It is common in all kinds of fever to acidulate the patient's drink. For this purpose cream of tartar, or the vegetable or vitriolic acid, is employed, and they are particularly useful in intermittents when the stomach and bowels are loaded with bile, the noxious properties of which they tend to correct. These, however, and the other medicines, which have been termed refrigerant, are improper in the cold stage.

The most effectual means of bringing on the hot fit, is the operation of an emetic. This, if the complaint be severe, should be exhibited as soon as the cold stage is formed, if it has not been

* Dr. Hunter on the Diseases of the Army in Jamaica.

† Dr. Cleghorn seldom permitted his patients to drink during the cold fit.

given before the commencement of the paroxysm, which we shall find is often entirely prevented by this means.* The antimonium tartarisatum is the best emetic in this case,† and should be given in pretty large doses. Nauseating doses of emetics are more properly indicated in the hot stage; the act of vomiting is of·more service in the cold. When spontaneous vomiting from bile or other irritating matter in the stomach supervenes, diluents only are necessary.

Purging in the cold stage is improper, and blood-letting altogether inadmissible. Blisters are proper in the cold fit, if coma or delirium attend. When these symptoms are considerable, the head should be shaved, and a large blister applied over it.‡

Such are the few directions to be attended to in treating the cold fit of an·intermittent. The practice in the hot stage is rather more complicated.

2. *Of the Means to be employed during the Hot Fit.*

The indication of cure in the hot stage of intermittents, I have already had occasion to observe, is to promote a flow of sweat. This is done,

1· By removing every cause of irritation.
2. By dilution.

* For the use of emetics in the cold fit, the reader may consult many of the authors who have been mentioned. See also a paper in the 4th volume of the Edinburgh Medical Essays and Observations, by Dr. Thompson.

† This medicine is generally used in the following manner:—Three or four grains are dissolved in as many ounces of water; and a table spoonful is given every half hour, till the desired effect is produced. In the present instance, however, this is often too tedious a way of inducing vomiting; it is therefore sometimes proper to repeat the dose every ten minutes or quarter of an hour. "If after exhibiting a few doses of tar- " tar emetic, (Mr. Clark observes) its operation does not proceed to our " wish, drinking acidulated liquors will not only render this preparation " of antimony, but almost every other, more active."

‡ There is a curious paper, by Mr. Kellie, in the 19th vol. of Dr. Duncan's Medical Commentaries, concerning the application of tourniquetes to the limbs, with a view to prevent or remove the cold fit of agues. From the few observations which he made, he drew the following conclusions:—1. That at any time during the cold fit of an intermittent, if tourniquetes be so applied as to obstruct the circulation in two of the extremities, in three minutes thereafter the hot stage will be induced.—2. That if the tourniquetes be applied previous to the accession of the paroxysm, the cold stage will be entirely prevented.—3. That where the cold stage of an ague is either thus shortened or prevented, the following hot stage is rendered both milder and shorter.—Mr. Kellie's observations deserve attention; they are too confined however to determine fully either the success or the safety of his proposal. I am informed that his experiments have been repeated at the infirmary of Edinburgh without success. Mr. Kellie has since published a work on the use of tourniquetes in various complaints.

3. By the use of sudorifics.

4. By supporting the strength when much debility attends; and

5. By moderating excitement when the symptoms of synocha prevail.

1. Every cause of irritation tends to protract the hot fit. The most common cause of irritation in intermitting fever, is bile in the stomach and intestines. When this occurs, these passages are in the first place to be cleared, which will have been done to a certain degree if the emetic has been exhibited in the cold fit, which it ought to be when the stomach is oppressed, unless spontaneous vomiting supervenes. Cathartics, it has just been observed, are improper in the cold fit, nor are they well suited to the hot stage of intermittents. The bowels should be cleared during the apyrexia, but not immediately before the fit is expected, for a reason which will afterwards appear. When the hot fit is of long duration, however, and the bowels much oppressed, a gentle cathartic becomes necessary.

Of cathartics, calomel has lately been much recommended in fevers of all kinds, especially by the practitioners of warm climates. Dr. Lysons,* and others, particularly recommend it in intermittents. It will presently appear that small doses of antimonium tartarisatum, or ipecacuanha, are often for another purpose exhibited with advantage in the hot stage of intermittents. These not being sufficient to excite vomiting, pass the pylorus, and generally render any other cathartics during the paroxysm unnecessary. If the action of these medicines indeed is determined to the skin, by means presently to be pointed out,† they generally induce sweat and not catharsis. When this happens, however, there is perhaps no case in which we should attempt to move the bowels ; nothing tending more effectually to check perspiration, and in these circumstances to protract the paroxysm.

The exhibition of emetics in this complaint sometimes renders that of other medicines troublesome. But as emetics are not so well suited to the second as the first stage of intermittents, the only difficulty arises from the operation of the emetic given in the cold fit still continuing. When this happens in cases where it is necessary to move the bowels in the hot stage, we must have recourse to clysters. These indeed are preferable to cathartics when the strength of the patient is much reduced, and the cause of irritation is chiefly confined to the large intestines, as in costiveness.‡

* Dr. Lysons' Treatise on the Use of Camphor and Calomel in Fevers.

† Chiefly opium and gentle warmth.

‡ It is not necessary or proper to make the clysters employed in this complaint very irritating ; they should be composed chiefly of an emulsion of oil, water, and mucilage, heated to the temperature of the body, and injected in considerable quantity. If this is not sufficient to move the

Other causes of irritation will be pointed out when we speak of continued fever ; and as far as these operate in the paroxysm of an ague, the observations which will then be made are applicable to the case before us, with this exception, that external heat is less to be dreaded in intermitting than in continued fever. We shall presently find that gentle warmth is among the means of shortening the hot as well as the cold stage of agues ; in the former, however, it is to be employed with more caution.

2. During the hot fit the patient should not be refused the use of diluent liquors. Many indeed do not permit him to drink till the sweating stage commences. There is nothing more distressing however, and few causes of irritation more apt to increase fever, than thirst : and unless the quantity be very large, mild liquors in the hot fit will not be found to increase the oppression, and they tend to promote sweat.

In the cold stage, and while the hot is forming, whatever drink the patient uses should be tepid ; when the hot stage is perfectly formed, cold drink is both more grateful, and generally more beneficial. When a moisture appears on the skin, the drink should again be tepid.

In the treatment of all fevers we should have in view that the evacuent and diluent plan is debilitating, and must therefore be used with caution, unless the excitement is considerable.' It is also to be remembered, in attempting to discharge the bile from the stomach and intestines, that purging, and still more vomiting, tend to emulge the biliary ducts, and seem often to excite the liver to a more copious secretion of bile. We might therefore endanger the patient's life, were we to persevere in attempting entirely to free his stomach and intestines of a matter which, in consequence of the very means we employ, is poured into these cavities in greater quantity.

In the hot as in the cold fit, when a vomiting and purging of bile occur spontaneously, diluents only are necessary, and if these motions prove obstinate, they must be allayed (when there is reason to suppose that the greater part of the bile is discharged) by opium ; which we shall presently see is otherwise useful at this period. Acids in this case, as in others, where the bile is prevalent, should be mixed with the drink.

3. The next means of promoting perspiration in the hot stage of intermittents, is the exhibition of sudorifics. I have already had occasion to observe that vomiting is not so well suited to the second as the first stage. Nauseating doses, particularly of antimonial emetics, are more serviceable in the hot fit, especial-

bowels, a small quantity of common salt, or any of the purging salts, may be added, or the clyster may be made with an infusion of senna instead of water.

ly when combined with opium, and when their operation is determined to the skin by gentle warmth.

As our view here is to promote perspiration, James's Powder,
which is supposed by many to be better calculated to promote
the action of the skin than the other preparations of antimony,
is generally preferred to tatar emetic.* Either of these medicines conjoined with opium is among the most powerful we possess in the hot fit of intermittents. Dover's Powder, in which
opium is combined with a small quantity of ipecacuanha, is used
with the same view, but seems inferior to the former. Opium
alone has been found one of the most successful means of shortening the hot fit.† This effect it seems chiefly to produce by
promoting the perspiration.

4. Wherever there is much debility, especially where those
symptoms appear denoting a great degree of debility in the natural functions, the paroxysm is protracted, and the patient in
danger of falling into typhus. I have already observed that
these symptoms are seldom present to a considerable degree till
the complaint more or less assumes the form of this fever. This
part of the treatment therefore will be considered at length when
we speak of continued fever; and as what will then be said is in
every respect applicable to the present case, it would occasion
needless repetition to enter on it here.

I am now, therefore, to consider the last set of means for shortening the hot stage of intermittents.

5. Wherever the inflammatory diathesis is considerable, not
only the duration of the paroxysm, but that of the fever, will be
protracted; and as this diathesis is the most frequent cause of ob-

* The preparation of James's Powder was long a secret, and procured
its inventor much reputation and gain. It is now known to be a preparation of antimony, and perhaps in few respects superior to tartar emetic.
Till lately James's Powder was supposed to be the calx antimonii nitrata.
Dr. Pearson's experiments, which have generally been supposed to place
the nature of those powders beyond a doubt, make it the pulvis antimonialis of the London Pharmacopeia. Some have suspected that Dr. Pearson's conclusions are not altogether to be depended on. Dr. William
Wright of Jamaica, a physician well known in the medical world, and
to whose works I shall have occasion to refer more than once in the course
of the present Treatise, informed me that for the purpose of making the
experiment he had given the pulvis antimonialis for James's Powder, and
that the patient, who was accustomed to use this powder, discovered the
deception merely from the effects of the medicine being different from those
he had formerly experienced—See Dr. Pearson's paper in the Philos.
Trans. for 1791.—Dr. Higgins used to observe in his lectures, that James's
Powder is prepared from a mixture of crude antimony pulverised and
chared bones, calcined in a reverberatory furnace.

It is said Dr. James generally gave his powder conjoined with calomel,
to which many attribute the success of this medicine in the hands of its
inventor.

† See the observations of several of the authors who have been mentioned, particularly Dr. Lind, for the use of opium in intermitting fever.

stinacy in intermittents, the means of relieving it may be regarded as the most important part of the treatment during the paroxysm ; and indeed when these are not indicated, little in general
need be done at this period, except what the feelings of the patient point out ; for although sudorifics certainly shorten the duration of the hot fit, they are not to be regarded, like the means
for removing the inflammatory diathesis, as essential to the cure
of the complaint.*

The first observation to be made respecting the treatment during the paroxysm of an ague in which this diathesis (that is, the
symptoms of synocha) prevails to a considerable degree, is, that
all stimulating medicines are hurtful, and consequently that opium, in other cases so beneficial, is then to be avoided.

The means for relieving the inflammatory diathesis are different, according to its degree. A variety of saline preparations is
recommended with this view, and they are often sufficient, when
the inflammatory symptoms are not considerable. Whatever other means we employ, indeed, these always make a useful addition
to them. The reader will find a great variety of them enumerated by the authors whom I have had occasion to mention. He
will find most of those employed by foreign practitioners in the
192d page of the 1st vol. of Burserius's Institutiones Medicinæ
Practicæ. The following chiefly deserve attention.

The saline mixtures are prepared by mixing a mild fixed alkali
with lemon juice, nearly in such proportion as to form a neutral
salt; care being taken, however, that there shall be an excess of
acid. This medicine should be taken during the effervescence,
and repeated every third or fourth hour. It is grateful to the
stomach, relieves the feverish heat, and tends gently to move
the body. The spiritus mindereri is a medicine of the same
kind, but not equal to the other where the inflammatory diathesis
is considerable.

To the same class of medicines belong the various acids, vegetable as well as mineral. The best of these are lemon juice,
and the sulphuric acid ; and the best way of using them is in the
drink as above recommended.

Nitre has long been a celebrated medicine in all cases of fever,
in which the symptoms of synocha prevail. The effects of this
drug upon the animal fluids, when out of the body, seem to have
had a principal share in raising the reputation of nitre in these
complaints ; for many have been inclined to account for the effects of medicines on chemical principles. Hoffman says, it is
better than the refrigerants of the acid kind, since it is not apt to
coagulate the juices ; for solutions of it dissolve recent thick
blood ; and in some degree, says Dr. Lewis,† preserve it from.

* This observation will be sufficiently illustrated in considering the use
of the bark in intermittents.
† Dr. Lewis's Materia Medica.

coagulation as well as corruption. Nitre changes dark blood to a red colour, and produces the same effect on the flesh of dead animals. But it is surely impossible to determine the effects of a medicine upon the living entire body, from any experiments made upon parts of it, either before or after death. If we estimate the virtues of nitre from its effects on the entire living body, we shall find it fall much short of the encomiums bestowed upon it. When given in the common dose of a few grains, it often produces little or no effect. Where its effects are obvious it diminishes excitement, and for this purpose is superior perhaps to most of the other medicines which have been mentioned ; given in larger doses it oppresses the stomach, and sometimes, not always, proves cathartic. Nitre should never perhaps be given in a solid form. In this state it is most apt to occasion oppression and sickness. When these symptoms occur from its use, they may generally be removed by plentiful dilution,* which is itself a powerful means of moderating excitement, and should always make a part of the treatment when the excitement runs high.

But wherever the excitement is considerable we must have recourse to more powerful remedies than any of these, namely, evacuations. I have already made some observations on the use of cathartics, in the hot stage of intermittents. In addition to these observations, it may now be remarked, that when the symptoms of synocha prevail, although there be no irritating matter in the stomach or bowels, it is proper to exhibit frequent diluent and gently cathartic clysters. It is to be kept in view, however, that when the excitement runs high we should not attempt to overcome it by cathartics.

The effect of evacuations in relieving this state of the system, is proportioned to the rapidity with which they are made. The evacuation procured by cathartics is slow ; and although a moderate catharsis will relieve the inflammatory diathesis when it does not run high, in order to relieve it when considerable, a long continued purging is necessary, by which the patient's strength would be much impaired. In this case, therefore, we must have recourse to some evacuation which can be made with more rapidity, and which, consequently, will relieve the symptoms without being pushed so far ; and then purging is only to be employed to procure an evacuation of the fæces or other irritating matter in the alimentary canal, or at most, very gentle cathartics are to be recommended to aid the more powerful remedy.

* For the use of nitre, in a variety of complaints, the reader may consult a treatise on this medicine, by the celebrated Stahl ; and the article nitre in the Materia Medicas of Lewis, Cullen, &c. In these authors he will find various formulæ for the exhibition of nitre ; but it is generally admitted, that the best way of using this medicine is in the drink, when the patient can be prevailed upon to take it in this manner. Sugar is one of the best articles for correcting its taste.

Of all the means with which we are acquainted, none so effectually diminishes excitement as blood-letting. This remedy demands particular attention, since there are few, perhaps none, by which more good or harm may be done.

The first remark to be made on blood-letting is, that strictly speaking it is not to be ranked among the curative means in the treatment of intermitting fever, but to be regarded as the remedy on which we chiefly depend for counteracting a certain diathesis that tends to protract the complaint. This observation must be kept in view, since it has been asserted by some that the cure of intermittents may be attempted by blood-letting alone; an opinion which has often led to improper modes of practice in these fevers. It is not to be denied indeed that mild vernal intermittents, which are generally more or less of an inflammatory nature, now and then yield to this remedy; but the only inference to be drawn from this is, that such fevers, being very mild, require no remedy after the inflammatory diathesis is removed.* So far indeed is blood-letting from being the remedy on which we depend for the cure of agues, the truth seems to be, that except in those cases where actual inflammation, or that diathesis which disposes to it, are present, it is universally hurtful in these complaints. Even Sydenham, who in general recommends venesection with so much freedom, observes, that in young people a quartan, which would have terminated in six months, is by blood-letting protracted to twice that period: and in old people the disease is not only protracted, but life endangered, by the rash use of the lancet.

It is impossible to lay down any rule respecting blood-letting, in the different species of intermittents, which will be found generally applicable. It is by authors having attempted to do this that the subject has been involved in so much perplexity. On reviewing, however, the works of those who have had extensive opportunities of treating this complaint, we may perceive, what the symptoms are which render blood-letting necessary; at what period of the disease it is proper to employ it; what the consequences to be dreaded from it are; and in what circumstances, these consequences are most apt to take place.†

* I use the terms inflammatory diathesis and increased excitement as nearly synonimous, for although a tendency to inflammation often exists without increased excitement, yet it is only when attended by the latter that we can with certainty determine its presence. There is reason, however, to suspect its presence in all cases in which an intermittent proves obstinate, if the epidemic be of an inflammatory nature, and the season of the year and state of the weather be such as dispose the body to inflammatory affections. In such cases although there be little increase of excitement a moderate blood-letting is generally attended with the best effects.

† In treating of continued fever I shall have occasion to speak of blood-letting in fevers at greater length; at present I am only to make such observations respecting it as relate particularly to the treatment of agues.

I shall make a few observations on each of these heads. In the
first place then we are to consider, what the symptoms are which
render blood-letting proper in intermitting fever.

Wherever the countenance is flushed, the head-ache considerable, or the delirium obstinate, with a full and hard pulse, blood-
letting is necessary. When along with this state of the pulse
the fever assumes more of the continued form, or the patient is
affected with dyspnœa, we must have recourse to this remedy.*

It is difficult to point out the degree of excitement which, independent of local affections, or the fever assuming a more
continued form, warrants the employment of blood-letting. The
use of this remedy in intermittents will be better understood, after
considering its exhibition in continued fever. One observation
must be kept in view, that, for two reasons, a less degree of excitement warrants blood-letting in intermitting than in continued fever. In the first place, the removal of increased excitement, that is, of the symptoms of synocha, is of more importance in the cure of the former than of the latter disease; and
because in the former we have less reason to dread the debilitating effects of blood-letting. This observation will be sufficiently
illustrated when speaking of the use of the bark in intermittents,
and of blood-letting in continued fever.

In those cases where there is no increase of excitement, and
still more where the pulse is small, frequent, and intermitting,
we cannot do a more improper thing than make use of the lancet.

With regard to the period of the disease at which it is proper
to employ blood-letting, it may be observed, that as the continuance of every disease tends to weaken, those symptoms which
indicate this remedy are seldom present after the complaint has
lasted for a considerable time. Except, therefore a new disease
requiring blood-letting supervene, it is seldom proper in protracted cases. At the first attack, on the contrary, it often proves
beneficial, particularly in the spring, or at other times when the
epidemic has an inflammatory tendency.

Blood-letting to a greater or less extent is generally necessary
at the beginning of intermittents in warm countries, especially
when the patient has lately arrived from a colder climate.† In

* When the difficulty of breathing is urgent, as sometimes happens,
with a low pulse, and in cases where the strength of the patient has been
much reduced, either by the continuance of the disease, or previous evacuations, local means are preferable to general blood-letting.

† See Dr. Curtin's letter to Dr. Duncan, in the 9th vol. of the Medical
Commentaries, and the observations indeed of most authors who treat of
the fevers of warm countries. " For my own part, (says Dr. Cleghorn,
" speaking of the tertians of Minorca) when I was called early enough
" in the beginning of these fevers, I used to take away some blood, unless
" there was a strong contra-indication, from people of all ages."

warm climates, however, this remedy is always to be employed with much caution.

Blood-letting in the hot fit of agues was regarded by the Ancients as a dangerous practice; succeeding experience however has contradicted this maxim; and it is now generally admitted, that the patient may be bled at all periods of the disease, except during the cold and sweating stages, and at the time the paroxysm is expected, that is, either in the hot fit, or during the intermission.

If we reflect upon the end we have in view when we prescribe blood-letting in intermitting fever, we shall find reason for confining this remedy to the hot fit alone. It has already been observed, that blood-letting is not to be regarded as one of the means of a radical cure. It has been a favourite opinion in medicine, and still is with many, that fevers depend upon a noxious matter existing in the fluids, and that this may be evacuated by blood-letting. We can perceive however, without very minute observation, that the effect of blood-letting in all kinds of simple fever, that is, of fever which is neither in any degree produced by, nor has itself caused, any local affection, is merely that of diminishing excitement,* which, if violent, threatens a dangerous degree of subsequent debility, and even when but little above the healthy standard, tends to render intermittents obstinate.

From this view of the subject, it appears that we ought not to employ blood-letting during the remission or apyrexia. The excitement is never considerable at this period, and blood-letting will not prevent it becoming so during the ensuing paroxysm with the same certainty, that it will relieve the increased excitement when present. Besides, when the excitement is morbidly increased, the patient bears the loss of blood better than at other times. Dr. Lind regretted that he had bled a patient during the apyrexia; the event was unfortunate, and he owns that an experienced physician thought it probably would not have been so, had the blood-letting been ordered during the paroxysm.

In intermitting fever, therefore, the most proper time for letting blood is during the hot fit of the first paroxysms. We are now to consider, the consequences to be dreaded from blood-letting.

The certain consequence of repeated blood-letting, especially when not employed with judgment, is debility, and this now and then is so sudden, even where the quantity of blood lost is not very considerable, that patients have sometimes expired almost immediately after venesection. This has not often happened; the powers of life, however, are frequently so impaired as to render the fever more obstinate and dangerous; or even to un-

* See what is said of blood-letting in the treatment of continued fever, in book ii. of this vol.

dermine the constitution, and induce dropsy or other lingering diseases.

Another consequence of blood-letting, not to be overlooked in diseases which are of long continuance, is plethora. It is well known that the frequent repetition of blood-letting induces a state of body which renders the discontinuance of the habit dangerous.

It only remains to take notice of the circumstances in which the bad effects of blood-letting are most to be dreaded. There are few remedies whose good and bad effects more frequently seem to balance each other than that I am now speaking of; so that cases occur in which the most experienced and acute physicians cannot positively determine whether it ought to be recommended or not.

The general rule is, that wherever debility is present, or with certainty expected, blood-letting is dangerous; and yet, in both these cases we must sometimes employ it. In idiopathic fevers, however, it is only the latter of the difficulties with which we have to struggle. For wherever debility is actually present in these fevers, blood-letting we shall find is decidedly improper.

In sultry climates fevers run their course rapidly, so that a patient who is labouring under a strong full pulse, and the other symptoms of synocha, will in a short time be reduced to the last stage of weakness, and the symptoms denoting a dangerous degree of debility in the various functions will make their appearance. In such cases the violent excitement at the commencement of the fever, if not relieved, will terminate in this state of debility; yet the only means we have of relieving it are themselves of all remedies the most debilitating.

Mr. Clark,* after relating the fatal termination of three cases in which blood-letting was employed to moderate the violence of the excitement at the commencement of the remittent of sultry climates, observes, that he has since found it necessary to lay aside blood-letting in such climates, both at sea and on shore, except when local inflammation was present.

What is best to be done in such cases, can only be determined by considering a variety of circumstances, for which I must refer to the observations that will be made, on the same difficulty, when we speak of continued fever; as these are in every respect applicable in the present case.

Blood-letting is to be cautiously employed, whatever be the excitement, at the beginning of the complaint, if the epidemic is of a putrid nature, particularly if the patient is, or has lately been, subjected to the action of other debilitating causes: It must be sparingly used, for instance, in hospitals, where patients are often

* On the Diseases of long Voyages to hot Climates.

exposed to a noxious atmosphere, and their bodies generally reduced by a scanty diet. For similar reasons, blood-letting is
more to be feared in large and populous cities, than in the country. In summer and autumn it is a more doubtful remedy than
in winter and spring; fevers in the former seasons being frequently attended with much debility, which is the source of all
their most alarming symptoms. " Æstate et autumno," Burserius observes, " sanguinis missio in intermittentibus minus con-
venit."

In all cases it is to be remembered, that blood-letting is more
or less pernicious according to the habit of the patient. Those
accustomed to this evacuation, bear it better than others. Our
judgment ought also to be much influenced by the age and habit
of the patient. People of a plethoric habit, and in the vigour of
youth, most frequently require blood-letting, and are least apt to
suffer from it.

It appears, then, from what has been said,

1. That the symptoms indicating blood-letting in agues are
those of increased excitement, if considerable, or such as denote
a tendency to local inflammation.

2. That the period most proper for the exhibition of this remedy, is the hot fit, especially during the first paroxysms of the
disease.

3. That the consequences to be dreaded from this remedy,
are debility and its attendants ; and

4. That, on this account. it is most to be dreaded where the body is at the same time exposed to other debilitating causes.

Upon the whole, blood-letting is a remedy which generally
produces some important effect. If it does no good, it proves
hurtful and often dangerous ; and, on the other hand, in many
cases where it is indicated, no other means can save the patient.
The proper employment of blood-letting, therefore, forms an
important branch of the practice of medicine.

A moderate blood-letting for an adult is ten or twelve ounces,
but its extent must vary according to a variety of circumstances,
afterwards to be pointed out at a greater length. I shall presently have occasion to make a few additional observations on the
use of blood-letting in intermitting fever, when I speak of the
exhibition of the bark.

Such are the means to be employed during the hot fit.

All that we have to attend to in the sweating stage is, to avoid
whatever might tend to check the sweat ; in particular, if it lasts
for a considerable time, to give the patient frequent changes of
warm linen, that he may not be chilled by wet clothes ; to lay
him in flannel indeed is the best plan, if he has no particular dis-

like to it. If he is much reduced, his strength should be supported by gentle cordials.

Before we leave the first part of the treatment of intermittents, it will be proper to make some observations on

The Modus Operandi of the Remedies employed during the Paroxysm. [*]

Of the modus operandi of emetics.

It is a law of the animal economy, that an irritation applied to any part of the system, generally tends to induce such motions as are calculated to remove it. When these motions are excited in the more minute parts of the animal body, they are traced with difficulty, and the manner in which they act is obscure. Thus an extraneous body introduced beneath the skin, excites inflammation and suppuration, by means of which it is expelled; but we cannot trace all the steps of this process. Where the larger parts of the animal machine, however, are thrown into action, we trace with more ease the different motions excited, and can often perceive distinctly in what manner they operate in removing the cause of irritation. Thus, an irritation of the nares produces a sudden and violent contraction in all those muscles which are brought into action when we expire forcibly. The consequence of which contraction is a sudden and strong expiration, by which the air being forced violently through the nares, any extraneous body, irritating this part, is removed. Thus coughing also is occasioned by any extraneous body lodged in and irritating the trachea. We see an instance of the same thing in the involuntary exertions excited by tickling the sides or the soles of the feet; so in vomiting, the irritation applied to the stomach induces the action of those muscles which are capable of expelling its contents.

Concerning the action of the muscles employed, some difference of opinion has arisen. It has generally been supposed that the abdominal muscles and diaphragm act together, by which the stomach being forcibly pressed between these muscles, its contents are thrown out by the œsophagus. An eminent professor observes, that as the patient must inspire if the diaphragm contracts in the act of vomiting, part of the contents of the stomach, in their passage over the wind-pipe, would be drawn in with the breath. He therefore supposes that the diaphragm im-

* If what is here said of the modus operandi of the remedies employed during the paroxysm of an intermittent, appear to the reader too long a digression in laying down the treatment of this complaint, he may pass to the next section, and read this, after he has perused the whole of the treatment in agues, along with the account given of the modus operandi of the means employed during the apyrexia. But the treatment during the paroxysm and apyrexia, are so little connected with each other, that the mode of arrangement I have followed appears to me the most distinct.

mediately before the act of vomiting, is fixed by a strong permanent contraction, and that the contents of the stomach are thrown
out in consequence of the sudden contraction of the abdominal
muscles pressing the stomach against the rigid diaphragm.

Concerning this theory of vomiting, it may be observed, that
we do not find a muscle acting in the way in which the diaphragm
is here supposed to do, in any analogous case. This alone must
make us hesitate in admitting it. The following observation, as
far as I am able to judge, altogether sets it aside : Both in this
and the common account of vomiting, one effect of the violent
contraction of the abdominal muscles is overlooked, that of drawing down the ribs. In the act of vomiting, the ribs are forcibly
drawn down, as any person will feel by applying the hand to the
side of the thorax (which I have frequently done) while under
the operation of an emetic. By the descent of the ribs then in
vomiting, the thorax is narrowed, so that if it is not at the same
time lengthened in the same proportion, an expiration must take
place. But we know that no expiration takes place in the act
of vomiting ; the thorax must therefore be lengthened in proportion as it is narrowed : but it can only be lengthened by the contraction of the diaphragm, and this contraction must be instanta-
neous, to correspond with the sudden descent of the ribs. That
neither expiration or inspiration may take place, the one motion
must counteract the effect of the other. We know that if the
ribs descend, the diaphragm must at the same moment either
contract or become flaccid, a state in which nobody can suppose
it to be during the act of vomiting. It would be prevented indeed
from becoming absolutely flaccid by the action of the abdominal
muscles pressing up the bowels ; but were this admitted, it must
be granted that the cavity of the thorax is both narrowed and
shortened in a case where no expiration takes place ; while we
must at the same time admit that the yielding diaphragm is but
ill adapted to the office which we know it performs in the act of
vomiting. All difficulties are removed by supposing that the
diaphragm and abdominal muscles contract at the same instant ;
the latter drawing down the ribs, lessen the capacity of the thorax
in one way, in proportion as the descent of the diaphragm enlarges
it in another. Expiration is forcibly prevented in vomiting to
assist in depressing the diaphragm.

With regard to the peculiar effects of vomiting, by which it
tends to put a period to the cold, and induce the hot, stage of intermittents, we cannot speak with the same certainty ; there is
reason to believe that it does so, both in consequence of the sympathy which is known to subsist between the stomach and the
surface, and because the agitation which vomiting occasions
proves a stimulus to the system in general.

With regard to cathartics. Catharsis is induced by a double
operation of these medicines, which still act, as in the case of
vomiting, by exciting such motions as tend to expel them from

the body. This they do partly by increasing the peristaltic motion of the intestines, and partly by increasing the secretion from their surface.

It is almost unnecessary to observe, that different medicines are fitted to excite different parts of the system. Peppers and aromatics strongly affect the taste, and excite a flow of saliva, but they neither occasion vomiting nor purging. The preparations of antimony which act so violently on the stomach and intestines, are almost insipid.

But the remedies employed during the paroxysm of an intermittent, whose modus operandi chiefly deserves attention, are opium and blood-letting.

In a treatise, entitled an experimental Essay on Opium, I have endeavoured, by comparing the numerous experiments which have been made on this subject, to give a view of the modus operandi of this remedy. It would be improper here to enter on any account of the experiments by which we arrive at this knowledge; I shall only quote from the treatise* the result of what I have there said.

* In a periodic work the following observation is made on this treatise: "From the experiments made in the treatise before us the author is led " to inferences widely different from those which have been drawn by for- " mer writers, but which it is to be feared are still remote from cer- " tainty." This observation can hardly be regarded as liberal, since the author of the analysis does not give the reasons which induced him to make it. As other authors had given a different account of the result of several experiments related in my treatise, I took an oppotunity in the summer of 1796, when I read a course of lectures on febrile diseases at Edinburgh, of publicly repeating these experiments. But as in a class the greater number of pupils sit at too great a distance to judge of the result of experiments of this kind with much accuracy, at my request many of the gentleman attended on a day on which there happened to be no lecture; they stood as near the table, on which the experiments were made, as their number would permit, and expressed their satisfaction with respect to the result. Many of them were men well acquainted with the subje t, and indeed with medicine in general. In the treatise alluded to I have mentioned several circumstances in the experiments in question, which may have occasioned to others, results different from those which occurred to me. A gentleman, however, present at the above meeting, Dr. Woolcomb, suggested a circumstance to which I am now inclined, almost wholly, to attribute this difference, namely, that the authors alluded to had not distinguished the spasms induced by an over-dose of opium, from the voluntary struggles of the animal. This admitted, explains the difference of result, in almost every case, in which I differ from others. And that the authors alluded to permitted themselves to be deceived in this way is probable, because they take no notice of the spasms occasioned by opium being of a peculiar kind, a circumstance which must have struck them had they properly distinguished these spasms, which; both in the warm and cold blooded animals, always assume the form of that species of tetanus which is termed the opisthotonos. Dr. Woolcomb indeed made the observation in consequence of having sometime before been present when one of these authors repeated the experiments without making this distinction; a want of attention to which now ap-

The effects of opium on the living animal body may be divided into three classes. The first, comprehending its action on the nerves of the part to which it is applied, does not differ essentially from that of any other local irritation. It is doubtful whether the first shock given to the system by the action of opium on the nerves of the part to which it is applied has ever been sufficient to destroy life.

A large quantity suddenly applied to a very extensive surface is capable, perhaps, of instantly killing animals less tenacious of life than frogs are, which were the subjects of the experiments above alluded to. A variety of strong impressions, that, for instance, produced by drinking a large quantity of spirits of wine, or of very cold water when the body is overheated, are well known to have occasioned sudden death. From all the facts with which I am acquainted, however, opium never occasions death in this way.

The second class of the effects of opium are those on the heart and blood vessels ; namely, that of increasing their action when it is applied in small quantity ;* and that of altogether destroying their action when applied more freely. In neither of these effects, however, does the action of opium differ essentially from that of other agents. Are not most substances, applied in small quantities, capable of exciting contractions in the muscular fibre, and of destroying its power when applied more freely? It does not appear, that the quantity of opium absorbed by the lacteals, from the largest dose, is sufficient to destroy the muscular power of the heart merely by its action on that organ. It may be safely asserted, that opium never kills by destroying the muscular power of the heart; except when a large quantity is injected into it or into the blood vessels. Opium received into the stomach, therefore, never induces death in this way.

It is ascertained, by the experiments related in this Treatise, that the action of the strongest solution of opium applied to the heart, is merely local ; it destroys the excitability of this organ, but it produces no other effect ; the excitability of all the other muscles of the body remaining unimpaired. It is almost unnecessary to observe, that I here speak of the effects of opium

pears to me to be the principal cause of all the confusion which has crept into the subject. I have not since found reason in any respect to alter, but have met with additional circumstances to confirm, the account of the modus operandi of opium, given in the above treatise. When I published my Essay on Opium I had not seen Dr. Crump's Treatise, which appeared about the same time: and not having devoted much time to the subject since, I have not examined it with the attention it deserves ; but, as far as I recollect, from a hurried perusal of it, it contains nothing which contradicts the results mentioned in the text, but several observations tending to confirm them.

* Compare a note in the 99th page of my Essay on Opium with Dr. Crump's experiments on the pulse.

when its application is confined to the heart ; if it is allowed in the course of circulation to pass to the brain, it then produces the effects which form the third class into which those of opium are divided.

The third class of the effects of opium comprehends those it produces when immediately applied to the brain : These are, when the dose is moderate, impaired sensibility, languor, sleep ; effects which are occasioned, in a greater or less degree, by all other gentle irritations of this organ, and which do not follow a moderate dose of opium till we know from the symptoms it produces, compared with the experiments which have been made on this subject, that it has been conveyed to the heart ; from which, in the course of circulation, it is sent to the brain, as well as to other parts of the body. What share its action on the latter parts has in producing these effects, it is impossible to say. We have reason to believe it but trifling, because opium directly applied and confined to the brain, produces the same effects as when permitted to circulate with the blood. It appears from the experiments just alluded to, that no part of these effects is to be ascribed to its action on the heart itself.

Opium applied to the brain more freely produces effects similar to those produced by other violent irritations of this organ— convulsions and death. And this is the way in which opium received into the stomach, occasions death : It is taken up by the lacteals, and in the course of circulation applied immediately to the brain. According to the quantity thus applied, it produces sleep, convulsions, or death ; for opium, even in the human body, does not always prove fatal when it induces convulsions.*

Of the manner in which opium acts in shortening the hot stage of intermittents, we cannot speak positively. There is reason to believe that it is chiefly by increasing the action of the heart and blood vessels. It is from this effect of opium that it is found hurtful wherever the inflammatory diathesis prevails, in which the action of these organs is already too great.

I shall seldom have occasion to say so much of the modus operandi of remedies. In this branch of medicine little upon the whole is ascertained, and nothing is more hurtful than hy-

---

* In some of the experiments alluded to in the Treatise I have been speaking of, convulsions were induced on rabbits by large doses of opium, which were not sufficient, however, to prove fatal ; and there are several cases on record in which this happened in the human body. See cases related by Mr. Dobson and an anonymous author in the Medical Museum. In all its effects on the living animal body, opium has much in common with other agents, but at the same time something in each peculiar to itself. It will appear (as far as I can judge) from what I shall afterwards have occasion to say, that the same observation applies to every thing capable of acting on living animals, whether acting immediately on the body, or affecting it through the medium of the mind.

potheses intermixed with the facts which are to conduct our practice.   On the other hand, when any thing certain is known
respecting the modus operandi of remedies, it is always of consequence to be acquainted with it.   If our knowledge in this
branch of medicine is confined, a physician is the less excusable
for not being acquainted with what is known

There is no remedy whose modus operandi demands more
attention than blood-letting, for two reasons; there are few concerning whose mode of action we can say so much with certainty; and there is none whose mode of action, particularly in fevers,
has been so much misrepresented, to which misrepresentation
the lives of thousands have been sacrificed.   I am now to point
out what is, as far as I am capable of judging from various observations, which will afterwards be considered more at length, the
only way in which blood-letting acts in relieving the symptoms
of idiopathic fever.

We know that the heart, deprived of the stimulus of the blood,
ceases to contract almost instantly in the human body, and in a
short time in all animals.   The presence of the blood is as necessary for the continued action of the heart, as the peculiar
structure by which it is fitted for contraction.   But every thing
capable of exciting contractions in the muscular fibre, produces
within certain limits more or less powerful contractions, in proportion to the quantity applied.

In the change from a state of health to that of synocha, one of
three things must take place; either the blood is driven towards
the heart in greater quantity than usual, or it becomes more
capable of stimulating the heart, or the heart itself becomes
more irritable, that is, more capable of being acted upon, and
thus contractions more powerful than those consistent with
health are excited.

But it has just been observed, that the effects of every stimulus
in exciting the muscular fibre are within certain limits proportioned to the quantity applied.   And whichever of the foregoing
circumstances be the cause of the stronger action of the heart in
synocha, this law still holds good.   Whether, therefore, the disease originates in the blood being propelled towards the heart in
greater quantity than usual, or in its having acquired morbid
properties, or in the heart having become more irritable, lessen-
ing the quantity of blood must diminish the force of its contractions.

The following experiment directly ascertains the point in question, which is otherwise so well established indeed as not to require this additional proof: Dr. Hales opened the blood vessels
of living animals, adapted glass tubes to their orifices, and observed to what height the blood rose in the tubes at each systole
of the heart; he then drew from the animals different quantities

of blood, and observed the force of the heart diminish in proportion as the blood was abstracted.

It must also happen, that the more suddenly the abstraction of
blood is made, the greater will be its effect in diminishing the
force of the heart. When it is gradually abstracted, the capacity
of the heart and vessels is readily adapted to the quantity of fluids
they contain. If it is suddenly drawn off, the change of capacity
is effected with more difficulty. The diminished action of the
powers supporting circulation, when the abstraction of blood is
made suddenly, is in a great measure to be attributed to this, that
the vessels not immediately adapting themselves to their contents,
the quantity of blood returned to the heart, is often more diminished than in proportion to the real loss of blood. It seems to
be in this way, that the loss of a few ounces of blood very suddenly
abstracted, often induces syncope, even in stout people who could
lose six times the quantity without inconvenience were it abstracted more slowly. Syncope from loss of blood in general indeed, must in a great measure depend on this cause. Did it
proceed from the absolute loss of blood it would be much more
fatal than we find it. It was common with the Ancients, in a
variety of diseases, to bleed the patient till he fainted.

If diminishing the action of the heart and blood vessels, be the
only effect of blood-letting in idiopathic fevers, it follows, that this
remedy can only be of service in these complaints when the
symptoms of synocha prevail. Till lately indeed it has been the
practice to have recourse to blood-letting in all kinds of fevers.
This practice was chiefly founded on mere hypothesis ; in part,
however, it was founded on a fact which I shall have occasion to
consider, more particularly, when speaking of the crises of fevers,
namely, that even in well marked typhus the loss of blood has
sometimes, though rarely, proved beneficial. There can be little
doubt that a spontaneous hemorrhagy has sometimes proved a
favourable crisis in all kinds of fevers. And there have been
some few cases perhaps, in which venesection was serviceable in
typhus. I have not, however, either in the course of practice or
reading met with any unequivocal case of this kind. If the state
of body in some rare cases of typhus be such, that the advantages
derived from venesection will more than compensate for the harm
done by its debilitating effects ; nobody has yet succeeded in
pointing out the means of detecting such a state.

We shall afterwards find the following observation sufficiently
illustrated ; that the symptoms, which are termed critical, a flow
of sweat, a hemorrhagy, a sediment in the urine, &c. are more
frequently the consequence than the cause of a favourable change
in the complaint ; and we may in vain induce such symptoms, if
we counteract that favourable change which often occasions their
spontaneous appearance.

It would be difficult to point out any other error in medicine, which has proved equally hurtful with the hypothesis, that led physicians to regard certain symptoms, which frequently attend the change from fever to health, as the sole cause of that change. From which source arose, among other hurtful species of practice, the indiscriminate use of blood-letting in this complaint.

SUCH is the plan of treatment during the paroxysm of an intermittent, and, as far as I can judge, the sum of what is known respecting the modus operandi of the principal means employed at this period. We are now to consider the remaining general division of the treatment of intermittents, namely, that during the remission or apyrexia.

SECT. II.

Of the Treatment of an Intermittent during the Apyrexia.

THIS is the most important part of the practice in agues, and that which, strictly speaking, can alone be regarded as curative.

The indications in the apyrexia or remissions are, to restore the patient's strength and to prevent the return of the paroxysm. The first is answered chiefly by an attention to diet and exercise; the other by medicines.

1. *Of the Diet and Exercise during the Apyrexia.*

This part of the treatment I shall consider at some length because it is that which is most generally neglected, and notwithstanding its simplicity, least generally understood.

Wherever there is much of the inflammatory diathesis, the patient's diet must be such as tends to counteract this habit of body. His food should consist of milk and vegetables, and even of these he should not be permitted to eat plentifully, if signs of plethora are evident. A spare diet is one of the few means we have of overcoming habitual fulness. While there is any tendency to inflammation in the system, fermented liquors must be avoided ; the patient's drink should consist of plain water, or some mild vegetable decoction.

When, on the other hand, much debility prevails, he must be allowed as full a diet as his stomach will bear. It often happens in debilitated states of the system, that the stronger kinds of animal food occasion a degree of irritation capable of exciting temporary fever. Beef, mutton, &c. ought therefore to be avoided; veal, lamb, and chicken, when the powers of digestion are not much weakened, will be found equally nourishing, and irritate less. Upon the whole, all that is necessary in this case is, to chuse that kind of food which affords most nourishment, with least irritation. The same rule applies to the drink : When the strength is much reduced, it should never consist of pure water, and in no case of any mixture containing distilled spirits, except where fermented liquors, which have not been distilled, cannot be procured. The best drink in cases where debility prevails is wine, particularly port, or, what is still better, claret, diluted with water; the quantity is easily regulated by attending to the constitution and habits of the patient, and the effects which the wine produces. Of the fermented liquors of this country, porter is generally found the best. This, or any others which the patient prefers, is always to be recommended in preference to any kind of distilled spirits, whether diluted or not.

While the digestive powers remain but little impaired, these few regulations are all that are necessary respecting the diet during the apyrexia of intermittents. But it is not uncommon for a considerable degree of dyspepsia to supervene in these fevers, and then a more particular attention to diet becomes necessary.

Acescent and oily articles of food, with a large proportion of liquid, compose the diet most apt to injure digestion. The opposite to this diet, therefore, is that which agrees best with dyspeptics. I have just had occasion to observe, that the flesh of old animals irritates more during digestion than that of young. By this, however, it is not m_ean_t that the latter is of more easy digestion. Just the contrary of this is true. The flesh of old animals in general is more easily digested than that of young, but irritates more while digestion goes on. Nearly the same may be said of the food derived from the whole animal world, compared with that composed of vegetables. The former is constantly found more irritating, more apt to induce fever; the latter more difficult to digest.

We must attend, therefore, to the state of the patient; and in particular to the tendency to fever or dyspepsia, and regulate his diet accordingly.

Where it is our view to obviate the symptoms of dyspepsia, a diet composed of the flesh of old animals, and bread toasted till it is hard, will be found the best. All kinds of soups, gravies, and fresh vegetables should be avoided, and every thing into the composition of which butter, or any other oily substance, enters. The same may be said of all hard animal substances, salted and smoked meat, cheese, &c. The harder animal substances are, the more difficult are they of digestion. This is not true of vegetables. There is perhaps no vegetable substance so easy of digestion as a hard sea-biscuit, provided it be properly masticated. The tough, thready, and membranous parts of vegetables are of most difficult digestion; next to these, the cold vegetables eat raw, melons, cucumbers, &c. Before a dyspeptic can shake off his complaints he must learn to resist the gratification of his taste, and he must endure this mortification not for days or weeks, but many months, or even years, if he is resolved not to be tormented by constant returns of the complaint; for when dyspepsia is occasioned by agues, or other lingering complaints, it often continues to barrass the patient long after every symptom of the primary disease is removed.

There is much difference of opinion respecting the proper drink in dyspeptic cases. I have just had occasion to observe, that the less the diet in this complaint consists of liquid the better. But there is generally present a considerable degree of thirst, and a certain quantity of fluid is necessary. The general opinion is, that every kind of distilled spirits, as less acescent, is preferable in dyspepsia to any of the fermented liquors, which have not been distilled. The truth is, that neither the one nor the other is a proper article of diet in dyspepsia. They are only to be given when it is of more consequence to support the patient's strength, than to adhere, in every respect, to that diet which is best suited to a weak stomach. But of the two, I have uniformly found (and I am acquainted with other practitioners, who have made this disease a particular study, that are of the same opinion) that fermented liquors, which have not been distilled, particularly the red wines, are less hurtful in dyspepsia than any kind of spirits, and that the more diluted they are, provided the patient does not take a very large quantity of fluid, they are the less injurious.

Wherever the patient's strength is not much reduced, the best drink in dyspepsia, is thin water gruel : this is neither very acescent, nor capable of hurting the digestive organs, by applying to them too strong a stimulus; and its mucilaginous property defends the stomach and bowels against any irritating matter they happen to contain.

The hurtful effects of taking the drink very warm in dyspepsia are generally admitted ; but most practitioners are not aware, that equal harm is done by taking it very cold. Even ice is sometimes prescribed as a tonic in cases of indigestion ; which I have known to be the means of inducing this complaint. There are many dyspeptics who cannot, without injury, take their drink of a temperature lower than 80° ; and there is no case of dyspepsia in which its temperature should be under 50°.

Whatever be the quality of the food, the dyspeptic must be restricted with respect to its quantity; particularly the quantity which he takes at one meal. This caution is the more necessary, because the appetite in dyspepsia is often morbidly increased. Nor is it proper for the interval between meals to be long. I do not know any rule of more importance in this complaint, than to eat frequently and not much at a time ; neither to permit the stomach to remain long empty, nor to oppress it with a load of food.

Such are the general observations by which the diet, during

the apyrexia of intermittents, is regulated. It would be tedious to enter into particulars which every one's reflection must suggest to him.

The exercise both of the mind and body, at this period, also demands particular attention. The degree of these must be suited to the strength of the patient. The different kinds of bodily exercise may be arranged under three divisions. That in which the body is moved by its own exertions, as in walking; that in which it is moved by any other power, as in the various modes of gestation; and that in which the circulation is promoted without moving the body, by friction for example, or merely by pressure.

Intermitting fever may induce such a degree of weakness, that friction may be the only kind of exercise which the patient can endure without fatigue. This, however, is seldom the case when the intermissions are considerable; but wherever the strength is much reduced, although the patient can bear a little of some rougher exercise, frictions are always useful. Friction is the principal exercise among the higher ranks of some Asiatic nations, and it was used both by the Greeks and Romans after they became luxurious.

As the total want of exercise is not more pernicious than that which occasions fatigue, the different kinds of gestation, even after the patient has recovered a considerable degree of strength, are often found preferable to those exercises, in which the body is moved by its own exertions.

The gentlest kind of gestation is sailing, which often proves serviceable in all cases of debility, and has been particularly recommended in weaknesses of the stomach and bowels.*

Next to sailing, the gentlest kind of exercise, commonly prescribed, is the motion of a carriage, and in those who are too weak to ride on horseback, it is often attended with the best effects. But in such climates as our own the patient must either be confined in a close carriage, or run the risk of being chilled. As a substitute for a carriage, but inferior to it, swings and spring chairs are frequently recommended with advantage. But none of these modes of exercise are equal to that on horseback, when the patient is strong enough not to be soon fatigued by it. It is particularly suited to those cases in which dyspepsia prevails. Of all kinds of exercise, Dr. Whytt observes, riding on horseback has been justly esteemed the best.† Sydenham is extravagant in his praise of this mode of exercise, and particularly recommends it in hypochondriacal and hysterical disorders. Riding, he observes, is preferable to walking, as it shakes the body more and fatigues it less. It is to be remembered, however, that

* See Dr. Gilchrist's Treatise on the Use of Sea Voyages in Medicine.
† See his Treatise on Nervous Complaints.

any rough exercise, and particularly riding on horseback, soon after meals, disturbs digestion.

Notwithstanding what has been said of riding on horseback; after the patient has acquired sufficient strength to walk for an hour or two without fatigue, this mode of exercise is found upon the whole preferable to all others; it is attended with a more uniform and general exertion of the muscles, and from the valvular structure of the veins is better fitted to promote circulation. It is often of service to combine the two last modes of exercise; riding on horseback being particularly adapted to restore the tone of the stomach and bowels, while walking is better fitted to strengthen the system in general.

In cases of debility we must regulate the exercise of the mind as well as that of the body. When the latter is debilitated, the former in general is languid and listless. This state of mind is more or less overcome by a proper degree of bodily exercise, but the occupation of the mind itself is the best means of removing it. The maxims which regulate the degree of bodily exercise, are also applicable to that of the mind. The great rule is to occupy without fatiguing it. Any study which fatigues is injurious, and the constant languor of a mind wholly unoccupied is no less so. Wherever the debility is considerable, the mind should be occupied by amusement alone; and even those amusements which interest the feelings much, or occasion any considerable exertion of mind, may be hurtful. When, on the other hand, the patient has recovered a considerable degree of strength, a moderate attention even to business is found serviceable. However varied our occupations are, if they tend only to present gratification, they soon become insipid. The mind must have something in view, some plan of bettering its condition, in order to arrest the attention for any length of time. I know of nothing of greater advantage to patients in a debilitated habit of body, than the conversation of friends who constantly present to them the fairest side of their future prospects.

The time of day, at which either the mind or body is exercised, is also a matter of considerable importance. Towards the evening every kind of exertion becomes irksome, and consequently hurtful. Besides, in those who are debilitated, a degree of fever (probably the consequence of the unavoidable irritations applied to the body throughout the day) comes on at this time, which is only to be relieved by repose; going early to bed, therefore, is of much consequence in such cases. Exposure to the night air is particularly hurtful to people in a debilitated state of body. This seems partly owing to the cause just mentioned, that all kinds of exertion are hurtful towards the end of the day, partly to the dampness of the night air, and partly perhaps to some less evident cause.

But although it is of consequence for the debilitated to go carly to bed, there are few things more hurtful than remaining in bed too long. After the degree of strength, of which the present state of the system is capable, is restored by sleep, any longer continuance in bed tends only to relax. Getting up an hour and an half earlier in the morning often gives a degree of vigour which nothing else can procure. I know people whose feet constantly become cold and damp if they remain in bed a few hours awake in the morning. It is remarkable, that the same effect is not produced, however long they remain in bed, provided they are asleep. For those who are not greatly debilitated, the best rule is to get out of bed as soon as they awake in the morning. This at first perhaps may be too early, for debilitated habits require more sleep than people in health; but the exertion of rising early will gradually prolong the sleep on the succeeding night, till the quantity which the patient enjoys is equal to his demand for it; thus, what at first sight may seem a paradox, getting out of bed early in the morning is one of the surest means of prolonging the time spent in sleep; an effect I have often known it have.

Lying late is not only hurtful by the relaxation it occasions, but also by occupying that time of the day at which exercise is most beneficial. As soon as the patient rises, he should have breakfast, because exertions of every kind are improper while the stomach is empty; nor are they proper during the first part of digestion, being apt to impede it; they ought to be delayed till about an hour after breakfast. From this time to two or three o'clock is the proper time of the day for the exercise both of the mind and body; after this the debilitated should lay aside every occupation which tends to fatigue; to which the exertions during the former part of the day will sufficiently incline them.

In every circumstance respecting diet and exercise much attention must constantly be paid to the patient's age, habits, and inclinations.

Old people are less subject to that diathesis which disposes to inflammation, than the young; in them debility is most to be dreaded, and when it occurs is removed with most difficulty. We seldom find occasion therefore to recommend a low diet to them. Wine, it has been said, is milk for old men, and this proverb contains one of the best maxims in medicine. In old age also, repose is more necessary, and exertions of every kind are less beneficial, and more apt to be hurtful.

With respect to diet, however, no general rule can be laid down; in old people we sometimes meet with the inflammatory diathesis, which must be treated in the manner just pointed out, but with the more caution the older the patient is. In young people, on the other hand, we often meet with a debilitated state of the system, which is more easily counteracted indeed at this period of life, but which even in youth often baffles all our endeavours.

In both old and young the inflammatory diathesis is most apt
to occur in an early stage of the disease ; the frequent repetition
of the paroxysms tends to overcome this diathesis and to produce
debility ; a poor diet, therefore, is generally hurtful in protracted cases.

‑ ‧ The patient's desires also lead us to form indications respecting
his diet and exercise.   When the remissions are but imperfect,
he has little or no desire for food or exercise, and nothing could
be more hurtful than to force him in such cases to take either
the one or the other ; any inclination to sleep, during the intermission, should be encouraged.   Sleep restores the strength after
the debilitating effects of the last paroxysm, and affords new
vigour to combat that which succeeds.   On the other hand, when
the patient has any inclination to eat or walk about, we are not
to insist on his keeping his bed, or abstaining from food, during
the intermission.   The necessity for sleep or food is best determined by the patient's feelings ; and nobody but himself can
judge of them.   Longings for particular articles of food, if not
very improper, should be indulged, since the irritation they occasion, when not gratified, does harm. ' It is common, in all kinds
of fever, for the patient to long for fresh fruits ; which tend
both to refresh in typhus, and allay the inflammatory symptoms
of synocha.   During the intermission of agues, however,
they prove hurtful, when the patient is troubled with dyspepsia,
or bowel complaints.

,‘ In regulating the diet, during the intermission, some attention
should be paid to the season of the year.   In spring it has been
observed, the inflammatory diathesis prevails more frequently than
in autumn.   In the latter season, especially at its commencement, we dread debility ; fevers are then more apt to become
malignant.   The warmer and moister the season is, the greater
reason is there to dread debility.   The inflammatory diathesis
is most apt to prevail when the weather is cold and changeable. ɩ

We must attend also to the nature of the prevailing epidemic.
When it is accompanied with inflammatory symptoms, the patient
should avoid animal food and fermented liquors ; when accompanied with those symptoms which have been termed putrescent,
every thing which debilitates must be shunned, and as full a diet
prescribed as the state of the patient admits of.

The most important part of the treatment in agues still remains to be considered, namely, the medicines employed during the remission or apyrexia.

2. *Of the Medicines employed during the Remission or Apyrexia.*'

These may be divided into two classes : such as are exhibited
during the whole, or at least a great part, of the apyrexia ; and
such ‧ as only prove beneficial when the paroxysm is expected. ‧

In the first place, of those exhibited during the whole or a great part of the apyrexia.

Of all the medicines, recommended in intermittents, none has been so generally employed as the Peruvian bark. On this me; dicine indeed the generality of practitioners wholly depend for the cure of these fevers. It therefore particularly demands attention.*

This valuable medicine is the bark of a middle sized tree, a native of Peru. The circumstance which led Europeans to pay attention to the Peruvian bark, was a remarkable cure performed by it on the countess del Cinchon, the Spanish viceroy's lady, in the year 1640. It is said, that the Indians were not ignorant of its virtues as early as the year 1500. In 1649, a jesuit brought a considerable quantity of it into Italy, which was distributed by the fathers of that order at a high price over a great part of Europe, from which circumstance it got the name of jesuit's bark ; and, about the same time, the cardinal de Lugo imported a quantity of it for the use of the poor at Rome. " When first in tro-" duced (Dr. Cullen† observes) it was found to cure intermittents " very readily ; but whether it was that a medicine of more " seeming efficacy was at the same time brought into Europe, " or whether timid practice lessened the dose, it went out of cre-" dit, and was not till 30 years afterwards restored by Talbot."

The bark is an astringent bitter, with some degree of aromatic flavour ; to none of these qualities, however, can its power of curing intermitting fever be attributed, since no combination of astringents, bitters, and aromatics, is found equally effectual.

A variety of prejudices respecting the bark prevailed for a long time after its introduction into Europe, and prevented its general use. The more ancient of these do not even deserve to be mentioned, such as, that those who use this medicine die within a year, or according to others within seven years, that it is particularly pernicious to fat people, &c. The prejudices which in many places still interfere to prevent the free employment of this medicine arose chiefly from the nature of the fevers in which the bark is recommended.

Intermitting fever, it has been observed, is often followed by obstructions of the viscera, dropsy, &c. ; these, which are the consequences of the disease, were, and in some places still are, attributed to the bark.‡

* This medicine is mentioned by authors under a variety of appellations, chincona, chinachina, chinchina, kina kina, kinkina, quina quina, quinquina, pulvis comitissæ, gentiana indica, antiquartium Peruvianum, jesuiticus pulvis, cardinal de Lugo's powder, &c.

† See his Materia Medica.

‡ It is now well ascertained, however, that there is no foundation whatever for this opinion. Dr. Millar (Account of the Diseases most preva-

Although almost all practitioners at present employ the bark in agues, at least when they are protracted beyond a few paroxysms, there is some difference of opinion concerning the period of the disease at which it ought to be exhibited, the preparation of the patient, &c.

We determine when and how the bark is to be given, by attending to the following circumstances.

1. The period of the disease.

2. The nature of the symptoms, particularly the presence of the inflammatory diathesis, or debility.

lent in Britain) declares it his opinion, contrary to what he once thought, that the fever, and not the bark, is the cause of the obstructions and dropsies which frequently supervene on agues, and that the bark is the best means of preventing these affections. Dr. Jackson (Account of the Diseases of Jamaica) remarks, that he always found dysentery, dropsy, and visceral obstructions, most common where the bark was most sparingly employed. When the ague, Dr. Lind observes, was stopped by the bark immediately after the first or second fit, as in my own case and that of 200 of my patients, neither a jaundice nor dropsy ensued ; whereas when the bark could not be administered on account of the imperfect remssions, of the fever, or when the patient had neglected to take it, either a dropsy, jaundice, or a constant head-ache were the certain consequences, and the degree of violence was proportioned to the number of the preceding fits, or to the continuance of the fever.

The bark indeed is by many regarded as among the best means we have of removing such affections, when they are the consequences of agues. Dr. Brocklesby (on the Diseases of the Army) recommends it in cases of visceral obstruction after the use of mild and repeated emetics and cathartics ; and Dr. Strack (De Febribus Intermittentibus) remarks, that he has found the bark more powerful than any other medicine in removing indurations of the spleen, and has observed it successful in the dropsical affections which supervene on intermittents.

It is also a prevalent opinion in many places, that agues cured by the bark more frequently return than those which leave the patient after running their full course. But Torti (Therapeutice Specialis) has justly observed, that if fevers cured by the bark sometimes return, those removed by other means are no less apt to do so ; and when overcome by the efforts of nature alone, they frequently attack the patient a second time or oftener. Since these fevers, he continues, in whatever manner they are cured have a tendency to return in autumn, but not in spring and the beginning of summer, we must, with Morton, conclude, that the disposition of, the fever, and not the nature of the remedy, is in fault. Numberless observations might be quoted to the same purpose. In short, amidst all the prejudices entertained against the bark, wherever it has been fairly tried, it has proved both a safe and successful medicine in intermittents. Never was there any medicine, D'Aquin observes, known to cure fevers so quickly, and with so much safety. The authority of Sydenham is not to be overlooked. " Vere affirmare possum non ob-" stante tam vulgi quam perpaucorum e doctis prejudicio, me nihil mali " Ægris accidesse ab ejus usu vidisse unquam, vel cum ratione suspicare " potuisse." If other authorities be required, I might here repeat the names of almost every author I have had occasion to mention. So generally indeed is the innocence of the bark admitted and confirmed by so extensive an experience, that no authority against it can now claim any attention.

3. The climate, and the season of the year.

4. The age and habit of the patient; and

5. The nature of the epidemic.

1. Of the period of the disease, most proper for the exhibition of the bark.

Where the debility is great, the symptoms consequently alarming, and much danger to be apprehended if the fever again recurs, especially where the apyrexia is short and imperfect, it is often adviseable to begin to give the bark about the end of the hot fit; for were it delayed till the remission takes place, it might be impossible to throw in a sufficient quantity before the succeeding paroxysm. And if the patient be much reduced, and the symptoms termed putrescent have made their appearance, the bark, as I shall presently have occasion to observe more particularly, is proper after the remissions have become so slight as to be hardly perceived. The general plan in intermitting and remitting fever, however, is not to give the bark till complete apyrexia, or an evident remission of the symptoms, takes place; it is then given in various doses and at different intervals,* as the state of the complaint requires.

There has been some dispute respecting the best time of the apyrexia for the exhibition of the bark. Many give it immediately after the paroxysm, and at intervals till the fever returns; others only during a few hours before the paroxysm. We must determine in which of these ways the bark is to be exhibited, by attending to the duration of the apyrexia, the quantity of bark required, and the quantity which the stomach is capable of receiving in one dose.†

When the apyrexia is short, and the quantity of bark required considerable, it must be given immediately after the paroxysms,

* While the intermitting form remains distinctly marked, it is universally admitted that the exhibition of the bark during the cold or hot fits is improper. Dr. Fordyce made a trial of the bark during the hot fit, and found that it both increased the length of the paroxysm, and rendered the crisis less perfect. Dr. Cleghorn also remarks, that when the bark was given during the paroxysm, the patient died; but he recovered often after his case seemed desperate, if the remissions were seized for the exhibition of this medicine.

† While the prejudices against the bark were prevalent, it was generally exhibited in the former of these ways, in all cases. The doses were small, and the intervals at which they were given long. Sydenham disapproved of giving the bark in large doses, and generally endeavoured to seize long intervals for throwing it very gradually into the body. He recommends mixing an ounce of bark with syrup of roses, and giving the patient the size of a nutmeg morning and evening, on the days of intermission, until the whole quantity is finished. The same quantity was repeated in 14 days, which was given a third time in the same manner. While such was the mode of prescribing the bark, we cannot be surprised that it was not found very successful.

and continued till the return of the succeeding fit at longer or shorter intervals, according as the case is more or less urgent, and the stomach able to bear it. On the other hand, when the apyrexia is long, and especially when a great quantity of the bark is not necessary, its exhibition should be delayed till within six or eight hours of the time at which the paroxysm is expected. For a considerable quantity given at this period is more likely to succeed, than the same quantity in smaller doses, throughout the whole of a long apyrexia.

From the observations that will be made on the modus operandi of the bark, it will appear probable, that in the cure of intermittents this medicine acts chiefly by its effects on the stomach and intestines, and that on this account our endeavours should be directed to have a proper quantity of bark in the primæ viæ, at the time the paroxysm is expected.

The period then at which the bark is to be exhibited in agues, is during the apyrexia, and particularly towards the end of it, if it be long. As soon as the fever returns, the exhibition of the bark should be discontinued.

Many attempt to determine the quantity of bark which will with certainty remove an intermittent;[*] this however depends on the severity of the disease, compared with other circumstances which will be pointed out as we proceed. It may be remarked upon the whole that tertians require more bark than quotidians, and quartans than tertians.

2. The next thing to be attended to in prescribing the bark, is the nature of the fever. When the pulse is strong and full, and still more when it is hard, when the face is flushed, and the heat considerable, especially when these symptoms are accompanied with rheumatic or pleuritic pains, or a difficulty of breathing, even although the apyrexia be complete and long, the bark must not be exhibited, till such symptoms are removed by the means already pointed out in the treatment of the paroxysm.[†]

* Dr. Millar observes, that he cannot recollect a case of remitting fever, in several years extensive practice, in which the patient died after taking two ounces of bark. And Mr. Reid, in his Account of the Diseases of the West Indies, makes the same observation.

† What is here said is well illustrated by Sir John Pringle's Account of the Intermittents prevalent among the British troops on the Continent, which were of an inflammatory nature. " The cure of these fevers (he " observes) depends chiefly on evacuations, and low diet. Neutral salts " and diluting acid liquors are assistants, and the bark is useful when " there are complete intermissions. These fevers (he observes in another " place) have such fair remissions, even with a breaking in the water, as " might persuade a physician unacquainted with their nature, that they " would always yield to that medicine, but he would be often disappointed. " Whether it be that some inflammation hinders the bark from taking " effect, or that these quotidians are not true intermittents, as not being " of a tertian or quartan form, certain it is, that they can be seldom safely

It is chiefly at the commencement of the disease that the inflammatory diathesis prevails, and when this is corrected, mild,
especially vernal intermittents, often yield spontaneously.* The

" stopped by it. For though the paroxyms have disappeared under its
" use, yet having so often seen the breast affected or a lurking fever re-
" main, after giving the febrifuge, at last I made it a rule to attempt the
" cure without it, or at least to delay giving any, till in the convalescent
" state the patient required it only as a strengthener." Sir John Pringle
generally found it necessary to begin with opening a vein, and to repeat
the blood-letting according to the urgency of the symptoms. Most of the
remittents which came under his care, either in spring or towards the
end of autumn, were accompanied with pleuritic or rheumatic pains; and
the use of the bark often changed them into continued inflammatory fevers.
It may be observed in confirmation of what was said of the proper period
for blood-letting in these fevers, that he particularly recommends the hot
fit for this purpose. He generally gave a cathartic immediately after the
blood-letting. From the observations made respecting the treatment during the paroxysm, the propriety of this mode of practice appears doubtful. There are few authors who treat of intermittents, who have not had
occasion to make observations similar to those of Sir John Pringle.—Dr.
Donald Munro, in particular, gives nearly the same account of the remittents which prevailed among the soldiers on the Continent.—When the
bark had failed on several trials, Dr. Rush observes, one or two moderate
blood-lettings generally secured its success; in these cases, he adds, the
pulse is full and a little hard, and the blood sizy. The bark is always unsuccessful, he justly remarks, when blood-letting is necessary, and he says
he has known many instances in which pounds of this medicine had been
given without effect, which yielded readily after ten or twelve ounces of
blood were taken away. Dr. Rush thinks that blisters often serve the
purpose of blood-letting in these cases; but they are not to be depended
upon. How different a mode of treatment is to be pursued, when our
practice in agues is not incumbered by the presence of the inflammatory
diathesis, will appear from comparing what is said by these authors, with
what Dr. Jackson says of the fevers which prevailed among the troops in
America. " Time, (he observes) is not to be spent in frivolous prepara-
" tions, or diseases attacked with feeble remedies, when the health of
" soldiers is concerned." In the autumnal months, when signs of malignity
and danger were present, he generally seized the first intermission for
exhibiting the bark, without premising either vomiting or purging, even
where the bowels were loaded. He gave two drams for a dose, and repeated it every two hours, while the fever was absent. Two ounces, he
observes, taken in the space of eight or ten hours, were often more effectual than double the quantity in small doses and at long intervals.

* Dr. Cleghorn seldom gave the bark in tertians till the fifth day. From
the paroxysm which took place on that day, he judged whether or not the
bark was necessary, and in what quantity it ought to be given. If this
paroxysm, namely the third, was not longer and attended with worse
symptoms than the second, if the patient preserved his strength, and if a
lateritious sediment appeared in the urine, he often ventured to trust the
cure to nature. As he judged from this paroxysm of the future treatment
of the disease, he was careful to premise such medicines as tended to moderate the complaint, and prepare the body for immediately receiving the
bark, in case the symptoms of the third paroxysm proved it necessary.
During the first three or four days, therefore, he ordered evacuations. It
was his custom, we have seen, to take away a little blood at the commencement of the disease, if the state of the patient admitted of it; and
he never failed to clear the primæ viæ of any irritating matter which they
happened to contain at this period; and to these means alone the com-

continuance of disease always tends to overcome the inflammatory diathesis; thus we constantly find, as was observed on a former occasion, 'that however well marked this diathesis is at the commencement of fever, it always disappears in its progress. On this account practitioners have found, that many intermittents yield to the bark with more ease, after they have run through several paroxysms, than at their commencement.*

Many, from this circumstance, have been led to lay it down as a general rule, that the bark is not to be given at the commencement of agues; and this rule they found the more useful, as it was often necessary to clear the primæ viæ before its exhibition. Such appear to be the sources of the prejudice against giving the bark at the commencement of intermittents; for a prejudice it certainly is, when made a general rule. If confined to those cases in which the inflammatory diathesis prevails, it is the result of universal experience.

We are not, however, in such cases, as Dr. Brocklesby and others recommend, to delay the use of the bark till the continuance of the disease has overcome this diathesis. This would often be attended with the worst consequences. We are only to delay it till by the proper use of the means above pointed out, we have corrected that state of the system which renders the exhibition of the bark improper. There is nothing in the nature of intermittents, except their being frequently attended by the inflammatory diathesis, which prevents the use of the bark at every commencement, that is, after the first paroxysm.

plaint sometimes yielded. But if the third paroxysm was the longest and most severe that had happened, if it was attended with any dangerous symptoms, if the sick became giddy, feeble, or languid, without delay he had recourse to the bark. As soon as the sweat ceased to flow, he ordered two scruples or a dram of it to be given every two or three hours, or every hour and an half, so that five or six drams might be taken before next day at noon. It is necessary, he remarks, that a considerable quantity of the bark be given at this period; since after it, the fits are often redoubled, so that we have not a proper opportunity of giving the medicine. It is to be remembered, however, that Cleghorn practised in the mild climate of Minorca. In general we shall find that the exhibition of the bark should not be delayed so long as he recommends, particularly in autumnal agues.

* When the patient was athletic, Dr. Brocklesby observes, he allowed the fever to run on for a little, before he gave the bark. Giving the bark too early, he remarks, in athletic habits, produced much pain of the head, yellowness of the eyes, and sometimes continued fever.—Hillary also observes, that he has frequently seen the early use of the bark render the fever continued, and mali moris. See Brocklesby on the Diseases of the Army, and Hillary's Account of the Diseases of Barbadoes.
In those cases where the tendency to inflammatory symptoms prevents us giving much of the bark, Dr. Brocklesby recommends giving small doses of it with myrrh, snakeroot, or some other such medicine, till the inflammatory diathesis is sufficiently removed to admit of giving the bark in larger doses.

Wherever 'the' pulse is feeble and quick, and the strength greatly reduced, the early exhibition of the bark is indispensable.* Nay it appears, from the observations of Mr. Clark, Just quoted in a note, as well as those of others, that where the symptoms of typhus are well marked, the bark is to be exhibited even during the paroxysm.†

While the inflammatory diathesis is present, the bark proves the more hurtful, the more the fever shows a tendency to become continued. The use of the bark in these circumstances' indeed often renders it so.

The contrary of this observation is true of the cases in which debility prevails; in these, provided the remissions are still distinctly marked, the greater tendency the fever shows to become continued, the greater is the quantity of bark required; and the more the patient is capable of receiving, the greater tendency the fever shews to resume the intermitting form. These observations, the truth of which must strike every one who peruses with care the works of the original authors on the subject, have been frequently overlooked, and much confusion has arisen from writers attempting to lay down, as generally applicable to the treatment of agues, the maxims of practice, which they found suited to the particular cases which fell under their own observation.

In the treatment of agues, more attention has been paid than seems proper, to the state of the stomach and bowels. It is a very prevalent opinion, that while the stomach and bowels are loaded,

* Dr. Brocklesby observes, that when the patient was weak and irritable, he gave the bark immediately, and then did not even wait for the previous exhibition of emetics and cathartics, whatever the state of the bowels might be. This part of Dr. Brocklesby's observations is well illustrated by those of Mr. Clark, on the Diseases in long Voyages to hot Climates, which in a striking manner point out the propriety of having immediate recourse to the bark wherever there is much debility; and particularly if the symptoms peculiar to typhus make their appearance. " If the remissions are distinct, (he observes) the bark will have a more " speedy effect; but even although the disease, (which was always at- " tended with symptoms of debility) is continued, by its use, it is effectu- " ally prevented from growing dangerous and malignant." When the patient was too weak to receive the bark in powder, he had recou⸱ ⸱ to the decoction, and when even this could not be retained alone, h⸱ ⸱⸱e along with it a large dose of solid opium; for the patient's life s⸱ ⸱ed to depend on the exhibition of the bark. In such cases he found ⸱ch benefit from giving wine along with the bark. This is not only serv⸱ ⸱ble by supporting the patient's strength, but also by rendering the ⸱ark more effectual; for in very debilitated states of the system much larger quantities of the bark are required, to prevent the return of the fever.

† The bark (says Raymond) should be given during the paroxysm, with much acid, particularly the vitriolic acid, when the patient has the facies hyprocratica, when he is subject to syncope or coma, when his pulse intermits, and his breathing is stertorous, and then, he adds, it is the best of all remedies, and often rescues the patient from the very jaws of death. See Raymond's paper on the Intermittents of Mettlin-burgh, in Baldinger's Sylloge Opusculorum.

whatever be the state of the symptoms, the bark ought not to be exhibited. Intermittents, Dr. Mead* observes, are not safely cured by the bark until the primæ viæ have been cleared, and al‑most every writer on the subject makes similar observations.

When the symptoms are not urgent, and especially when there is any degree of the inflammatory diathesis, if there is reason to suspect the presence of irritating matter in the stomach and bowels, it is proper to delay the use of the bark till after the op‑eration of an emetic and cathartic.

But in urgent cases, and where there is no inflammatory dia‑thesis, the bark ought not to be delayed an hour on account of the state of the stomach and bowels. Nay it even appears from the observations of Dr. Jackson,† Dr. Donald Munro, and others, that actual vomiting and purging should not induce us to delay the exhibition of the bark, when the state of the fever requires it. "I may remark," says the former of these authors, "that the "bark was often rejected by the stomach, and in some cases past "off almost instantly by stool, yet the course of the fever seem‑ "ed to be no less effectually checked by it than when such effects "did not occur."—"In violent cases," Dr. Donald Munro‡ ob‑serves, "where it was necessary to give the bark before emetics "and cathartics could be exhibited, I often gave it along with a ca‑ "thartic, and found that keeping up a catharsis did not prevent the "bark curing the ague." From these and similar observations it appears, that the remark of Dr. Millar‖ and others, that the exhibition of the bark can be of no service while a diarrhœa con‑tinues, is unfounded ; or at least not to be admitted in its full extent.

From the same observations also, we must infer that the com‑mon practice of giving large doses of opium, and other medi‑cines, to allay spontaneous vomiting and purging, in order to exhibit the bark early in urgent cases, is often improper; since the continuance of these will not prevent the effects of the bark, if it can be made to lie on the stomach only for a short time, and the dose be constantly repeated ; and by checking them we lay up a fruitful source of irritation, which never fails to increase the fever.

In less urgent cases, where the immediate exhibition of the bark is not necessary, if spontaneous vomiting and purging occur, the proper treatment is to promote these evacuations by diluents, till the primæ viæ are sufficiently freed from the irritating con‑tents ; and then to allay the commotion excited by opiates, be‑fore we order the bark.

* Monita et Præcepta Medica.
† See his Account of the Diseases of Jamaica.
‡ See his Account of the Diseases of the Army.
‖ See his Work on the Diseases most prevalent in Great Britain.

3. The climate and season of the year influence our practice in the use of the bark. As in sultry climates, diseases run their course rapidly, and the change from a state of increased excitement to that of debility, in' the fevers of such climates, is often very sudden ; evacuations, although they seem necessary at their commencement, often prove fatal by increasing the subsequent debility. In these climates therefore, when the symptoms are not very urgent, but a full pulse and other signs of the inflammatory diathesis present, instead of preparing the patient for ·the bark by blood-letting,[*] it is often safer to defer the febrifuge till a few paroxysms of the fever have removed this diathesis, and at most to promote this effect by cooling laxatives, and diluent clysters.[†]

In this, as in many other instances, much depends on the discernment of the practitioner, even after he is made acquainted with every circumstance which ought to influence his judgment. When the inflammatory symptoms run so high as to bring the life of the patient into immediate danger, we must in every part of the world have recourse to blood-letting. And we are also to remember that the continuance of violent excitement, even where life is not in immediate danger, is itself a highly debilitating cause, and will often debilitate more than a well timed blood-letting, which relieves it.[‡]

[*] Dr. Lind, in his account of the Remitting Fever of Bengal, relates a remarkable instance of the bad effects of blood-letting in tropical climates, even when employed with caution. A patient of his, convinced that the operation would relieve him, insisted on being bled. Dr. Lind in vain dissuaded him from it. Only five or six ounces were taken from him, the consequence of which was, that he lost his strength, and in less than an hour, during which he made his will, he was carried off by the next fit. Dr. Lind candidly adds; "a certain able physician is of " opinion that if this man had been bled during the hot fit, and not be- " tween the fits, it might perhaps have been attended with a happier " issue." Mr. Badinock and the surgeon of the Ponsborne, he observes, bled each of them two patients; each lost one.

[†] It is on account of the tendency to debility in the fevers of sultry climates, that we find authors insisting particularly on the necessity of having recourse to the bark in these fevers at an early period. I have already quoted the observations of Dr. Jackson. The early use of the bark, Dr. Brocklesby observes, is particularly necessary in the fevers of the West Indies, especially in those which appear in the rainy season. It was observed, when speaking of the causes of intermittents, that it is during the rainy season of sultry climates that the most dangerous fevers prevail.

[‡] In a treatise just alluded to, Dr. Lind on the Remitting Fever of Bengal, we find an instance of the good effects of blood-letting when judiciously employed even in this dreadful fever. " The first mate," he observes, " complained of a violent pain in his head with a full and hard " pulse. I took about four or five ounces of blood from him, and he was " not only greatly eased by it for the present, but his recovery was not " in the least checked by it, nay, the fever after it became less irregular." In such cases the utmost caution is required ; for even where the inflammatory symptoms appear considerable, the sudden sinking after blood-letting is often wonderful.

In cold climates, fevers of all kinds are more generally accompanied with inflammatory symptoms, and none more frequently
than agues ; evacuations previous to the use of the bark, therefore, are more necessary in these climates, and must often be
carried to a greater extent. It is fortunate that in such climates
they are not attended with the same danger.

℅ Even the season of the year in the same climate influences the
exhibition of the bark. In vernal agues, from the greater prevalence of inflammatory symptoms, evacuations previous to the exhibition of the bark are more necessary than in autumnal intermittents ; and they are also safer. It is in the latter season that
debilitating causes are most apt to change these fevers to the
continued form, and the early exhibition of the bark is less frequently improper, and more generally necessary.

4. In prescribing the bark we must also attend to the age and
habit of the patient. If he be young and plethoric, the pulse will
often be full ; and evacuations, previous to giving the bark, will
frequently be found necessary. When the patient is old or reduced by low diet, previous disease, or any other cause ; it is seldom necessary in agues unaccompanied by any tendency to local
inflammation, to prepare him for the bark in any other way, than
by a gentle emetic and cathartic when the stomach and bowels
happen to be loaded. In these cases the bark should be given in
considerable quantity during the first or second remission, not
only because in debilitated habits the continuance of the fever is
most to be dreaded, but also because wherever there is much debility a greater quantity of bark is required for the removal of the
fever. It is to this circumstance, together with the power of habit, that we are to attribute the obstinacy of protracted cases.

5. One circumstance to be constantly kept in view in the treatment of agues, is the nature of the prevailing epidemic. When
it is frequently attended with local inflammation, or when the inflammatory symptoms of the fever itself run high, the bark must
be used with caution ; and never where there is any appearance
of the inflammatory diathesis till after proper evacuations. When,
instead of these symptoms, the epidemic is accompanied with
much debility and a tendency to assume the form of typhus, the
bark must be given early, and in large quantity, and evacuations
of every kind cautiously advised.

Such are the principal circumstances to be attended to respecting the exhibition of the bark in agues. It will be proper,
before we leave this part of the subject, to say something of the
different forms in which this medicine has been prescribed.

It may be used in extract, tincture, infusion, or decoction ; but
it is now generally granted that the simple powder is the best
preparation of it. It never succeeds so well as when given in
substance.

Although we ought never to have recourse to the decoction, infusion, tincture, or extract, when the stomach will bear the powder; yet when it will not, we often find some of these preparations useful. The infusion is prepared by allowing the bark to remain in about six or eight times its weight of cold water for about 24 hours.

Many prefer this to the decoction, which is prepared by boiling the bark in water for a short time. The former of these, Dr. Lewis* observes, strikes a deeper colour with chalybeates than the latter. Skeete prefers the decoction, but he thinks the infusion prepared with magnesia, in the manner pointed out in his Treatise on the Red and Pale Bark, preferable to either.

The extract is prepared by boiling the bark with water for a short time, filtrating the mixture, and inspissating it by evaporation. Proof spirit extracts more of the virtues of the bark than water; rectified spirit more than either. The gummy part is extracted by the water, the resinous by the spirit; so that the best preparation of the bark, next to the simple powder, seems to be a combination of the tincture and the infusion.† After the bark has undergone the action of these two menstrua, it remains perfectly insipid to the taste, and deprived of its odour. The resinous part of the bark seems to contain the astringency. When it is boiled with water, the turbid decoction is bitter and astringent; but when the matter rendering it turbid is deposited, the astringency is no longer perceived; while the bitter taste remains unimpaired. What has been called the resina corticis Peruviani, and which is chiefly if not altogether a pure resin, is obtained by precipitation from the tincture by water. This preparation is more exceptionable than any of the others which have been mentioned.

When the patient is a child, and we cannot persuade him to take the bark by the mouth, it may be injected per anum. It may be worth while also to try this method when the powder will not remain on the stomach. This however is a much less efficacious way of giving the bark. When it is given, in clysters, some prefer the extract to the powder, supposing it to contain much of the virtues of this medicine in small bulk; there seems however to be no foundation for this preference.

The external use of the bark has also been recommended, and has sometimes proved serviceable. It is not however to be depended on. This mode of giving the bark, like the last, is only to be had recourse to when it cannot be taken by the mouth, and it is only to children, who require a smaller dose, that we can expect it to prove beneficial. The mode of applying it is sewing

* See his Materia Medica.

† Skeete recommends adding a little of the tincture to the infusion. See his Treatise on the Red and Pale Bark.

the powder into that part of the clothes, which is wrapt about the body. It is sometimes made into poultices, and applied to the stomach and wrists, or the decoction is used as a bath for children.*

·In some cases it is proper to give other medicines along with the bark. When the strength is much reduced, the powder may be given in wine, and more or less of the wine taken as the state of the patient requires it between the doses of the bark. When the stomach is very irritable, a dose of solid opium, or opium and camphire given with the bark, often enables the patient to retain it. There is nothing which is of more service in preventing the nausea and oppression which frequently attend the use of the bark, than a few drops of the vitriolic acid given along with it.†

In soldiers, sailors, and others, who have been accustomed to the use of distilled spirits, brandy is often the most convenient vehicle in which we can give this medicine. Porter was recommended by Morton and Dr. Lind in the fever of Bengal. Lime water is particularly recommended by Skeete, as increasing the virtues of the bark. It is generally proper to add a little gum arabic to any vehicle we employ, that the powder may be the more readily suspended in it.

When the stomach is habitually weak, aromatics, bitters or astringents joined with the bark are often beneficial, they are recommended by Mead, Brocklesby, and others.‡

. When the bark occasions purging, we must have recourse to opiates and astringents ; the gum kino and extract of logwood is one of the best astringents in this case. If there is reason to suspect that the purging proceeds from acidity, which is frequently occasioned by the bark deranging the digestive powers, we must then combine with it some absorbent powder. If on the other hand the bark occasions costiveness, it is necessary to give along with it a gentle laxative ; for this purpose rhubarb is particularly recommended by Dr. Mead ; it has the double advantage of moving the body and tending to restore tone to the stomach and bowels.

In prescribing the bark, we often find it necessary to join to it

* For the external use of the bark see the 2d vol. of London Medical Observations.

† Dr. Lind properly recommends all kinds of acids, saline draughts and crystals of tartar, as proper additions to the bark when the thirst is urgent, and the stomach oppressed with bile.

‡ Dr. Lysons particularly recommends the snakeroot ; he gave two parts of the bark and one of snakeroot. The dose of this mixture was only a drachm, and the author asserts that two or three doses will rarely fail to stop any distinct tertian or quartan. He also maintains that the disorder is less apt to return when cured in this way, than by the bark alone. See Dr. Lysons' Practical Essays on Continual and Remitting Fever, &c.

something capable of concealing its taste. Milk is very generally known to possess this property. The various aromatic waters may be employed for the same purpose. " Among the materi- " als I have tried," Dr. Lewis observes, " for covering the taste " of the bark, liquorice or its extract was found to answer the " purpose most effectully, whether in a liquid form, or in that of " an electuary." Liquorice and butter-milk have been particularly recommended for this purpose.

Some prefer the bark in pills. This mode of giving it is very troublesome, as the pills must always be taken soon after they are prepared; if they are allowed to become hard, which they are apt to do, from the quantity of gum necessary to make the powder cohere, they occasion nausea and oppression. When they become hard, they must be ground again to powder, and then by the addition of a little water they readily form a mass, which is as proper as at first for being made into pills.

There are two kinds of bark at present in common use, the red and the pale. The genuine red bark is more bitter and astringent to the taste than the pale, and shews a greater degree of astringency when tried with chalybeate solutions. The red bark likewise contains more resin than the pale. But the proportion of the resin differs in different parcels of it. Rubbing the pale bark with calcined magnesia, while we prepare the infusion of it, is said to increase the deepness of the colour, the astringency, bitterness, and antiseptic power of the infusion. Calcined magnesia used in the same way with the red bark, produces none of these effects on it.[*] There can be little doubt of the genuine red bark having been found more powerful in the cure of agues than the pale, as appears from the observations of Saunders[†] and Rigby[‡] on this bark, and Skeete's treatise on the red and pale bark. Dr. John Hunter[§] says, he often found the red bark more effectual than the pale in removing agues, but thought it was more apt to affect the bowels.

But whatever be the efficacy of the genuine red bark, it is very doubtful whether that now sold in the shops be at all superior to the pale. Many are of opinion that it is not, and that it owes its deeper colour to being dyed. A quantity of the genuine red bark was first brought to England in a Spanish prize, captured in 1781, and it is very doubtful if any more of it ever came to this country.

I have treated of the bark at considerable length, because in fact the cure of most intermittents is now almost entirely trusted to this medicine; and where it has met with a fair trial, it has

[*] See Dr. Skeete's Treatise.
[†] See Saunders on the Red Peruvian Bark.
[‡] See Rigby on the Red Peruvian Bark.
[§] See his Account of the Diseases of the West-Indies.

been attended with a degree of success in these fevers which sufficiently justifies the general partiality in its favour. Circumstances may occur however to prevent our employing this medicine; in some places it cannot be easily procured; in others its
high price often prevents the poorer ranks of people from using
it in sufficient quantity. It is therefore necessary to be acquainted with the articles which may with the greatest probability of
success be used in its stead. Besides, although there are few of
the articles I am about to point out upon the whole so successful
in agues as the Peruvian bark, yet it has often happened that in
cases where this bark has failed, some of these have succeeded.

I shall in the first place make some observations on the other
barks which have been found capable of removing intermittent
fever.

The Angustura bark was first imported from the West Indies
in 1788. It has been found successful though inferior to the Peruvian bark in the cure of agues. We are not acquainted with
the tree which produces it, its place of growth, &c. Respecting
these points Mr. Brand, in a treatise on it, the second edition of
which appeared in 1793, makes some conjectures. The Angustura is given in smaller doses than the Peruvian bark; about 15
or 20 grains are a moderate dose. It is less apt to disorder the
bowels than the Peruvian bark, and has succeeded in agues where
both the red and pale bark had failed. It is to be observed that
an intermittent's yielding now and then to a second remedy, after
the first has failed, is no proof of the second being upon the whole
preferable. There are many instances of simple bitters having
succeeded in the cure of agues, after the bark had failed. The
change, although to a medicine upon the whole less efficacious,
seems often beneficial. The reader will find an account of the
Angustura bark in the treatise just mentioned, and in several papers referred to in that treatise.

The cinchona Jamaicensis, discovered by Dr. William Wright,
has also been used with success in intermittents; it seems inferior however to the bark last mentioned. Dr. Wright's account
of the cinchona Jamaicensis is in the Philosophical Transactions
for the year 1772. There are also some observations on it in
Skeete's Treatise on the quilled and red Peruvian bark.

The St. Lucia bark or cinchona Caribbœa has also been found
successful in these fevers. Dr. Kentish has published some experiments made with it, and Mr. Wilson, of St. Lucia, wrote a
paper on it, which appeared in the Philosophical Transactions.
Dr. Skeete thinks it probable, that a similar bark is produced in
all the West India Islands. This is perhaps superior to the cinchona Jamaicensis.

The bark of the mahogany tree, Dr. Wright informed me, has
often been used with success in intermittents. But from the

trials he has made he considers it as much inferior to the Peruvian bark. It is so like the latter that it is often fraudulently mixed with it, or even sold for it unmixed.*

The Tellicherry bark, or as it is called in the East Indies, the corte de Pala, has also been found successful in intermittents.

The bark termed Swietenia febrifuga, an account of which the reader will find in a thesis, published at Edinburgh in 1794, by Dr. Andrew Duncan, jun. has also been recommended in agues. This bark was discovered and sent from the East Indies by Dr. Roxburgh. Dr. Duncan terms it Swietenia soymida. Soymida from the Indian name of the tree from which it is procured. It often succeeds in removing agues. But from the trials made with it, both at Edinburgh and in other places, its virtues seem to be considerably inferior to those of the Peruvian bark.

A new species of bark has lately engaged the attention of medical men, termed the yellow Peruvian, which was hardly known in this country before the year 1793. Dr. Relph, physician to Guy's Hospital, has published some observations on it. It seems, from the trials that have been made in different places, to be superior, in the cure of agues, to any of the barks which have been mentioned, the common Peruvian bark itself not excepted.

Such are the principal barks which have proved successful in intermittents. A great variety of other articles have occasionally been used.

The lignum quassiæ is particularly recommended by Linnæus and Aurivillius. It has not however come into general use; so that, contrary to the opinion of these authors, we have every reason to believe it is much inferior to the bark. The faba sancti Ignatii has also been used with success. " Two grains of it," Dr. Lind observes, " infused in two ounces of boiling water, " made a nauseous bitter, which repeated twice a day cured four " patients of quartan agues, and failed in double that number." Bitters in general indeed have been found a more or less successful substitute for the bark in intermittents. Those just mentioned, wormwood, carduus benedictus, cammomile flowers, gentian, Virginian snakeroot, the lesser centaury, and the bitter orange peel, may be considered among the chief of this class of medicines.†

A variety of astringents have also been used with success; oak bark and galls, alum, the various preparations of iron, &c. As-

* Dr. Wright shewed me a specimen of this bark, sent him by a person who had bought a large quantity of it for Peruvian bark.

† The following is Dr. Morton's celebrated ague powder.
R. Pulver. Flor. Chamæmeli scrup. unum.
   Antimonii Diaphor.
   Salis Absinthii sing. semiscrup.
This was given every 4th hour during the apyrexia.

tringents in general are inferior to bitters in these complaints.
The combinations of astringents and bitters seem to be more
powerful than either singly.

· A variety of aromatics also have been recommended; camphire,
musk, myrrh, &c. Dr. Lysons sometimes used a bolus of camphire and nitre.

There are many other articles mentioned by authors as occasionally successful in intermittents. Sal ammoniac has sometimes been used with success. It has been regarded as more
beneficial, however, when given with a view to assist the bark.
This mode of using it is particularly recommended by Dr. Brocklesby. The reader may consult a paper by Mr. Collins, in the
2d volume of the Medical Communications, for the use of the
capsicum in agues.

A variety of metallic preparations have occasionally proved
successful in these fevers. There are some observations on the
use of the flowers of zink and white vitriol, particularly of the
former, in the cure of agues; by Dr. Blane, in his work on the
diseases incident to seamen. Mercury in various forms has also
been exhibited, and has sometimes proved successful. The
reader will find instances of agues cured by mercury in the 6th
volume of the Edinburgh Medical Essays and Observations. In
one instance, related by Dr. Donald Monro in the 2d volume of
the Medical Transactions, this fever yielded to no remedy that
could be thought of, till after a course of mercury, which had no
apparent effect but that of reducing the patient's strength. It
then yielded readily to the bark. Hoffman and Willis[*] have also
recommended mercury in intermitting fevers. Its powers however in these fevers are but inconsiderable. Van Swieten[†] says,
he has seen a quartan last through the whole of a very complete
mercurial salivation; and De Meza[‡] even alledges, that mercury
sometimes increases the malignity of intermittents.

A metallic oxyd, of greater activity than any of the medicines
which have been mentioned, has lately been recommended in the
intermittents; I mean the white arsenic. The success which
attended the use of this mineral in the cure of agues, drew the
attention of empirics, who have done much harm by distributing a
medicine that often proved successful but the bad effects of which
have, in their hands at least, perhaps more than counterbalanced
its advantages. The Ague Drops owe their efficacy to arsenic,
and possess all the dangerous properties of this mineral.

The use of arsenic in agues however has not been confined to

* See Willis, Opera Omnia; published at Geneva in 1782.
† See his Comment. in Aph. Boerhaavii.
‡ See the first vol. of the Acta Societat. Med. Havniensis.
See also a paper by Schulze and Grævius on the Use of Mercury in
Quartans, in the 5th vol. of Haller's Disput. ad Morb. Hist. et Cur. Pertin.

the practice of empirics. Many regular practitioners recommend it. In their own practice they employ it freely, and they say
without any bad'consequences. It would require a very extensive experience to determine the propriety of having recourse
to arsenic, before safer means have failed. The following consideration alone must for a long time render the employment of
arsenic, at least the throwing any considerable quantity into the
system, even in small doses, a doubtful, practice. It is well
known that lead, mercury, and perhaps other metals, seem to
lurk in the body, so that their effects do not appear for some time ;
but when they do, they are proportioned, not to the quantity
taken in any one dose, but to that which has upon the whole
been received into the body. Thus it sometimes happens that
repeated doses of mercury fail to produce a salivation, which at
length occurs, if the use of the mercury be continued, with a
degree of violence that endangers life ; as if all that had been
given exerted its whole force at once. As mercury may be
given in a hundred cases without the occurrence of such an accident, it requires a very extensive experience to determine
whether or not any other medicine is subject to the same objection. Thus it also happens in the lead mines and smelting-
houses, that the small quantity of lead daily received into the
body is attended with no bad effects, till the workman after having been engaged in the business for a considerable time, is suddenly seized with a complaint known to be the effect of the lead,
which often proves fatal.

It is not to be denied, however, that agues, which have resisted
the most assidious use of the bark and other medicines, have
yielded to arsenic. I have already had occasion to observe, that
an intermittent's yielding to a second remedy after the first had
failed, is no proof that the second is upon the whole preferable.
From the observations which have been made on the use of arsenic in agues, however, we have reason to believe it the most powerful of all the medicines which have been recommended in these
complaints. In the medical reports of the use of arsenic in the
cure of remitting fevers and periodic head-aches, by Dr. Fowler,
of Stafford, we have ample proof of its success, and as far as his
experience goes, of its safety.[*]

In the 19th volume of Dr. Duncan's Medical Commentaries
there are a few additional observations on the same subject, by
the same author. From some letters subjoined to Dr. Fowler's

---

[*] The following is his mode of giving it :—64 grains of white arsenic
reduced to a very fine powder, and mixed with as much vegetable alkali,
is added to half a pound of distilled water, and gently boiled in a Florence
flask, in a sand heat, till the arsenic is completely dissolved ; half a pound
of compound spirit of lavender is then added to it, and as much more distilled water as makes the whole solution amount to a pound. The dose
of this is from two to twelve drops once, twice, or oftener in the day, according to the age, strength, &c. of the patient.

Treatise it appears, that many respectable practitioners have used arsenic in intermittents with safety.

The bad effects which small doses are apt to produce, even when given with caution, are disorders of the stomach and bowels, swellings of the face, or other parts of the body, an increased or diminished flow of urine, slight eruptions, head-ache, sweating, and tremors. These symptoms may generally be removed by gentle laxatives and emetics, or merely by discontinuing the use of the arsenic. Combining with it small doses of opium has been found in some measure to obviate these effects. Dr. Wilson of Lincolnshire, who had extensive opportunities of practice in these fevers, informed me, that he, and other practitioners in that country, had always treated them with arsenic, and had never experienced any bad effects from it, but on the contrary almost uniform success.*

* It may be proper here to remind the reader of the means to be employed when a dose of arsenic capable of endangering life has been taken. When any poisonous matter is received into the stomach, we have three things in view; first to evacuate the offending matter by vomiting; secondly, as much as possible to defend the stomach and intestines against the action of what still remains in these cavities; and lastly, to exhibit such medicines as tend to correct its noxious properties. When we find it impossible to discover the nature of the poison received into the stomach, or what comes nearly to the same thing, when we are aware of its nature but ignorant of any thing capable of correcting its noxious properties, the first of these means is indicated. We must instantly have recourse to an emetic, and there is none which answers better, because there is none which operates more quickly, than white vitriol; a scruple of which is a proper dose.

We must at the same time, as far as the operation of the emetic permits, have recourse to the second set of means; which are the more necessary, if from the time which the poison has been taken there is reason to fear that part of it has passed the pyloris. The only means we have of defending the stomach and bowels against the irritation of their contents, is making the patient drink and throwing in by clyster large quantities of oily and mucilaginous fluids. Dr. M'Bride, in his introduction to the Practice of Medicine, observes, that a large quantity of new milk or fresh melted butter has been known to save the patient's life, even where arsenic had been taken; and Eller, in his Observationes de Cognoscendis et Curandis Morbis, relates the case of a man saved by oily fluids, who had taken two drams of the red precipitate of mercury.

With respect to the third set of means, we are not possessed of any medicine capable of correcting the noxious properties of the oxyd of arsenic, the state in which this metal is generally taken. Arsenic itself, like other metals, when neither oxydified nor combined with an acid, is said to be innocent.

The calces of arsenic, in which this metal is combined with a large proportion of sulphur, as in the red and yellow arsenics, the native orpiments as they are termed, seem to be innocent. Sulphur equally deprives the oxyds of arsenic, antimony, and mercury, of their active properties. On this account the calcarious or alkaline hepar sulphuris is recommended in cases where arsenic has been taken, and this along with other means should not be neglected. It is very doubtful however whether the hepar sulphuris and oxyd of arsenic will sufficiently combine in the stomach and intestines to be of much service.

Other medicines have been employed, chiefly by the vulgar, and have occasionally succeeded in removing agues; such as bay leaves dried and powdered, in the quantity of a dram, three times a day; half a dram of the inner bark of the ash, half an ounce of sulphur in a glass of strong beer, &c. To these may be added such as seem to operate chiefly, if not wholly, by the effect which they have on the mind, such as camphire and saffron hung in a bag at the pit of the stomach, cobwebs mixed with crumbs of bread taken in pills, &c. It is a practice among the vulgar in some places for the cure of agues to take half a pint of their own urine three mornings successively, which is said to be a very effectual remedy. Any thing capable of making a strong impression on the mind, whether by exciting horror, superstitious dread, or confidence, occasionally proves successful. I shall have occasion to mention some other medicines of this kind among that class of remedies which still remains to be considered, namely, those which are only successful when given at the time the paroxysm is expected. The means to be employed at this period form the last division of those employed during the apyrexia.

When the fit is expected, the patient should avoid exposure to cold, should be put to bed and kept warm. Some have recommended the use of the warm bath. He should avoid taking much food or drink; and if there is no tendency to the inflammatory diathesis, what he takes should be stimulating. Diaphoretics are frequently serviceable, given a little before the fit is expected; for if we succeed in keeping up a sweat, the accession of the paroxysm is often prevented. " Intermittentes tertianas ", autumnales," Sydenham observes, " hoc pacto aggredior Ægro " in lectulo composito et stragulis undique cooperto sudores pro-" voco, sero lactis cerevisiato, cui salviæ folia incocta fuere, qua-" tuor circiter horis ante paroxysmi adventum."

In cases where metallic salts, that is, metals combined with acids, have been taken, corrosive sublimate or sugar of lead for example; drinking immediately a large quantity of a weak alkaline solution is the best means of preventing bad consequences. In this case the metallic salt is decomposed by the alkali as soon as it is received into the stomach, the alkali combining with the acid, and leaving the metal in a less active or wholly inert state. It has been proposed, instead of using the oxyd of arsenic in intermittents, to employ an arsenical salt, which would be more easily dissolved in water, and such a salt has been prepared by Mr. Milner, Professor of Chymistry at Cambridge, and has been used it is said with success in intermittents. The bad effects of an over dose of this as of other metallic salts would probably be obviated by the above alkaline solution. This solution is prepared by dissolving an ounce of vegetable alkali in a gallon of water, of which the patient is to drink as much as he is able. It is said, that the acid of arsenic is as innocent as the metal itself, so that it is only when combined with a small proportion of oxygen or with an acid that it is poisonous. A Treatise was published abroad a few years ago, containing observations on the effects of arsenic combined with different proportions of oxygen. The fact just mentioned (I have been informed) is ascertained by these observations, which I have not been able to meet with.

It is the general opinion, that the stomach and bowels if loaded should be cleared at this period, by the operation of an emetic and cathartic. Few medicines more powerfully promote perspiration than emetics, and to this their effects in preventing the paroxysm of agues must in part be ascribed. Emetics however seem here to operate also in another way. Any thing capable of making a strong impression on the nervous system, is occasionally found to prevent the recurrence of the paroxysm." There are few things which more powerfully affect every part of the system than the operation of an emetic.

The employment of cathartics at this period is a more doubtful practice, and seems to have been rather the result of hypothesis than observation. Should the acrid contents of the bowels produce spontaneous diarrhœa, it may be proper to encourage it by warm diluting liquors. Checking the purging would lay up a fruitful source of irritation to aggravate the symptoms of the ensuing paroxysm ; but if purging do not spontaneously occur, it ought not to be induced at this period, that is, a little before the paroxysm is expected.

The means which prove successful in preventing the paroxysm of agues in the way I am speaking of, produce one of three effects : They make a sudden and strong impression on the nervous system, or they quicken the circulation, or they induce sweat. Some medicines are capable of producing more than one of these effects, and some all three ; any one of them however is often capable of preventing the paroxysm of an ague.

Purging produces none of these effects, but rather their opposites. It makes no powerful impression on the nervous system ; it retards the circulation, by enfeebling the powers which support it ; and so far from promoting sweat, it even checks it when it has been induced by other means. From every thing we know of the nature of agues, purging seems to be one of the most powerful means that could be thought of for inducing the paroxysm. Sydenham indeed recommended purging along with sweating at this period ; but insists particularly on this, that the sweating be not checked by the stools ; and adds, that the cathartic ought to be omitted when the patient is reduced by the continuance of the disease or any other cause.

The reasons which Sydenham gives for employing cathartics in any case at this period, are such as sufficiently point out the hypothetical foundation on which the practice rests. When the two opposite motions of sweating and purging, he observes, are excited at the same time, they confound and disturb the ordinary course of the paroxysm. Notwithstanding his opinion, we can perceive from what Sydenham says, that his extensive experience sufficiently pointed out the error of this practice. He often found it necessary, he informs us, to give a dose of opium after the operation of the cathartic ; and before the accession of the paroxysm ; thus doing what he could to remove for the time the debilitating effects of the cathartic, and dispose to sweat.

For similar reasons he properly recommends opium after the operation of the emetic, if this be over before the fit commences. Opium not only makes a strong impression on the nervous system, but also gives a temporary vigour to the powers supporting circulation ; and is upon the whole the most powerful diaphoretic of which we are possessed ; so that there are few medicines better calculated to prevent the accession of the paroxysm. It may be used with advantage at this period, perhaps, (as we have seen it in the hot fit) combined with nauseating doses of emetics. It is doubtful, however, whether the debilitating effects of nausea are proper when the fit is expected.

In whatever manner we use opium with a view to prevent the fit, the patient under its operation should be put to bed, kept warm, and supplied with tepid diluting liquors. When we have endeavoured in vain during the first paroxysms of the complaint to prevent their accession, by inducing vomiting or sweat, we are not to persevere in the use of these means ; since if they do not soon remove the disease by their debilitating effects, they render it more obstinate. Dr. Cullen remarks, that endeavouring to prevent the paroxysm by keeping out a sweat, has often changed the fever to the continued form, which he justly observes is always dangerous.

Many medicines however have been employed with the same view, which instead of weakening tend to restore the tone of the system. The chief of these is a medicine which I have already had occasion to speak of at considerable length. It has been found that a large quantity of the bark received into the stomach immediately before the paroxysm is expected, frequently prevents its return. Dr. Millar and others have observed, that an ounce of the bark taken at a single dose when the fit is expected not only often prevents the paroxysm, but sometimes wholly removes the complaint. This however is far from being the best mode of giving the bark. Few stomachs can bear so large a dose of it, and it seems to answer better when given at intervals for some time before the accession of the paroxysm. In this way not only a greater quantity may be accumulated in the stomach and intestines at the time of accession; but by giving it at intervals its effects appear to be accumulated in the system, for those of each dose continue for a considerable time after it is taken ; some suppose, and not without reason, while any part of the medicine remains in the alimentary canal.

A vast variety of articles have been employed at this period, chiefly by the vulgar, and have occasionally succeeded in preventing ague fits. These are, either such as make a strong impression on the stomach, as spirit of turpentine, wine, warm strong beer, brandy, &c. with a variety of peppers and other acrid sub-

stances; or such as strongly impress the mind, swallowing a living spider, a powder prepared from human bones, and a thousand other things of this kind.

By regular practitioners the powder of cammomile flowers,
wormwood, or other strong bitters, have been used in the same
way. The foetid gums have also occasionally been found serviceable; and some recommend a variety of external irritating applications, salt mixed with the white of eggs applied to the
wrists, &c.

SUCH are the means of cure to be employed at the various
periods of intermitting fever, between the accession of one
paroxysm and that of the next; between which and the third paroxysm the same mode of practice, varied as the symptoms vary,
is to be repeated; and so on through every interval till the fever
is removed.

If the bark be immediately discontinued on the removal of
agues, they are apt to return; especially if they have lasted for a
considerable time, and the patient has been much reduced. It
is therefore proper in general to continue the bark for some time
longer, gradually diminishing the dose, and giving it at the periods at which the fever, had it lasted, would have recurred.

It is also proper for those who have lately laboured under
agues, not only to avoid exposure to marsh miasma, but all those
circumstances above enumerated as favourable to the operation
of marsh miasma in producing agues. Exposure to cold, irregu-
larities in diet, or any other cause which debilitates, is capable of
renewing these fevers. When exposure to such causes is unavoidable, as in the rainy seasons of sultry climates, the bark ought
to be used as a preventive.* In all cases the rules respecting
diet and exercise in the apyrexia must be attended to for some
time after the removal of agues, both in order to prevent their return, and to restore the patient's strength.

*Of the Modus Operandi of the Medicines employed during the
Apyrexia of Intermittents.*

ON this part of the subject I have only to remind the reader of
a few observations which have already been made.

I have just had occasion to point out the way in which the medicines given at the time the fit is expected, seem to act in preventing its accession. The effects of many of these can only be
ascribed to the impression made on the nervous system, since
they are are too sudden to be attributed to any change induced on
the fluids. It is only in this way that we can account for the

* See the 47th and following pages of Dr. Lind's Essay on the Means
of preserving the Health of Seamen.

effects of the bark, when the paroxysm is prevented by this medicine given only half an hour before the time at which it should have appeared. And when we reflect on the observation of Dr. Jackson, Dr. Monro and others, that if we persevere in giving the bark, the fever will be removed, although the medicine is constantly discharged by vomiting and stool, we have every reason to believe, that in whatever way the bark is exhibited, its effects in the cure of agues are to be attributed to its action on the nerves of the stomach and intestines.

The hypothesis of the bark removing agues by its antiseptic power, were it not maintained by some late respectable authors, and very generally blended with medical writings, would not deserve to be mentioned. Is there any species of ague, in which the fluids have been proved to be in a state of putrescency? Are there not many, in which such a state of the fluids has not even been suspected? Or, if it did exist, have we not every reason to regard it as the consequence, and not the cause, of the fever? But admitting both these points, admitting, in the face of the most direct evidence, that in agues the fluids are in a state of putrescency, and that this state of the fluids is the cause of the fever; will it be seriously asserted, that a quantity of bark is ever received into the mass of circulating fluids, sufficient by its antiseptic power to correct their putrescency?

BOOK II.

OF CONTINUED FEVER.

CONTINUED Fever is defined in the Introduction, an Idiopathic Fever with slight remissions and exacerbations.

For the sake of perspicuity, this fever was divided into two species, the Synocha, and Typhus.

The Synocha was defined, that species of fever in which the temperature of the body is greatly raised, the pulse frequent, strong, and hard, the urine high coloured, and the sensorial functions but little disturbed.

Typhus, it was observed, is characterised by being a contagious disease, by the temperature being little raised, the pulse small, weak, and generally frequent, the urine little changed, the sensorial functions much disturbed, and the strength greatly reduced.

It was observed, however, that although this division is useful in practice, and still more in acquiring a knowledge of continued fever, yet it cannot be regarded as accurate, since we scarcely ever meet with simple Synocha or Typhus; almost every continued fever assuming the form of the Synochus, that is, being a combination of the Synocha and Typhus, beginning with the symptoms of the former, and terminating in those of the latter. In the proportional degree in which either set of symptoms prevails, there is infinite variety; and it is convenient to apply the terms Synocha, or Typhus, according as the symptoms of the one or the other predominate.

CHAP. I.

Of the Symptoms of Continued Fever.

THE symptoms of continued fever are less regular and more protracted than those of agues. The cold stage is more frequently absent in continued, than intermitting fever, and generally consists of irregular chills, frequently interrupted and renewed, or of short fits of cold and heat, which succeed each other alternately for the first day or two, and often continue to do so, after the temperature of the body, measured by the thermometer or the feeling of another person, is uniformly raised.

The cold and shaking are never so severe as in agues, but the attending symptoms, langour, weariness, soreness of the flesh and bones, head-ach, &c. are upon the whole more so. The pulse during the chills in typhus, as in the cold stage of agues, is small and frequent ;* but in synocha, even during the chills, it is often strong, regular, and full.

These symptoms are at length succeeded by more permanent heat, often partial at first, soon becoming general. But the change from the cold to the hot stage is both more gradual and less striking, than in intermitting fever. The strength and fullness of the pulse increase as the chills abate ; but this change is seldom so considerable as at the same period in agues ; for the pulse from the first is generally pretty full and strong, if the fever be synocha ; and if it be well-marked typhus, it seldom acquires a great degree of strength, even after the heat is generally diffused. In this respect, however, there is much variety. It has already been observed, that all fevers, at their commencement, assume more or less of the form of synocha ; and it generally happens, in contagious fevers, that although the debility is considerable while the chills continue, yet after these, the pulse acquires a considerable degree of strength, which it often retains during the first days of the complaint.

As the hot stage advances, the various functions are affected in the same way as in agues ; but the heat, except in well-marked synocha, is generally less in continued, than in intermitting, fever. It is not, as in the latter, relieved in few hours by sweat, but continues along with the other symptoms of the hot stage, suffering more or less evident remissions, once or twice in the day, often for weeks, or even months ; and at length frequently leaves the patient gradually, without a remarkable increase of any of the excretions.† In other cases, the symptoms of continued fever

---

* The pulse is generally less frequent at the commencement of continued, than that of intermitting fever.

" The pulse during the first 24 hours beats seldom less than ninety " times in a minute, and very seldom more than one hundred and five in " a minute ; whereas in an ephemera, or in the first paroxysm of an in- " termittent, it very often rises to one hundred and twenty or thirty pul- " sations." See Dr. Fordyce's third Dissertation on Fever. Part I.

† During the exacerbations the heat generally rises one or two degrees above the mean heat of the fever in the trunk, and more in the extremities. See Dr. Currie's Med. Reports on the effects of water, cold and warm, &c. In the cold stage of continued fever, Dr. Currie observed the heat under the tongue as low as 92° of Farenheit, and he mentions 105° as the highest degree of febrile heat generally observed ; but he takes notice of one case of continued fever, in which it was as high as 108°. While the cold stage is changing to the hot, he remarks, some parts of the body are above, while at the same time others are below, the healthy degree ; nor is the heat diffused with any regularity, but is sometimes greater in one place, sometimes in another, and this irregularity continues till by degrees the heat becomes general and steady. Dr. Currie seems to be wrong however in supposing that the irregularity in the real temperature is the sole cause of the irregular sensations of heat and cold of which the patient at this period complains, which often continue after the heat,

are more suddenly relieved in various ways, afterwards to be pointed out.

During the first days of the complaint the symptoms generally return with increased violence after the slight remissions which take place ; if they do so for many days the danger is great. When they return with less violence after each remission, the fever is said to have taken a turn, and the prognosis is favourable.

It frequently happens, however, that the symptoms continue to return with nearly the same degree of violence for many days, or even for weeks ; and then, if they are not alarming, and the patient bears them without a remarkable diminution of strength, although the disease will prove lingering, the event will probably be favourable.

Such are the general course of continued fever, and the principal circumstances in which it differs from agues., It is necessary to consider its symptoms at greater length ; and it will be the most distinct plan, to give separately those of the two species, into which it has been divided, namely, the Synocha, that species in which the excitement is above, and the Typhus, in which it is below the healthy degree.

SECT. I.

Of the Symptoms of Synocha.

THE symptoms of synocha are as simple, as those of typhus are complicated. The prostration of strength, which precedes the attack of fevers, is generally less considerable ; and the cold stage is more frequently absent in synocha, than in typhus.

The pulse, even in the cold stage of synocha, is seldom small or very frequent ; after the heat commences, it becomes full, rapid, equal, or as it has been termed, vibrating ; still however its frequency is less than in those fevers in which debility prevails.

The respiration is frequent, hurried, generally oppressed, and attended with a dry cough.

The heat is greater than in other continued fevers, and of that kind which has been termed burning, in contradistinction to acrid.*. The face is full and florid, the eyes inflamed and incapable of bearing the light.

The secreting powers are more completely suspended than in most cases of typhus. The skin, mouth, and throat are dry, and the mucus covering the tongue becomes foul and viscid. The urine is scanty and high coloured, and the bowels costive.

measured by the thermometer, remains in the extremities as well as in the trunk uniformly above the healthy degree.

* See the observations on the heat in typhus, in sect. ii. of this chapter.

The head-ach is generally considerable, accompanied with throbbing of the temples or tinnitus aurium. The depravation of the senses however is less frequent in synocha than in typhus, nor is delirium a common symptom of this fever; but when it does occur in synocha, it rises to a degree which from the debilitated state of the system we hardly ever meet with in typhus. The patient becomes frantic, and is with difficulty retained in bed.

When the delirium is obstinate in synocha, we have reason to suspect an inflammatory affection of the brain; which there is still more reason to dread, if the patient is oppressed with coma. In enumerating the symptoms of phrenitis, I shall have occasion to point out the circumstances which form the very imperfect diagnosis we are possessed of between this complaint and synocha.

When synocha proves fatal within a few days of its commencement, (which, if it ever happen, is a rare occurrence) the pulse, it is said, does not become weak or intermitting before death; the patient seems to be carried off by the violence of the excitement.

When the disease continues for a longer time however, and the remissions are at all evident, the pulse during these (although the fever has not yet assumed the form of typhus) becomes weak and languid, the patient appearing to be exhausted by the foregoing paroxysm; which is renewed however in a short time, with all its former violence, or even stronger marks of excitement.

The hemorrhagies, which frequently occur in this fever, are generally from the nose, ears, lungs, rectum (if the patient happen to labour under the hemorrhoids) or from the uterus; and are almost always favourable; the blood discharged has the healthy appearance, except that the coagulum is frequently covered with the buffy coat.* Hemorrhagies from the higher parts of the intestines, kidneys, urethra, skin, eyes, &c. are rarely, the two last perhaps never, observed in synocha.

Such are the symptoms of well marked synocha. They vary in different cases from those just enumerated, to the mild febrile symptoms attending a common catarrh.

After the symptoms of synocha have continued for some time, if they do not terminate the patient's life, they always, at least in this country, begin to be changed to those of typhus; so that the whole disease is a synochus. The proportional duration, as well as violence, of the synocha and typhus in this, which has been termed the mixed fever, is different in different cases; and proves an endless source of variety. The manner in which the

* I shall afterwards have occasion to explain the nature of this appearance.

symptoms of synocha are changed into those of debility, also varies much. The duration of fevers in general is shorter, their symptoms more violent, and their changes more rapid, in the warm, than in the cold, and temperate climates. The symptoms which follow the state of increased excitement, are the most dangerous, as well as most varied part of the fever. These I am now to lay before the reader; where they predominate, the complaint is termed typhus.

SECT. II.

Of the Symptoms of Typhus.

AN uneasy and peculiar sensation in the stomach, sometimes attended with nausea and giddiness, frequently denotes the approach of those fevers, in which the symptoms of debility prevail.* In many cases, however, this sensation is scarcely, or not at all perceived; and the fever comes on with lassitude, anxiety about the præcordia, alternate heats and chills, or a sense of creeping in different parts of the body, which has been termed horripilatio.

The patient complains of uneasiness of the head, and fixes his attention with more difficulty than usual; is dejected and wishes to be alone. His appetite is impaired, he becomes restless, or if he remains long in the same posture, it is rather a sensation of languor, than of ease, which prevents him from changing it. He is disinclined to every exertion both of body and mind.

Either sleep forsakes him, or he is more inclined to sleep than usual, and then his sleep is such as does not refresh, disturbed by groans and starts.

At this period the pulse for the most part is frequent, small, and easily compressed; in other cases it is nearly natural, and the patient often labours for some days under more or fewer of these symptoms, not well enough to engage in business, nor sufficiently indisposed to be confined to bed.

The first symptoms of typhus are often more severe. The patient is attacked with a troublesome head-ach, acute pains in the back, loins, and extremities, which often resemble a general rheumatic affection, a distressing sense of weariness, much thirst, and nausea; sometimes attended with a burning pain of the stomach; more frequently by vomiting, vertigo, dimness of sight, or numbness of the extremities.

In some instances, this fever attacks with still more violence. The rigors from the first are strong, the pulse soft, small, fre-

---

* This peculiar sensation is taken notice of by a variety of authors, Dr. Jackson in his Account of the Fevers of Jamaica, Dr. Smith in his Account of the Jail Fever of Winchester, &c.

quent, and sometimes irregular. The general uneasiness, confusion of head, and dejection of spirits excessive. At the very
commencement the debility is often extreme, the tongue trembles
impeding the speech, the limbs shake, and the patient with difficulty supports himself. There are even instances of people, on
the first attack of typhus, falling suddenly to the ground, as if
thunderstruck.*

There are few complaints in which the symptoms are more
varied, than in typhus, whether we regard its accession or its
progress.

Of the State of the Animal Functions in the Progress of Typhus.

As the complaint advances, the debility of the muscles of voluntary motion increases.

In the advanced stage, the patient, incapable of any exertion,
lies on the back, and if turned on either side, soon resumes this
posture, he even slides insensibly towards the foot of the bed, and
has not power, although he understands what is said to him, to
put out his tongue, which is affected with a tremulous motion.
In other cases, but rarely in the fevers of this country, the patient, tormented with extreme anxiety, is constantly changing his
posture, and in some fevers, particularly in the plague, this symptom is often so violent, that it occasions a perpetual writhing of
the body, so that the patient seems to be in agony, but is generally
quite incapable of giving any account of his feelings.† When he
is less restless, the limbs, as death approaches, are sometimes
affected with numbness or palsy, more frequently they are moved
by a constant twitching of the muscles, often the forerunner of
general convulsions, in which he expires; sometimes in the first
attack, more generally after several returns of them. In some
cases, the muscles of the limbs are affected with more permanent
spasms, and cases are on record, in which complete tetanus has
supervened towards the fatal termination of malignant fevers.‡

The head-ach is sometimes confined to the under part of the
orbits, sometimes to the orbit of one eye, attended with strong
throbbing of the temples ; the carotid and temporal arteries often
beating strongly, while the pulse at the wrist is small and weak.||

---

* This sometimes happened in the late dreadful fever of Grenada, described by Dr. Chisholm.

† This symptom, which is a very fatal one, has been termed a mortal
inquietude.

‡ See Vogel, De Cog. et Cur. Morh.

|| When this symptom is obstinate, and accompanied with an acute or
deep seated pain of the head, or with a considerable degree of coma or
delirium, it generally denotes an inflammatory affection of the brain or its
membranes. In these cases, abscesses are often found in the encephalon
after death. Cases of this kind are related by Sir John Pringle and others.
Dr. Fordyce has justly observed however, that abscesses of the brain very

The uneasiness and confusion of head increase with the debility, and often on the second or third night a degree of delirium comes on, which goes off, however, on the succeeding day, and continues to return in the evening for several days. As the symptoms increase, a wandering of the mind remains throughout the day, and often increases at night to a degree of phrenzy, resembling the delirium of synocha. More frequently, however, the exacerbation of the delirium at night is less remarkable, and the patient is rather stupid than violent. At a more advanced period he continues uniformly sullen and sad, muttering to himself as if brooding over some heavy misfortune. The countenance is dejected, and the eyes heavy and inflamed. When the evening exacerbations are remarkable, the countenance appears more lively, the dull appearance of the eyes especially is less observable, and the patient is then easily irritated, speaks quick and answers hastily.

rarely occur in the fevers of this country. The same throbbing, also frequently indicating an inflammatory affection, is sometimes observed in other parts of the body, particularly in the fevers of warm climates. " In " the yellow fever," Dr. Linning observes, " there is a remarkable throb-" bing in the temporal arteries and hypochondria; in the latter sometimes " so great as to cause a constant tremulous motion of the abdomen."

* The ideas presented to us by the memory and imagination succeed each other with such rapidity, that unless we employ some means for the purpose of detaining them, we are unable to compare them together, and consequently to draw any inference from them. The means commonly employed to detain our ideas for a sufficient length of time are words. We have associated every idea with some particular sound, and by recollecting the associated sound we can detain the idea for any length of time. When we wish to compare two ideas in order to draw an inference from them, by recollecting the sounds with which they are associated we detain them till the comparison is made. Let any one endeavour to pursue a train of reasoning without recollecting the words associated with the ideas passing through the mind and he will find it impossible. In those cases, where the number of ideas to be compared is great, and the reasoning consequently complicated, we have found it necessary to invent means still more effectual of detaining our ideas, by applying to some of the external organs of sense an object which shall constantly excite the ideas which we wish to detain. Thus in mathematical demonstrations the ideas of curves, lines, angles, and of their relative positions, are detained in the mind by keeping the eye fixed on a diagram, or if the person be blind, the same purpose is answered by means of the sense of touch and a diagram made of wood. And it seems to form the chief difference between the intellectual powers of a man and brute animals, that the latter are neither possessed of language nor any other means of detaining their ideas; in consequence of which they are incapable of comparing them, and consequently of reasoning, to any extent. This is generally the state of our own minds in dreaming; we do not then employ words to arrest our ideas, and they pass through the mind with a rapidity which prevents us from comparing them. The rapidity with which ideas often pass through the mind in sleep appears at first view incredible. Dr. Gregory used in his Physiological Lectures to relate the case of a lady, who was subject to dreams while engaged in the common occupations of life; their duration was so short, that they often passed unobserved by those who conversed with her, yet it required many hours to give an account of the crowd of ideas which in so short a time had passed through her mind. " The rapidity of the succession of trans-

In other cases a considerable degree of coma comes on;[*] if this state increases, the jaw at length falls, and complete apoplexy supervenes. It goes off, however, ...

The different organs of sense are variously affected in the progress of typhus. Deafness is generally, not always, a favourable symptom.[†] A depravation of the sight, on the other hand,

"actions in our dreams," Dr. Darwin observes, Zoonomia, vol. i, p. 205, "is almost inconceivable; insomuch that when we are accidentally "awakened by the jarring of a door, which is opened into our bedcham- "ber, we sometimes dream a whole history of thieves or fire in the very "instant of waking." Our, seldom using the ordinary means to detain our ideas in sleep may account for many of the phenomena peculiar to dreaming. The most incongruous appearances do not seem to us at all wonderful; because it is only in consequence of comparing the present idea with former ideas that it can seem so. Were we deprived of all those ideas with which experience has furnished our minds, nothing would seem wonderful. A miracle only surprises because it contradicts the common course of nature; but were we ignorant of the common course of nature, we could not perceive the contradiction. It is the same thing, whether we have no fund of ideas laid up in the mind or are prevented from making use of them.

To the same cause we may attribute many of the phenomena of delirium. But there seems to be the following difference between dreaming and delirium: If in dreaming any cause occur to detain our ideas, we compare them and reason from them with as much accuracy as when awake. Thus I have frequently observed, that when I dreamt I was engaged in conversation, in which case of course I employed words, the train of thought was as consistent with experience as in my waking hours. I mentioned this circumstance to a gentleman, who told me, he also had observed that when he dreamt that he was speaking, his ideas were never inconsistent. In delirium, on the contrary, although the ideas are detained in the mind for a sufficient length of time, we are incapable of comparing them together so as to draw the proper inference. Delirium also differs from dreaming in the ideas themselves being generally confused and indistinct.

The foregoing observations respecting language strictly apply only to the first use of it, for by habit words come to be used without suggesting the ideas with which they were at first associated, in the same manner that figures are used in arithmetic without any reference in the mind to the numbers which they represent. The relations which the words bear to each other at length supersede those which they originally bore to the ideas with which they were associated. We certainly say that two and two make four, without the ideas originally associated with two and four being suggested to the mind. It is evident that in whatever way we use words, either for the purpose of suggesting and retaining the original ideas, or of suggesting and retaining the relations which the words bear to each other, the foregoing observations respecting dreaming are equally applicable.

[*] In this state the patient often receives into his mouth any thing presented to him, but seems as if he had forgot to swallow it, so that it remains in the mouth or runs out on the bed clothes.

"If the medicine or drink be presented a second time while the first "quantity still remains in the mouth, the patient often swallows this to re- "ceive what is offered, when no other means can induce him to do so." See Moore's Medical Sketches.

[†] Dr. Rush and others mention fevers in which deafness was found to be a very unfavourable symptom.

is among the worst symptoms of the complaint. The patient, as the fatal termination approaches, frequently starts up, catching at things which he sees passing before him, or picks the bed clothes, which appear to him striped or covered with black spots; sometimes every thing appears indistinct as if seen through a mist. The eyes indeed are variously affected throughout the disease; and some assert, that from their appearance alone they can determine the state of the patient. In the commencement of typhus they are dull and languid; the tunica albuginea having a bluer, and sometimes whiter, appearance than ordinary. In the furious delirium they are red, quick, and piercing; in the comatose, they are generally inflamed also, but heavy, half shut, and as if glazed. The last of these appearances indicates much danger; but the prognosis is still worse, if blood be extravasated in them. For some time before death they appear hollow, involuntary tears sometimes flow from them, and they become fixed and glossy. The sensibility of the skin seems often much impaired; and the taste and smell are sometimes almost wholly lost. The former is often otherwise vitiated, the patient complaining of a nauseous bitter taste, which mixes itself with every thing he takes.

Of the State of the Vital Functions in the Progress of Typhus.

THE pulse continues soft, weak, small, generally very frequent,* and if the symptoms increase, often becomes intermitting

* In tedious nervous fevers, in which the symptoms are moderate, the pulse is often as slow as natural, for some hours during the day; and in the more malignant forms of typhus, it has sometimes been observed a great deal slower. I mean even in those of this country. In the fevers of some tropical climates, this is much more frequently the case. This state of the pulse in malignant fevers is taken notice of by a variety of authors, particularly by those who give an account of the fevers of the West Indies. Dr. Fordyce in one of his Dissertations on Fever observes, that the pulse is sometimes as low as 50 or even 45. In the late dreadful fever of Philadelphia, Dr. Rush found the pulse at 44, and in one instance as low as 30. The pulse at a certain period of the yellow fever becomes as slow or slower than natural, and continues so till within a short time of the patient's death; for recovery is rare after this change of the pulse takes place. When the pulse becomes slow, the heat at the same time sinks to the natural standard, and sometimes below it. This and the other peculiarities of the fevers of sultry latitudes depend on some local affection. The slow pulse indicates an affection of the brain, which is farther indicated in many cases of the yellow fever by a dilatation of the pupil and squinting. Dr. Chisholm particularly takes notice of the slow pulse and dilatation of the pupil in the fever of Grenada, and found water in the ventricles of the brain in those whom he examined after death. The yellow fever is so called from the skin being tinged with yellow; when the yellowness is late in appearing, it sometimes comes on so suddenly that the patient almost instantly becomes of a yellow, deep orange, or copper colour. This circumstance, together with the urine and discharge from blistered parts not always appearing yellow when the skin is so, demonstrate, contrary to what was once supposed, that the yellow

or otherwise irregular. As death approaches, its weakness and irregularity become more remarkable, till at length the extremities grow cold and the pulse cannot be felt. This sometimes happens ten or twelve hours before death. There is a tendency to syncope on the slightest exertion, particularly in the erect posture; and for some time before death the debilitated state of the circulation occasions a shrinking of the features, and conspires with the relaxation of the muscles of voluntary motion to give that peculiar expression of countenance termed *Facies Hippocratica*, a presage that cannot be misinterpreted by the most inexperienced. The countenance assumes a livid, cadaverous appearance, the nose is sharpened, and the cheeks become hollow. The face however, during the progress of typhus, is sometimes flushed, and more frequently bloated.

The state of the breathing corresponds to that of the circulation; it is weak, generally frequent and interrupted with sighing or a dry cough; but as the debility increases, it often becomes calm and less frequent than natural, sometimes rattling.

The voice is low, weak, often shriller or hoarser than natural, and sometimes wheezing. Its being much affected in any of these ways affords an unfavourable prognosis. It is always a favourable sign when it again becomes natural.

The heat of the body at the commencement of typhus is seldom much increased, and has been observed even in the progress of the complaint to be little more than natural.* But in general, after the first days, especially when the worst symptoms shew themselves, a person touching a patient in typhus perceives a heat of a penetrating kind, which remains in the hand for some time after it is removed from the patient.†

colour in this fever is not owing to the presence of bile in the circulating fluids.

It sometimes happens towards the fatal termination of malignant fevers, that the pulse at the wrist, before it is wholly lost, beats for some time with less frequency than the heart.

* This is often the case in what has been termed the nervous fever, the Typhus Mitior. "Calor non raro naturalem vix superans," Frank observes, in describing this fever. It is not uncommon in malignant fevers, particularly those of warm climates, for the extremities to be considerably below the natural temperature, while there is a burning heat in the breast and other parts of the trunk.

† This peculiarity of the heat in typhus has been remarked by a variety of authors. "In the beginning," Sir John Pringle observes, "the heat is " moderate, and even in the advanced state, on first touching the patient, " seems inconsiderable; but upon feeling the pulse for some time, I have " been sensible of an uncommon ardour, leaving an unpleasant sensation " in my fingers for a few minutes after. The first time I observed this," he continues, "I referred it to the force of imagination; but I was assured " of the reality by repeated experiments, and by the testimony of others, " who, without knowing my observations, had made the same remark." " On pressing the skin of the patient," says Dr. Moore, " a sensation of

Of the State of the Natural Functions in the Progress of Typhus.

THE tongue at the beginning of the fever is covered with a thin white mucus; as the disease advances, this mucus becomes thicker and of a brownish colour, and the clammyness of the mouth and brown colour of the tongue generally increase with the fever. In the advanced stage deep chops often form in the tongue, the mucus covering it becomes fetid, dry, and firm, and a corresponding change taking place in that which besmears the teeth and other parts of the mouth, and probably also in the mucus of the trachea and bronchiæ, the breath becomes offensive, and the deficiency of moisture renders the speech inarticulate.

Sometimes however the tongue continues moist to the end of the disease and then, particularly in the middle, it often assumes a yellowish or greenish appearance In other cases it is dry and smooth, of a shining dark red, which at last becomes brown or almost black, while at the same time a black furring covers the lips and teeth. The last appearance of the tongue sometimes supervenes in the progress of fever, although at an earlier period it has been covered with mucus.

There is often a difficulty of swallowing from the dryness, sometimes from a paralytic affection, now and then from convulsive* contractions of the throat; the fauces are often covered, particularly towards the end 'of the disease, with aphthæ, that is, specks of a white, brown, or blackish colour, often becoming ulcerous: and when they occur in the worst kinds of fever, very commonly the forerunner of mortification.† We shall have occasion to consider this eruption more particularly when I come to speak of it as characterising a species of synochus.

" a peculiar penetrating heat remains on the hand for some minutes after;
" whereas the heat communicated by the skin of a patient in the inflammatory fever, is more transient."
Dr. Huxham, in his work on the ulcerous Sore-Throat, has also taken notice of this peculiarity of the heat in typhus. " There is a peculiar biting
" heat," he observes, " in persons labouring under malignant fevers. 'On
" first touching the skin the heat seems very little if at all above natural;
" but by continuing the finger a longer time on it, you are sensible of a
" disagreeable scalding in it, which sensation remains in the finger for a
" short time after you have quite removed it from the sick person. This,
" he adds, Quesney calls la chaleur d'acrimonic, and very justly distin-
" guishes it from la chaleur d'inflammation. The sensation in truth is as
" different as touching a very hot piece of dry wood and dipping your
" finger into tepid spirit of hartshorn."
Frank also observes of the heat in typhus, " sæpe manifeste acer digi-
" tosque urens."
Dr. Wright calls it a biting heat. (Annals of Med. vol. 2.) It was remarked, when speaking of intermittents, that Galen makes a similar observation respecting the heat in some of them.

* Even the hydrophobia has been known to supervene towards the termination of malignant fevers.

† If the respiration and deglutition be free, Dr. Fosdyce observes, the
prognosis is seldom bad, although the other symptoms appear alarming.

The patient complains of thirst,* the appetite is impaired or wholly lost; and nausea and vomiting are frequent symptoms at an early period. The matter rejected is frequently a viscid, colourless transparent fluid, without much taste or smell; an astonishing quantity of which is often discharged in fevers. It is frequently mixed with, and sometimes the matter discharged almost wholly consists of, bile; often in a very acrid state, especially in the fevers of warm countries.†

The body, as in other fevers, is generally costive, except there be irritating matter present in the intestines, and the patient is often troubled with flatulence and spasmodic contractions of the bowels. A little before death indeed, an ichorous or bloody diarrhœa frequently occurs, without any evident cause; this is always one of the worst symptoms. The prognosis is desperate, if from the highly putrid and offensive nature of the stools compared with other symptoms,‡ we have reason to believe that some part of the intestines is mortified; a frequent accident in the worst forms of typhus.

The appearances of the urine as the fever advances, are various. Sometimes it is pale or limpid, which is never a favourable appearance; sometimes high coloured, and turbid, often giving a good deal of uneasiness while it is discharged, which is sometimes a favourable appearance, and is never to be regarded as unfavourable. The same cannot be said of the urine when it appears brown, and deposits a matter like coffee grounds. This is owing to an admixture of blood, and is uniformly a bad symptom. The urine is sometimes tinged with yellow, the effect of bile in the circulating system. It sometimes deposits a lateritious, or branny sediment; these have been termed the critical sediments, and their appearance is generally, though not universally, a favourable symptom. It has sometimes, indeed, been found, a very fatal one.|| These sediments have obtained much

* Not to complain of thirst, when the mouth and fauces are very dry, is an unfavourable symptom, as it generally denotes a considerable degree of insensibility. In the low nervous fever however, even when the sensibility is not impaired, there is often no thirst. There is often no thirst, Frank observes, except for wine, which all patients in this fever desire.

† The black vomiting, a symptom so much dreaded in the fevers of sultry climates, in which the matter discharged resembles coffee grounds, is the consequence of a very vitiated state of the bile, which assumes this appearance. When the progress of the fever is rapid, Dr. Jackson observes, this matter is often as black as soot. When the progress is more gradual, it is not so dark, and often of a greenish colour. The bile in these fevers also is often passed by stool in so acrid a state as to inflame and excoriate the anus and parts in its neighbourhood. Towards the fatal termination, the stools in the yellow fever of the West-Indies often assume much of the appearance of tar or molasses.

‡ These will be pointed out at length when we consider symptomatic fevers.

|| See Dr. Linning's Observations on the Yellow Fever of America, in the 2d vol. of Essays and Observations, Physical and Literary.

of the attention of physicians, and have given rise to some very ill-founded hypotheses. I shall have occasion to speak of them at greater length, in considering the crises of fevers.[*]

It sometimes happens in typhus, that the urine is suppressed, or passed in small quantity, although the bladder is distended. This is an unfortunate accident, as it always proves the cause of much irritation. Sometimes it is suppressed without pain or distension of the bladder, which denotes a suspension of the secreting powers of the kidneys, and affords a more unfavourable prognosis.

The skin for the most part is dry ; sometimes a moisture is observed on it, particularly in the morning, and while this continues, the symptoms often suffer an abatement.[†] In some cases a freer discharge by the skin takes place, but this symptom with the manner in which we form the prognosis from it, will also be considered at some length when we speak of the crises of fevers. It may, according to the circumstances which attend it, afford a very good, or very bad, prognosis.

I have already had occasion to observe, that hemorrhagies are generally to be regarded as unfavourable in typhus. Hemorrhagies from the eyes and kidneys have already been mentioned.[‡] It is not a much better symptom when blood flows from the stomach and intestines, occasioning a vomiting of blood, and tinging the stools with a dark red, or blackish colour. There is, perhaps, no hemorrhagy which may be regarded as affording a more unfavourable prognosis in typhus, than that from the pores of the skin ; which is not an uncommon occurrence in the worst forms of the complaint. The blood in these cases is particularly apt to flow from blistered parts, from old sores, or wounds, although quite healed up, from the holes, for instance, made in the ears, for earrings ; from places where the patient on former occasions,

* In particular epidemics the urine has assumed a variety of uncommon appearances, probably depending on some affection of the urinary organs, but none of these have been very distinctly marked. Thus, Dr. Chisholm observes, the urine was sometimes green, sometimes inclining to black, and of an oily consistence. Those which have been mentioned are the more common changes which happen in the urine in the progress of fever. Dr. Fordyce has attempted to describe a state of the urine which he regards as peculiar to malignant fevers, and his account is probably accurate ; but the circumstances which characterise this state of the urine do not admit of being sufficiently defined to enable common observers to distinguish it. "The urine has a more viscid appearance than common; is " frothy, browner, and not absolutely transparent, although there is no " cloud or sediment." Dr. Fordyce's 3d Diss. on Fever, part 1.

† In malignant fevers " the sweat if there be any tinges the linen with a dilute ichorous appearance." Fordyce's 3d Diss. on Fever.

‡ Dr. Linning observes of the bloody urine in typhus, that he always found the admixture of blood become less, when the pulse acquired any degree of fulness, and again increase as the pulse sunk ; denoting how much such hemorrhagies depend on a debilitated state of the system.

had been let blood, &c. In the worst cases of malignant fever, indeed, blood, or rather a thin serum, in which more or fewer of the red globules are broken down and suspended, seems sometimes to run from almost every surface of the body, whether external or internal.

There are certain hemorrhagies, however, which now and then even in typhus prove salutary ; the most favourable of these is the epistaxis. This indeed is often a bad symptom, as well as the hemorrhagies just mentioned, especially when the blood falls only in drops ; when it flows more freely, it has sometimes been attended with a sudden and favourable change in the complaint.

Other hemorrhagies, enumerated among the symptoms of synocha, also occur, though less frequently, in typhus. These are not so often favourable as the epistaxis, but they are never so much to be dreaded as those which more peculiarly belong to typhus.* Hemorrhagies will be considered among the other crises of fever.

It sometimes happens in typhus, that the blood which flows from the vessels of the skin is detained beneath the cuticle, giving the appearance of small round spots, which have been termed petechiæ. So frequent are petechiæ in the typhus gravior, that this fever has got the appellation of typhus petechialis, But typhus, (it was observed more particularly in the Introduction) often appears in its very worst forms, unaccompanied by this symptom. Petechiæ occasion no elevation of the cuticle, so that they are seen, but not felt. They are red, brown, or blackish ; the darker the colour, the more danger they indicate. Their shape is also various; in general they are circular, at other times running into

---

* Dr. Fordyce, in his 3d Dissertation on Fever, gives the following account of the state of the blood in malignant fevers. It is the best I have met with. "At the beginning, when the putrefaction has not gone to any "great length, if blood should happen to have been taken from the arm, "the coagulum is loose and easily broken, the serum being hardly of a "browner colour than common. Sometimes, when the depression of "strength is not very great, the blood retains this appearance during the "whole course of the disease.

"If there is greater depression of strength, and by consequence putre- "faction is in a greater degree, the serum becomes of a browner colour. "In a still greater degree, it is red ; in this case, on examining the red par- "ticles with a microscope, many of them are found diminished in size, and "not regular spheres, or oblate spheroids ; some have the appearance of "being broken in two, and look like half moons ; but most of them retain "their healthy appearance. If the putrefaction goes on still further, there "is hardly any distinction between serum and coagulum ; if still further, "the coagulable lymph forms a kind of bag, leaving the serum on the "outside distinct. In the substance of the bag itself there is no intermix- "ture of red particles, so that it looks like the buff which is on the surface "of the coagulum in cases of general inflammation ; but within this bag a "red fluid is contained, which upon being examined with a microscope, "shews the red particles of a variety of forms."

each other they assume various forms. They vary from a size scarcely perceptible to that of a shilling, and are sometimes even larger. Petechiæ generally make their first appearance on the neck, breast, and back; they more rarely appear on the face and extremities, except on the inside of the arm, where the skin is tender, and about the wrist. They are sometimes so crowded together, that at a little distance the skin appears uniformly reddish. In other cases they are thinly scattered. Petechiæ generally appear before the end of the second week. They are generally, but not universally, an unfavourable symptom. There are instances of the febrile symptoms abating on their appearance.*

Instead of petechiæ the skin is sometimes covered with blotches of a larger size, and generally of a purplish colour, termed vibices; at other times it is marked with streaks, or stains of different colours, which sometimes cover almost the whole body, particularly the breast, and often give it the appearance of marble, variously coloured.

These are symptoms which indicate much danger. The danger however is not always proportioned to the number of the petechiæ or vibices. It is usually the greater, the earlier they appear. Ramazzini observes, that those of his patients in whom they appeared on the first day, almost all died. Petechiæ do not always continue through the whole course of the disease, but sometimes disappear in a few days; in other cases they disappear for a short time, and then return. They have been observed to continue, however, not only during the whole course of the disease, but for a considerable time after every other symptom of it had disappeared. There are some petechiæ (Strack remarks) which vanish in three days; others remain during the whole disease and after death; while others remain for a considerable time after the fever has been happily terminated.

Petechiæ sometimes, though much more rarely, appear in synocha. The reader will find cases of this kind in Eller de Cognos. et Curand. Morbis, and Dr. Grant's Treatise on the Fevers most frequent in London.†

* I shall afterwards have occasion to make some observations on the particular species of synochus, which this symptom characterises.

† Petechiæ sometimes appear unaccompanied by fever of any kind. For cases of this kind the reader may consult the inaugural Dissertations of Dr. Edward Graaf and Dr. Adair, Dr. Grant's Treatise just alluded to, Dr. Duncan's Medical Facts and Observations, and the last vol. of his Commentaries in which there are four cases of this complaint. It is also mentioned by other writers. It has only lately been known in this country. This disease has received a variety of appellations: Petechiæ sine febre, Petechianosos, &c. It belongs to the third order of Dr. Cullen's third class of diseases, the Impetigines. It is often accompanied with a tendency to hemorrhagy in different parts of the body; the complaint itself indeed is to be regarded as very nearly allied to hemorrhagy. It has sometimes disappeared with a flow of sweat, lasting for several days, more frequently without any remarkable crisis. In some cases it has proved fatal.

When Petechiæ and the worst kinds of hemorrhagies or other symptoms denoting extreme debility appear, there is generally a considerable tendency to mortification. The sweat and other secretions have a putrid smell, and even gangrene occurs spontaneously. It is then most apt to appear on the nose, lips, cheeks, fingers, and sometimes attacks a whole limb the hands or feet becoming black,* and the gangrene now and then extending as high as the elbow or knee. The extremities thus affected become cold, and often remain in this state for many days before death. In general however mortification is not spontaneous in typhus, but the consequence of slight injuries and then it may occur in any part of the body, although it is still, most apt to appear in the extremities.

I need hardly observe, that this tendency to mortification, or in other words to the extinction of the powers of life, affords a very unfavourable prognosis. Notwithstanding Dr. Miller, in his account of the diseases most prevalent in Great Britain, and some others, have maintained that a degree of mortification appearing on the ends of the fingers, is to be regared as a favourable symptom in bad kinds of typhus.†

Patients in this fever often groan, and seem uneasy, yet are unable to explain or point out the seat of their uneasiness. This is an unfavourable symptom, not only denoting a considerable degree of stupor, but indicating the presence of an irritation, which cannot fail to increase the danger. It is the business of the attendants to discover the source of this irritation, and if possible to remove it. It often proceeds from the urine or fæces being too long retained, but very frequently from excoriations, in consequence of the patient having lain too long in the same posture. This, in cases where the tendency to mortification is considerable, is often attended with very melancholy effects. Instances occur, in which, after escaping from a dreadful fever, the patient at a time when he begins to consider himself out of danger, discovers a mortified sore on some part of the body, which baffles all the succeeding care of his physician. Accidents of this kind warn us, to have the parts on which the patient rests examined from time to time, and when any degree of redness appears, if possible to make him change his posture. When he is so weak that he can lie only on the back, all that can be done is, to make the bed as soft as possible, and defend the parts on which he chiefly rests by proper plasters. But such is the proneness to mortification in many cases of typhus, that no care can prevent it.

* Huxham on Fevers, Frank's Epitome de Curand. Hom. Morb. Vogel de Cog. et Cnr. Morb. &c. Vogel particularly notices spontaneous mortification in typhus, and points out the parts of the body it is most apt to attack.

† It must be admitted, that in some rare cases the appearance of gangrene has been attended with a favourable change, the fever abating soon after it.

Typhus sometimes terminates in ten or twelve days, or within that period; if it be protracted for a longer time, the symptoms usually suffer but little change during a considerable part of the disease. When it is protracted beyond the 14th day, without the more alarming symptoms of debility shewing themselves, the prognosis is generally good.

Dreadful as this fever often is, it sometimes appears in a very mild form. Those who have been exposed to the contagion or other causes of typhus, are sometimes affected with alternate heats and chills, listlessness and debility; yet are never so ill as to be confined to bed; and these symptoms, after teazing the patient for days, sometimes for weeks, often wholly disappear. The mildness of the disease however at its first appearance, by no means assures us that it will not become serious. The worst forms of typhus are often preceded for several days by very mild symptoms.* Between the worst and mildest forms there are innumerable degrees of this complaint, which insensibly run into each other.

If the case is about to terminate fatally, the symptoms which have been enumerated denoting extreme debility, shew themselves gradually. Cold viscid sweats appear on different parts of the body, or the colliquative diarrhœa, which has been mentioned as a frequent forerunner of death, supervenes; and the patient, reduced to the last stage of weakness, either calmly expires, or is carried off by convulsions.

When, on the contrary the event is about to prove favourable, the worst symptoms either do not appear, or if they have appeared begin to abate; and the state of the patient is sometimes evidently changed for the better in the space of a few hours.† After each succeeding remission, the symptoms return with diminished violence, till the fever is wholly removed, leaving the various functions in a state of debility, from which in general they soon recover, and often acquire a degree of vigour superiour to what they possessed before the attack of the fever.

In many cases however the debility which remains after long protracted fevers is the source of fatal diseases, of the various

---

* " But I can discover no symptom which may at all times be regarded " as a certain and infallible forerunner of this complaint; for at first it " often appears very trifling, and its symptoms at an early period are " sometimes so slight, that even the sick themselves cannot be persuaded " that they labour under any disorder, but continue to walk about for several days." See a paper by Henricus Maius, in Haller's Disp. ad Morb. Hist. et Cur. Pert. There are many good observations in several papers on fever in the fifth volume of this work.

† It sometimes happens, though much more rarely, that the fever from being alarming is wholly removed in the space of a few hours. When the change is so sudden, it is generally attended with some of the symptoms that have been termed critical, which will presently be considered.

kinds of dropsy, of phthisis, or any other complaint to which the patient happens from other causes to be predisposed. For the circumstances which usually act as predisposing causes of a variety of complaints, often become exciting causes in debilitated states of body, however induced.

It is not uncommon for those fevers, in which much debility prevails, to be followed by a permanent derangement of some of the functions. The patient has been known to remain deaf or blind. More frequently these senses are only impaired. The voice also is sometimes so much altered, that it never recovers its usual tone, and is now and then wholly lost. It is not uncommon for the judgment to remain deranged, particularly after fevers in which the delirium has been obstinate. From this melancholy consequence the patient frequently recovers, unless there be an hereditary disposition to mental derangement.

A set of symptoms common to all kinds of fevers still remains to be considered; those which attend the more sudden changes from fever to a state of health,* and which have on that account been termed critical.

SECT. III.

Of the Crises of Fevers.

OF the symptoms which attend the more sudden changes from fever to health, the most common is what has been called the critical deposition of the urine.

During continued fever the urine is usually passed in small quantity, is sometimes high coloured, more frequently pale, and for the most part without much cloud or sediment. As the symptoms abate, it is passed in greater quantity, and generally deposits a more or less copious sediment. This sediment consists either of red crystals, which usually do not appear till from 4 to 24 hours after the urine is passed, and fall to the bottom, leaving it limpid; or the sediment consists of a reddish or whitish matter which generally appears within an hour or two after the urine is passed, and only falls in part to the bottom, the urine remaining turbid. The latter of these sediments has been termed furfuraceous or branny;† the former, from its resemblance

* It is only at an early period that fevers terminate suddenly, either favourably or otherwise. The termination of protracted fevers is usually gradual. "When the nervous fever," Dr. Moore observes, "terminates "favourably before or at the end of the second week the crisis is gene- "rally obvious; but when that happens at a later period, particularly if "after the third week, the favourable term is less evident, and sometimes "several days pass during which the disease abates so gradually, that the "most experienced are in doubt whether it abates or not."

† The white sediment when dried is also found to consist of minute crystals.

to brick-dust, lateritious ; but the last term has not been used in a very definite sense. Sometimes both these depositions take place from the same portion of urine. But when there is much of the one, there is generally but little of the other.

These sediments have long been and still are by some regarded as a morbific matter, which was the cause of the fever, and to the discharge of which the abatement of the symptoms is to be attributed. But the truth is, that both sediments are almost constantly met with in greater or less quantity in the urine of persons in health.

I had occasion some years ago to make observations on the urine, with a view to determine the modes of life which dispose this fluid to deposit what Scheele calls the lithic acid, which is the same with the brick coloured sediment which appears in the urine of febrile patients.* From these observations it appears, that the red coloured sediment is most copious when, from an acescent diet or a debilitated state of the digestive powers, there is much acidity in the primæ viæ, or when the perspiration is checked, in consequence of which, the acid, which ought to have passed by the skin,† is thrown upon the kidneys.

It is farther shewn, that if while the perspiration is checked, the action of the kidneys is also debilitated, the acid causing the deposition of this matter from the urine accumulates in the system, and is thrown off by the skin and kidneys when their vigour is restored; and that in proportion as the perspiration is free, the less of this acid passes by urine. Thus the appearance of the lateritious sediment in the urine is merely a symptom of returning health, but generally indicating a less free perspiration than natural.

'The other, the cream-coloured or furfuraceous sediment, which also now and then assumes more or less of a red or rather a pink colour, but has an appearance very different from the former, was found most copious in the urine of those who used an alkalescent diet, or in whom the perspiration was unusually free, so that any acid received into, or generated in, the body was passed chiefly by the skin.

This sediment therefore, like the former, is merely a symptom of returning health, and particularly indicates the renewal of a free secretion by the skin, which in fevers is generally a favourable symptom.

But whether a favourable symptom or not, it is still attended with the same deposition from the urine. In some fevers terminating fatally there is an unusual tendency to sweat, which only

* An account of these observations was published in 1792.
† It is ascertained by experiment, in the Treatise alluded to, that an acid passes off even by insensible perspiration.

exhausts the strength. In these, the critical deposition of the urine is constantly present, but without bringing relief. This is the case in hectic fever. I have observed this deposition in other cases where there were night sweats without any fever. Nay I have found on repeated trials, that I could at pleasure occasion the appearance of the furfuraceous sediment in the urine of healthy people, by promoting the perspiration by small doses of tartar emetic or Dover's powder. In short all that we can infer from it in fevers is, that a relaxation of the skin has taken place, that the secretion by this organ is restored. These appearances in the urine therefore, at the favourable termination of fevers, are certainly not the cause, but the consequence, of recovery.*

Next to the critical deposition of the urine, there is no symptom which so generally attends the change from fever to health as sweating. This we found to be the crisis of intermittents, accompanied however as sweating generally is, whether in health or disease, with a sediment in the urine. Even continued fever is seldom terminated favourably without some degree of moisture appearing on the skin. The crisis in synocha, says Hoffman, is in most cases a profuse sweat. Dr. Grant remarks of the synochus, " Nor do I find the crisis ever perfect till the night kindly " sweats begin to flow ; and Dr. Huxham declares, that he never saw, " a malignant typhus cured till more or less of sweat had issued." It is surprising that the best effects are sometimes produced, even in those fevers in which debility prevails most, by profuse and long continued sweats. Dr. Donald Munro remarks, that in the petechial fever the sweat often continued for three or four days with the best effects. Another remarkable peculiarity of this fever (the petechial) says Hoffman, is the profuse cold sweats, of an acid smell, continuing for several days and nights, and proving a salutary crisis.†

* The following are the only appearances of the urine, if we except those it assumes in consequence of morbid affections of the urinary organs, which can be distinctly marked, namely, the pale urine without cloud or sediment; the pale urine with a light cloud appearing a few hours after it has been passed ; the high-coloured urine remaining clear or having a light cloud formed in it without sediment; the high-coloured urine remaining clear or having a light cloud formed in it and depositing usually a considerable time (from 4 to 24 hours) after it has been passed a red crystalised sediment; the high coloured urine becoming turbid after it has been passed for a short time, (from one to five or six hours) and depositing a light coloured sometimes reddish sediment, now and then (after the urine has stood for a longer time) mixed with more or less, never with much, of the red crystalised sediment; and in almost every complaint, as well as in perfect health, the urine occasionally assumes all these appearances. Such is the foundation of the practice of those empirics, who pretend to determine the complaint under which their patient labours by inspecting the urine.

† He adds however, that these sweats, although proving critical, always indicate much debility, and that if the patient's strength be not supported while under them, he frequently sinks when on the brink of recovery.

From these facts however we are not to draw an inference, which long misled physicians, and proved a source of much mischief; that the solution of the fever is to be wholly attributed to the flow of sweat, and that could this symptom by any means be induced, it would always prove equally beneficial. To this hypothesis, besides other erroneous parts of practice, we may trace the employment of the hot regimen in fevers; an error so fatal, that it may be seriously questioned, whether the medical art, during its prevalence, did more good or harm in these complaints. It has just been shewn that the critical sediments in the urine are to be regarded, not as the cause, but the consequence, of recovery. Critical sweats are to be viewed in nearly the same light. Nothing would be more hurtful than any means tending to check a sweat which is attended with an abatement of the symptoms, and it is even proper, as will be pointed out more particularly in considering the treatment of fevers, to use innocent means to promote such sweats; but to endeavour to force out sweats by warmth and heating medicines, is universally prejudicial. The wished for crisis is never obtained in this way, and the attempt has often cost the patient his life.

Even spontaneous sweats in fevers are not always to be encouraged. When, as sometimes happens, they occur at an early period of the disease, and continue without relieving the symptoms, they indicate danger, exhausting the strength without proving critical. Nor are those sweats to be encouraged which are viscid and partial. Unless the sweat be thin and universal, it rarely proves beneficial.

Sweating not only does not always afford a favourable prognosis, but is sometimes among the most fatal symptoms in fevers. Sweat running copiously from the head and neck is mentioned as a frequent forerunner of death in the yellow fever.* It is of the same fever that Dr. Linning observes, that the urine often shews the critical sediment on the very first day, which he uniformly found a bad symptom, and the more copious the sediment was, the worse, he observes, was the prognosis.†

One of the most fatal fevers of which we have any account is the Ephemera Britanica, described by Caius; the chief symptom of which was a profuse flow of sweat, from which it received the appellation of Sudor Anglicus.‡

Except the critical deposition from the urine and sweating, there is no symptom which oftener attends the more sudden changes from fever to health than diarrhœa. If a diarrhœa super-

* See Dr. Jackson's observations on this fever.

† See Dr. Linning's letter to Dr. Whytt, on the yellow fever of South America, in the 2d vol. of the Essays and Observations, Physical and Literary.

‡ See Caius de Ephemera Britanica.

vene on any of the critical days, Hassenhorl* observes, we must be careful to do nothing that may check it ; and Hoffman remarks, that in his practice he has more frequently observed a diarrhœa critical in the petechial fever than either sweat or hemorrhagy.

In many epidemics there is a peculiar tendency to terminate in this way, and then the discharge is generally more or less dysenteric. It is in autumn, the season in which dysenteric affections are apt to appear, that fevers are most frequently terminated by a discharge from the intestines.†

This crisis is generally for some time preceded by flatulence, gripes, and pains of the loins.

Spontaneous diarrhœa, however, is far from being universally favourable in fevers. If it occurs in typhus, while the other symptoms are alarming, if the symptoms are not relieved by it, and particularly if the discharge is attended with much loss of strength, it is among the worst symptoms of the complaint, often baffling all our endeavours to check it, and proving the forerunner of death. This diarrhœa, which by medical writers is emphatically termed colliquative, I have already had occasion to notice.

Although we are never to expect the same effects from the exhibition of cathartics, which sometimes attend a spontaneous diarrhœa in fevers, it is often useful in the synocha, for reasons which will afterwards appear, to keep up a moderate catharsis. This is never to be attempted in typhus, in which the bowels ought only to be moved, for the regular expulsion of the fæces.

Vomiting may also be enumerated among the crises of fevers ; it never proves critical, however, except at, or very soon after, the commencement of the disease ; then, whether spontaneous or induced by art, it sometimes stops the progress of fever.

The crisis which next deserves attention is that by hemorrhagy. A spontaneous flow of blood from the different parts of the body is frequently attended with an abatement, or total removal of the symptoms of synocha ; and, what may appear surprising, sometimes of those of typhus, that is, of those fevers whose characteristic feature is debility.

As physicians inferred from the critical deposition of the urine, that fever is owing to the presence of a morbific matter in the blood, and that this morbific matter must be thrown out of the body before the fever can be removed ; and as they inferred from the relief obtained during critical sweats, that this matter may be thrown off by the skin ; so they inferred, from the abatement of the symptoms which frequently attends hemorrhagies, that it

* See his Historia Febris Petechialis.

† In autumn, Quarin observes, fevers are more frequently relieved by a spontaneous purging than at other seasons.

may be thrown out of the body by venesection. Nor did the very obvious objection, that although fever be admitted to arise from the presence of morbific matter in the blood, a partial abstraction of this fluid cannot free the system of a matter diffused through the whole mass, prevent them from recommending venesection in all kinds of fever.

If there be any practice which has been more baneful than the hot regimen, it is the indiscriminate use of blood-letting in these complaints. This subject it will soon be necessary to consider more particularly ; it is sufficient here to observe, that repeated experience has at length convinced physicians, (at least those physicians who condescend to take experience for their guide,) that the effects of venesection and a spontaneous hemorrhagy in fevers, are often so different, that the favourable change, which frequently attends the latter, must be attributed to something else than the mere loss of blood. And as we certainly know that the critical depositions of the urine, and have often reason to believe that critical sweats are the consequence, and not the cause, of the favourable change which attends them ; so we have reason to believe of spontaneous hemorrhagy, that partly, at least, it is owing to the general relaxation of the extreme parts of the vascular system, which takes place in the change from fever to health. The loss of blood in critical hemorrhagies, indeed, is often too trifling to be supposed capable of any considerable effect.

Of hemorrhagies, that from the nose is most frequently critical. It is generally preceded by some of the following symptoms. An unusual redness of the eyes, sometimes an increased secretion of tears, a sense of weight in the temples, dimness of sight, pain of the head, generally, Quarin observes, of the occiput, itching of the nose, and the *pulsus dicrotus*, regarded by physicians as one of the chief symptoms portending a critical hemorrhagy in fevers. In this state of the pulse, which is also called rebounding, the artery seems to strike the finger double.

Before hemorrhagies in general, the patient usually complains of heat, tension or pain in the part from which the blood is about to flow. The worst species of hemorrhagies which occur in malignant fevers, however, are not preceded by any other symptoms than those of general debility, and never prove critical.

Critical hemorrhagies, it has been observed, are most frequent in those fevers, which arise from gluttony, the abuse of intoxicating liquors, or suppressed discharges.

Eruptions of various kinds now and then prove critical in fevers ;. this is sometimes, but not often, the case with the eruptions enumerated in the Introduction as characterising particular species of synochus. Even the appearance of petechiæ is sometimes attended with an abatement of the febrile symptoms. Of these eruptions the aphthæ most frequently bring relief.*

* " Ad Aphthas," Sydenham observes of a continued fever which raged

Aphthæ, however, are far from always being a favourable appearance in fevers. When light coloured, and accompanied with a considerable flow of saliva, they are often attended with an abatement of the symptoms. But when there is little flow of saliva, and particularly when the aphthæ are of a dark colour, they are never a favourable, and often a very fatal symptom. An increased secretion of mucus from the fauces, or of saliva, although there are no aphthæ, is often a favourable symptom in fevers.* The latter sometimes amounts to a salivation, and has been known to prove critical. Both Sydenham† and Huxham‡ relate cases of this kind.

An eruption of another kind, more frequently than any of these just alluded to, attends the favourable termination of fevers; a scabby eruption appearing about the mouth or behind the ears.||

One of the most remarkable crises of fevers, is a swelling and suppuration of glandular and other parts of the body. This crisis rarely happens in the synocha. The parotid glands are the parts most commonly affected. They swell and become inflamed, and the event of the fever seems often to depend on the discharge of the matter generated in them.

It has generally been found the most successful practice to lay them open as soon as, or even before, any fluctuation can be perceived in them. " If the disease," Sir John Pringle observes of typhus, " terminates in a suppuration of the parotid glands, " one caution only is needful, which is to open the abscess soon " without waiting for a fluctuation, or even a softness of the " tumor, which may never happen. The pus being here so very " viscid, that, after it is ripe the part will feel as bard, as if the " suppuration had not begun."§

I have heard Sir Walter Farquhar observe, that when he at-

in London in 1669, 70, 71, 72, " cum jam discessum meditaretur, erat " propensior." (See Sydenham De Febribus Continuis). The favourable termination of that species of synochus, which is attended with the miliary eruption, is often preceded by the appearance of aphthæ. Sometimes, Dr. Mead observes, (see Mead's Monita et Precepta Medica) the matter of the fever occupies the fauces in the form of aphthæ, at the same time that it appears in the miliary eruption on the skin. If they are white, and attended with a copious flow of saliva, they do not portend danger but safety. Dr. Grant repeatedly cautions against repelling aphthæ when they appear in fevers, and thinks that even astringent gargles are hurtful.

* The former of these is mentioned as having generally been attended with an abatement of the symptoms in the late dreadful fever of Philadelphia.

† See Sydenham de Febribus Continuis.

‡ See Huxham on Fevers. Vogel observes, that intermittents are sometimes cured by a salivation.

|| Rush on the Yellow Fever of Philadelphia, and Chisholm on that of Grenada, &c.

§ Sir John Pringle's Observations on the Diseases of the Army.

tended a regiment on the continent, there appeared among the troops a violent fever accompanied with a swelling of the parotid glands, which never came to suppuration. Almost every patient attacked with this fever died, till it occurred to him that an incision of the enlarged gland might prove serviceable; from which he experienced the best effects.

Several cases related by Dr. Donald Monro,[*] prove in the most satisfactory manner the advantage derived in fevers from the free suppuration of the parotid glands when swelled and inflamed. "Swellings of the parotid glands," he observes, "appeared in many subjects towards the decline of the fever, which "came to suppuration and proved critical. In two only, out of "those I attended while in Germany, they came on early in the "fever, but did not suppurate; both patients died. All the rest "recovered, except an old man, an invalid of Bremen."[†]

Dr. Monro applied poultices and gummous plasters to the inflamed glands, and as soon as the presence of matter could be perceived, he laid them open. The cases in which the patients died before this happened seem to point out Sir John Pringle's mode of treatment to be preferable, as it does not appear that any bad consequences followed the laying open of the inflamed glands at an early period.

In some epidemics, however it has proved otherwise, as appears from the observations of Acrel, in the Memoirs of the Royal Academy of Sciences at Stockholm. He often met with abscesses in different parts of the body in malignant fevers. At first he opened them as soon as matter was formed, the consequences of which were, that the strength sunk, the fever became worse, and the patient generally died within eight days.

In some cases, after the fluctuation of the matter was distinctly perceived, a purulent discharge from the intestines, fauces, or nose supervening, the tumors subsided, and the patient got well. The physicians endeavoured to promote the termination which nature pointed out. They gave gentle laxatives as soon as the matter was formed, during the operation of the third of which, it is observed, the stools were generally mixed with purulent matter, the tumors subsided, and the fever disappeared.

These swellings sometimes appear in the arm-pits, or in the groin, and sometimes in the testicle. Instances of all of which the reader will find in Dr. Donald Monro's Observations on the

[*] See Dr. Monro's Treatise on the Diseases of the Army.

[†] This case demonstrates in a striking manner the connection between the suppuration of the parotids and the solution of the fever. A swelling appeared on the right side, which came to suppuration and proved critical. The fever in a short time returned; another swelling appeared on the other side, which came also to suppuration, and the fever again ceased. The patient afterwards died hectic, in consequence of the profuse secretion from the sores.

Diseases of the Army. Dr. Rush observes, that glandular swellings frequently accompany the yellow fever. He never saw them come to suppuration, but generally found, that they tended to afford a favourable prognosis. Dr. Chisholm however observes, that they were among the unfavourable symptoms of the late dreadful fever of the West Indies, which differed in many respects from the common yellow fever, particularly in being accompanied, at least in Grenada, with pestilential eruptions.*

The last symptom I shall mention, as deserving a place among the crises of fever, is shivering. When this occurs in the progress of continued fever, it is sometimes followed by the hot stage, and other symptoms of a paroxysm of an intermittent, which proves the termination of the continued fever, and often the commencement of an ague. "The certain sign," Dr. Grant† observes, "of turgid matter after decoction, is that sensation, which " we distinguish by the name of a chilly fit. After this, the pulse " will rise and the heat increase ; nothing ought then to be at- " tempted but dilution, which nature commonly points out by an " increase of thirst. This state frequently lasts a considerable " time, but gives no cause for uneasiness ; some evacuation will " certainly follow, and that evacuation, whether it be sweat, saliva, " urine, stools, or eruption, will infallibly prove, in some measure, " critical."

As it was formerly observed, that when an ague becomes a continued fever, it is to be treated in the same way as if it had been so from the beginning ; it may now be observed, that when a continued fever becomes an intermittent, it is to be treated like other intermittents, without any regard to the form it at first assumed.

* A symptom of a very peculiar kind sometimes appeared in this fever, and often proved critical. " About the same time," Dr. Chisholm observes, " another symptom appeared in many instances, which, were it " not for its singularity, might be considered too minute to be mentioned " among those which distinguish the disease. Its singularity arises from " the silence of other writers concerning it, and from its appearing in the " present instance to be critical. About the end of the second day the " patient begins to complain of a violent pain in his testicles ; he says he " feels a contraction of the spermatic cord. On examining the testi- " cles they appear much lessened in size, and drawn up towards the " abdomen, and the scrotum appears remarkably flaccid and empty. " The surface of the scrotum becomes soon after very painful, and an ex- " coriation takes place chiefly at the most depending part, from which a " considerable quantity of very offensive purulent matter issues ; at the " same time a similar discharge from the urethra takes place, which cea- " ses with the disease when the event is favourable, or becomes ichorous " or bloody and insufferably fetid when death is the consequence. In " cases which terminate favourably, the scrotum in a few days is covered " with a coat of hardened pus ; which, in the convalescent state, comes " away very easily by means of a warm bath. In fatal cases, this affec- " tion of the scrotum always terminates in gangrene a few hours before " death." See farther information on this subject, in the 122d and following pages of Dr. Chisholm's treatise.

† On the Fevers most common in London.

There is a variety of other symptoms said by authors to be critical in fevers, but most of them have been observed so rarely that their occurrence may rather be regarded as accidental, than as particularly connected with the solution of the fever ; some of them indeed may be regarded as the consequences of the fever. Suppurations in different parts of the body happening a considerable time after its termination, rheumatism, catarrhus vesicæ, or common catarrh, occurring about the time when the fever goes off, indolent swellings, schirrus of the different viscera, various affections of the teeth, jaws, joints, and bones,* spasmodic and other nervous affections, &c.

SECT. IV.

Of the Prognosis in Continued Fever.

THE prognosis in continued fever has been delivered in what has been said of the symptoms and crises of this complaint, and of the prognosis of intermittents.

The danger in fevers arises from two causes, increased excitement, and debility. In the synocha, the former is to be dreaded ; in the different varieties of typhus, the danger is very generally proportioned to the loss of strength. The symptoms of increased excitement are less to be dreaded than those of debility, because we are possessed of more certain means of removing them.

There is a third head, to which authors refer many of the symptoms of typhus, namely putrescency. " From all this it " appears," Dr. Cullen observes of the prognosis in fevers, " that " the symptoms shewing a tendency to death may be discovered " by their being either the symptoms
" Of violent reaction ;
" Of great debility ;
" Or of a strong tendency to putrefaction in the fluids."†

In the 105th paragrsph he observes, " the symptoms denoting " a putrescent state of the fluids are,

" 1. With respect to the stomach ; the loathing of animal " food, nausea and vomiting, great thirst, and a desire of acids.

" 2. With respect to the fluids ; 1. The blood drawn out of " the veins not coagulating as usual. 2. Hemorrhagy from dif- " ferent parts, without marks of increased impetus. 3. Effu- " sions under the skin or cuticle, forming petechiæ, maculæ and " vibices. 4. Effusions of a yellow serum, under the cuticle.

* Some of these perhaps have a better claim to be regarded as connected with the solution of the fever. See Vogel de Cog. et Cur. Morb.

† See Dr. Cullen's First Lines, vol. i. p. 160.

"3. With respect to the state of the excretions ; fetid breath, "frequent loose and fetid stools, high coloured turbid urine, fetid "sweats, and the fetor and livid colour of blistered places.

"4. The cadaverous smell of the whole body."

The first set of symptoms, the loathing of animal food, nausea and vomiting, thirst, and a desire of acids, are common to all kinds of fever, and as strongly marked in synocha, in which no putrescency of the fluids can be suspected, as in typhus.

Of the second set of symptoms it may be observed, that the hemorrhagies and effusions so common in malignant fevers are readily accounted for, and might have been foreseen from the relaxed state of the solids independently of any change induced on the fluids. We know, however, that in such fevers the blood is thinner and consequently more apt to be extravasated than in health, but in a machine so complicated as the animal body, may not this change be owing to many other causes than putrescency ? Are not the debilitated state of the various functions in typhus, particularly that of the secreting organs, sufficient to account for it ? If so, why attribute it to any other cause ? That the blood is in no degree actually putrid, even in the worst forms of typhus, we are well assured. It does not indeed coagulate so readily as usual, but never has any fetor.

The remaining symptoms seem, at first view, to afford a better argument for the opinion of a putrescency of the fluids. When more closely examined, however, they also will all be found referable to the head of debility.

When the various functions of the system are much impaired, the contents of the stomach and alimentary canal stagnate. These form no part of the living body. They are as apt to ferment as the same matter out of the body exposed to the same degree of heat and moisture, unless the antiseptic liquors of these cavities are supplied to check this tendency. Thus it happens, where the powers of life are much exhausted, that the contents of the stomach and intestines become putrid, especially if there be present a large proportion of bile, which is a septic. The same thing takes place on the surface of the body. The failure of the due secretion and absorption there causes a stagnation and putrefaction of the natural moisture. Hence the putrid smell of the sweat. This also happens in parts which have been blistered, in ulcers, &c. so that it is not difficult to account for the cadaverous smell of the body, without supposing any degree of putrefaction in the circulating fluids. And if those labouring under typhus, are more subject to gangrene than people in health, all that this proves is, that in them the vital powers are more languid and apt to fail.

The various symptoms therefore arranged by authors under the head of putrescency, come under that of debility. And in con-

sidering the treatment of fever, we shall find that all the means
employed with a view to obviate what are called the symptoms of
putrescency are such as tend to strengthen the system.

CHAP. II.

Of the remote Causes of Continued Fever.

I HAVE more than once had occasion to observe that I would not
always attempt a division of the remote causes into predisposing
and exciting : Because there are many complaints, none of whose
causes belong properly to either of these heads, all of them acting
sometimes as predisposing, sometimes as exciting causes. This
is true of the remote causes of continued fever. There are two
causes of continued fever indeed which act in general as exciting
causes. The one, the application of cold, occasioning the fevers
characterised by an increase of excitement ; the other, contagion,
occasioning those in which debility chiefly prevails. We shall
find, however, that both of these act sometimes merely as predisposing causes, and that the other circumstances, about to be pointed out, acting usually as predisposing, act sometimes as exciting
causes. As the remote causes of intermittents were arranged under the head of marsh miasma, I shall arrange those of continued
fevers under the two heads of cold and contagion ; because in considering these, we shall have occasion to take a view of the various circumstances capable of producing, or favourable to the production of, this order of fevers.

SECT. I.

Of Cold as a Cause of Fever.

THIS part of the subject Dr. Cullen has considered fully in
his First Lines ; and to what he has said, there is little of importance to be added. I shall therefore quote his observations, omit-
ting however such as appear to be hypothetical.

" The operation of cold on a living body is so different in dif-
" ferent circumstances as to be of difficult explanation ; it is here
" therefore attempted with some diffidence.

" The power of cold may be considered as absolute or relative.

" The absolute power is, that by which it can diminish the tem-
" perature of the body to which it is applied. And thus, if the
" natural temperature of the human body, is as we suppose it to be,
" that of 98 degrees of Farenheit's thermometer ; every degree
" of temperature less than that, may be considered as cold with
" respect to the human body ; and in proportion to its degree

" will have a tendency to diminish the temperature of the body.
" But as the living human body has in itself a power of genera-
" ting heat, so it can sustain its own proper heat to the degree
" above-mentioned, though surrounded by air, or other bodies
" of lower temperature than itself ; and it appears from observa-
" tion, that in this climate, air, or other bodies, applied to the li-
" ving man, do not diminish the temperature of his body, unless
" the temperature of the bodies applied be below 62 degrees.
" From hence it appears, that the absolute cold in this climate
" does not act on the living human body, unless the cold applied
" be below the degree just now mentioned.*

" It appears also, that the living body being surrounded by air
" of a lower temperature than itself, is necessary to its being re-
" tained in its proper temperature of 98 degress ; for in this cli-
" mate every temperature of the air above 62 degrees applied to
" the human body, though still of a lower temperature than itself,
" is found to increase the heat of it.† And from all this it ap-
" pears, that the absolute power of cold with respect to the hu-
" man body is very different from what it is with respect to inani-
" mate bodies.

" The relative power of cold, with respect to the living body,
" is, that power by which it produces a sensation of cold in it ;
" and with respect to this it is agreeable to the general principle

* There is an evident inaccuracy in this statement, because the velocity
with which caloric is abstracted by any medium, is not only in an inverse
ratio to its temperature, but also in a direct ratio to its density. The temperature of the body is not diminished by air at the temperature of 62° ;
but it is diminished by water or quicksilver at the same temperature, be
cause their density is greater than that of air.

I shall here, and in other places, follow chemical writers in the use of
the term caloric ; confining that of heat to the sensation produced by caloric. Expressing by the same term both the sensation and that which
causes it, is a constant source of inaccuracy. The same objection applies
to the common use of the term cold. We want a term expressive of the
abstraction of caloric.

† There is also an inaccuracy in this statement. For the increase of temperature in this case is almost wholly confined to the surface. It appears
from a variety of experiments, particularly those of Dr. Crawford, Dr.
Fordyce, and Mr. Hunter, that the living body resists an increase as well
as a diminution of its temperature, and that there is no temperature to
which we can venture to expose the human body, which will raise the internal parts more than a very few degrees above the natural temperature.
See an account of Dr. Crawford's experiments in his Treatise on Animal
Heat ; of those of Dr. Fordyce, Sir C. Blagden, and others, in the LXVth
volume of the Philosophical Transactions ; and of those of Mr. Hunter,
in his work on the Animal Economy. Mr. Hunter's experiments, if accurate, are the most conclusive in favour of the body possessing a peculiar
power of resisting an increase of temperature, as in them the result cannot be attributed to the effects of evaporation. Dr. Crawford's experiments prove, that an animal disengages a less quantity of caloric in a
high than in a low temperature ; but if Mr. Hunter's experiments are accurate, our bodies must possess a power of combining, as well as disenga-
ging, caloric.

" of sensation, that the sensation produced is not in proportion
" to the absolute force of impression, but according as the new
" impression is stronger or weaker than that which had been ap-
" plied immediately before. Accordingly, with respect to tem-
" perature, the sensation produced by any degree of this, de-
" pends upon the temperature to which the body had been imme-
" diately before exposed; so that whatever is higher than this
" feels warm, and whatever is lower than it feels cold; and it
" will therefore happen that the opposite sensations of heat and
" cold, may, on different occasions, arise from the same tempe-
" rature as marked by the thermometer.

" With respect to this, however, it is to be observed, that al-
" though every change of temperature gives a sensation of cold
" or heat as it is lower or higher than the temperature applied
" immediately before, the sensation is in different cases of dif-
" ferent duration. If the temperature at any time applied is un-
" der 62 degrees,* every increase of temperature applied will
" give a sensation of heat; but if the increase of temperature
" does not arrive to 62 degrees, the sensation produced will not
" continue long, but be soon changed to a sensation of cold. In
" like manner, any temperature applied to the human body, lower
" than that of the body itself, gives a sensation of cold; but if
" the temperature applied does not go below 62 degrees, the sen-
" sation of cold will not continue long, but be soon changed to a
" sensation of heat." The paragraphs which follow in Dr. Cullen's First Lines, respecting the manner in which cold acts on
the living animal body, are omitted, as not only hypothetical but
in some parts inconsistent. In the 92d paragraph Dr. Cullen enumerates the morbid effects of cold.

" 1. A general inflammatory disposition of the system, which
" is commonly accompanied with rheumatism or other phlegma-
" siæ.

" 2. The same inflammatory disposition accompanied by
" catarrh.

" 3. A gangrene of particular parts.

" 4. A palsy of a single member.

" 5. A fever, or fever properly so called, which it often pro-
" duces by its own power alone, but more commonly it is only
" an exciting cause of fever by concurring with the operation of
" human or marsh effluvia.

" Cold is often applied to the human body without producing
" any of these morbid effects, and it is difficult to determine in
" what circumstances it especially operates in producing them.
" It appears to me, that the morbid effects of cold depend partly
" upon certain circumstances of the cold itself, and partly on cer-
" tain circumstances of the person to whom it is applied.

* See note in page 171.

" The circumstances of the cold applied which seem to give it
" effect are, 1. The intensity or degree of the cold. 2. The
" length of time during which it is applied., 3. The degree of
" moisture at the same time accompanying it. 4. Its being ap-
" plied by a wind or current of air. 5. Its being a vicissitude,
" or sudden and considerable change from heat to cold.

" The circumstances of persons rendering them more liable to
" be affected by cold, seem to be, 1. The weakness of the system,
" and particularly the lessened vigour of the circulation, occasioned
" by fasting, by evacuations, by fatigue, by a last night's debauch,
" by excess in venery, by long watching, by much study, by rest
" immediately after great exercise, by sleep, and by preceding
" disease. 2. The body, or its parts, being deprived of their
" accustomed coverings. 3. One part of the body being exposed
" to cold, while the rest is kept in the usual or a greater warmth.

" The power of these circumstances is demonstrated by the
" circumstances enabling persons to resist cold. These are, a
" certain vigour of constitution, exercise of the body, the pre-
" sence of active passions, and the use of cordials.

" Beside these, there are other circumstances which, by a dif-
" ferent operation, enable persons to resist cold, acting as a sen-
" sation ; such as passions, engaging a close attention to one ob-
" ject, the use of narcotics, and that state of the body in which
" sensibility is greatly diminished, as in maniacs. To all which
" is to be added, the power of habit with respect to those parts
" of the body to which cold is more constantly applied, which
" both diminishes sensibility, and increases the power of the ac-
" tivity generating heat."

There is little to be added to these observations on cold, considered as an exciting cause of fever. Except that when cold acts
as the exciting cause, the fever is generally of that species which
has been termed synocha. It is chiefly when cold concurs with
the marsh miasma or contagion in producing intermitting fever
or typhus, that it acts as a predisposing cause.

SECT. II.

Of Contagion.

WITHOUT detaining the reader, by remarks on the indefinite manner in which the terms contagion and infection have often been employed ; it will be sufficient to define the sense in
which I shall use them.

If it can be proved that the plague, or any other disease, is
communicated to a healthy person, not only by the sick themselves, (in which case it is possible to ascribe the spreading of
such complaints to the effects of imagination) but also by any
thing which has been in contact with the sick, although the per-

son infected is ignorant of its having been so ; I say, if these are established facts, it is then ascertained, that matter of some kind passes from the sick, or something which has been in contact with the sick, to the person receiving the disease. This is then as thoroughly ascertained as if we could detect the matter in its passage. This matter I shall call contagion; and its action on the person on whom it induces the disease shall be termed infection.

The following observations on contagion, may be divided into three parts.

In the first we shall consider the source from which contagious fever springs.

In the second, the different ways in which it spreads ; and

In the last, (what depends on a knowledge of the other branches of the subject) the means of preventing its appearance and checking its progress.

There are few parts of medicine involved in greater obscurity, than the nature of contagion. Universal experience only could convince us, that the application of a matter, which cannot in general be detected, and which is often applied in very small quantity, should almost constantly produce nearly the same train of symptoms whatever the state of the body be at the time it is received into it. Such is the property of the contagion of small-pox, of the plague, of lues venerea, and other contagious diseases.

Many have attempted to determine the origin of these complaints. But such inquiries have generally proved fruitless, and often led those engaged in them to very absurd opinions, which do not even deserve to be mentioned. In the history of medicine we observe contagious diseases which had long prevailed suddenly disappearing, and others arising in their stead. But the facts preserved, concerning the production and disappearance of these diseases, throw no light on the sources from which they arose.

The leprosy of the Jews, and other species of leprosy which raged in Europe in the 12th and 13th centuries, are scarcely now to be met with. We find Celsus speaking of the hydrophobia as a new complaint ; and we have a remarkable instance both of the production and disappearance of a contagious disease in the Ephemera Britanica, or, as it was termed, the Sudor Anglicus, described by Caius* and others. The gangrenous sore throat, Allionius† observes, was scarcely known before 1610, since which time it has made dreadful havoc in almost every country of Europe. The Plica Polonica seems to have made its appearance only in the last century. The address of the Polish physicians to the university of Paris is still extant, in which the disease is

* Caius de Ephemera Britanica.
† Allionius de Miliarium Origine.

described as new, extremely contagious, and quite incurable by
any means which they could think of. After quoting the observation of Glisson, that the rickets were only known in England
30 years before he wrote, Dr. Ferriar* observes, " the yaws, the
" sibbens, and other national infectious disorders afford strong
" proofs of the variety of animal poisons; and Mr. Hunter in his
" excellent work on the Lues, has given good reason for believing
" that new poisons are constantly produced among the poor of
" great cities." From these and many similar observations, it
appears that Dr. Cullen is wrong in attempting to limit the number of contagions to a very few species.

., Concerning the source of the above and other contagious diseases, there is but one conjecture which appears at all probable.
That each, though afterwards propagated by contagion, is at
first produced independently of contagion, by a concurrence of
causes which rarely takes place. And when, at any period, it
happens, that no person labors under the disease, it must of course
cease to exist ; and cannot be reproduced unless a sufficient quantity of the contagion is preserved in fomites,† till the same causes,
which first gave rise to it, again conspire. Thus contagious diseases may for a long time disappear, while a different combination
of causes may give rise to other disorders, which will in like
manner spread by their peculiar contagions. The probability of
this conjecture will be strengthened by what I am about to say
of typhus.

. Whatever be the difficulty of tracing the source of other contagious diseases, it is no difficult matter to detect that of typhus.
The combination of a very few circumstances, and those of frequent occurrence, is sufficient to produce this complaint.

... Typhus, that is, fever in which debility prevails, may arise in
any ill ventilated and crowded place. Mr. Howel and others,
who escaped from the black hole of Calcutta, were seized with
this fever. Thus Dr. Lind ascribes the production of many contagious fevers on shipboard to keeping the hatchway shut. Typhus
frequently arises in hospitals, jails, transport ships, &c. when due
care has not been paid to ventilation. It is evident, therefore,
that the effluvia of the living body, become putrid by stagnation,
are capable of producing this fever.‡

Putrid effluvia, from any other source, also produce typhus.
Thus uncleanliness of all kinds is favourable to the production of
this complaint ; and on this account such fevers generally take
their rise among the poor, and among them are most fatal. " I

* Dr. Ferriar's Medical Observations and Reflections.
† Matters impregnated with contagion.
‡ It is observed, by Dr. Fordyce and others, that many brute animals
are subject to typhus, when crowded together in ill-ventilated places.
This fever has been observed to break out among hogs, and more frequently
among sheep.

" have known a nervous fever," Dr. Ferriar observes, " which
" was putrid also in many instances, preserved in a small town for
" almost two years, among the poor alone." But one of the most
" satisfactory cases of this sort," he remarks a little lower,
" was observed, by Dr. Heysham, at Carlisle. In 1778 and 1779,
" a fever of the nervous kind raged in that city, which did not
" seem to have been introduced from any neighbouring place.
" Dr. Heysham with great industry traced its origin to one of the
" gates which was tenanted by five or six very poor families." This
" disorder," Sir John Pringle observes, " is incidental to every
" place, ill aired and kept dirty, that is filled with animal steams
" from foul and diseased bodies ; and on this account, jails and
" military hospitals are most exposed to this kind of pestilential
" infection. As the first are in a constant state of impurity, and
" the latter are so much filled with the poisonous effluvia of sores,
" mortifications, dysenteric, and other putrid excrements. Nay,
" there is reason to apprehend, that when a single person is taken
" ill of any putrid disease, such as the small-pox, dysentery, or
" the like, and lies in a small close apartment, he may fall into
" this malignant fever."

The confinement of the putrid effluvia is not always necessary
for the production of typhus. When the cause is sufficiently
powerful, the whole air of a neighbourhood may be so loaded with
putrid effluvia, as to be capable of producing this fever.

Senac gives an account of a malignant fever occasioned by the
offal of a city being accumulated without the walls. It was received into a ditch filled with water, and while it was covered
with the water, was not attended with any bad consequence ; but
when the quantity increased so that it rose above the surface, a
dreadful fever spread through the city and its neighbourhood, and
in the same place, where four hundred used to die yearly, the
deaths were increased to two thousand.* It often happens that
typhus spreads itself over the adjacent country, when the dead
are left unburied on the field of battle. And Forestus mentions a
fever of the same kind, which raged at Egmont, in North Holland, occasioned by a whale which had been left on the shore.
Many more instances of the same kind might be adduced.

The putrifying effluvia of animal and vegetable matters produce continued fever when the situation and air are dry, and intermittents when they are damp.†

. Such is the p n a source of typhus ; but in the causes of
every species of fever we find a source of this ; for from whatever
cause fever arises, and whatever appearance it at first assumes,
it may by various accidents be protracted, and become a contagious typhus.

---

* The air was so loaded with putrid effluvia, that those who lived near
the heap of putrifying matter could not keep flesh sweet for three hours.

† Compare what is here said with what was said of the remote causes
of intermitting fever, b. 1, c. iii.

It is said, that typhus has been found more apt to arise among people who live much on animal food, particularly if salted, than among those who use a large proportion of fresh vegetables. This opinion, however, the result of hypothesis rather than observation, appears to be ill founded. Typhus is least apt to arise when the diet is such as best preserves the vigour of the system ; and this diet is different in different circumstances. Peculiarity of constitution and habit influence it much. I shall presently have occasion to point out the states of body which predispose to, or tend to prevent, infection.

It has been a favourite opinion, that certain states of the air, independently of the circumstances which have been pointed out as the sources of typhus, often produce this, as well as other contagious fevers. This induced Sydenham to mark attentively the state of the weather, in different years, during which epidemics of different kinds raged. But after the most careful observation he was obliged to confess that he could perceive no difference in seasons in which very different contagious diseases prevailed.

Van Swieten made a similar set of observations, which led him to the same conclusion. He marked down for ten successive years, three times a day, the height of the barometer and thermometer, the direction and strength of the wind. He also marked the quantity of rain that fell, the various changes of the air, diseases, number of the sick, and of those who died. These observations, like those made by every other person in the course of his own experience, prove, that certain complaints, pleurisies, quinsies, &c. are most frequent in certain kinds of weather ; but they throw no light on the source of contagious diseases.

Of the Ways in which Typhus spreads.

In whatever manner typhus is produced, it is always, I may say, (instances of the contrary are so rare*) propagated by contagion.

There are three ways in which a contagious disease may spread.

1. By actual contact.

2. Through the medium of the air.

3. By means of substances which have been in contact with, or near the sick.

Concerning the first of these, little need be said. It is probable, that the larger the surface which has been in contact with the sick, and the longer it has been so, the less will be the chance

* It is remarkable indeed, that we sometimes meet with malignant fevers, which do not appear to be at all contagious. "Sometimes," Dr. Lind observes, " one man may be seized with the petechial, or with the " yellow fever, while the rest continue unaffected." Dr. Lind gives several instances in support of this observation.

of escaping infection. ' Of the other ways in which contagious diseases spread, it will be necessary to speak at greater length.

The air is the medium through which contagion in most instances perhaps is applied to the body ; since it is common for people to be attacked with contagious diseases in consequence of approaching the sick, without touching them or any thing which has been in contact with them.

' It appears, from a variety of observations, however, that the contagious atmosphere, that is, the air sufficiently impregnated with the contagion to produce the disease, extends only for a short distance around the sick, not only in typhus, but in all other contagious disorders, certainly not above a few yards, probably not above a few feet.

Contagion, however, may be conveyed from place to place by the wind, and thus the disease may be communicated at a considerable distance from the sick. In proof of this, many facts might be adduced ; one of the most striking on record happened on the 11th of May, 1750, at the Old Bailey.

. The prisoners were kept for nearly a whole day in small, ill-ventilated, and crowded apartments ; some of them also laboured under the jail fever. When they were brought into court, the windows at the end of the hall, opposite to the place where the judges sat, were thrown open ; the people on the left of the court, on whom the wind blew, were infected with a malignant fever, while those on the opposite side escaped. The lord chief justice and the recorder, who sat on the lord mayor's right hand, escaped ; while the lord mayor and the rest of the bench who sat on his left, were seized with the distemper. Many of the Middlesex jury, on the left side of the court, died of it, while the London jury, who sat opposite to them, received no injury.*

Some maintain, that we may often detect the presence of contagion in the air ; that it may be perceived by the sight or smell. Of this, however, there seems to be no proof, and much of what has been said on this subject may be ascribed to the effects of imagination. To this at least may be attributed what has been said of a mist surrounding those who labour under the worst kinds of fever, or of a cloud hanging over a city where such disorders rage. Caius observes of the Sudor Anglicus, that a disagreeable smell preceded the distemper, and a black cloud was seen to move from place to place as if driven by the wind, the distemper following the course of the cloud. Concerning the accu-

* It may be owing to contagion being conveyed by the wind, that contagious diseases are most malignant in calm weather, the wind being a principal means of preventing the accumulation of the contagion. It is said, that during a plague at Vienna the wind did not blow for three months ; at the end of this time a breeze arose, by which the distemper was evidently alleviated. See Van Swieten's Comment. in Aph. Boerhaa-vii.

racy of observations, which so many have had the same opportunity of making, and so few have made, there must be much doubt.

The smell of patients labouring under fever seems, from a variety of facts, to depend on something distinct from the contagion. Fomites may be highly impregnated with contagion without having any particular smell ; where the smell of the patient is strongest the contagion is often weakest, and vice versa. Upon the whole we have reason to conclude, with Dr. Fordyce, that the presence of contagion in the air is not to be detected by any of the senses.

It has just been remarked, that there is no particular state of the weather, which, independently of the circumstances pointed out as the sources of typhus, are capable of producing this fever. It has been observed, however, that while contagious distempers rage, certain states of the air are more or less favourable to their progress. The plague has been observed to spread more rapidly in damp foggy, than in clear dry weather. Dr. Lind observes of typhus, that a damp air seems to increase the strength of its contagion ; Dr. Smith makes a similar observation. This has been ascribed to the contagion being diffused through the air with greater difficulty when loaded with watery vapour. It is more probably owing to the sickly state of body which a damp air induces ; it checks the perspiration, disorders the stomach; and often renews febrile and other complaints.*

It is generally supposed, that hot weather is favourable, and cold weather unfavourable, to the spreading of contagious diseases ; and this, with some exceptions, is true. It is common for contagious diseases to suffer a check, or cease altogether, when the winter sets in. But the worst fevers have often raged at the coldest seasons. The plague did so in London, and there have been instances of the plague suffering a check as the weather grew warmer.

There seem to be particular states of the air, not to be distinguished by the senses, which are favourable to the spreading of contagious diseases. It appears, from the observations of Dr. Linning on the yellow fever of North America, that although this fever infects readily the inhabitants of a town where it rages, and particularly those lately come from the country, yet if the sick retire to the country, they do not communicate the fever. Dr. Lind mentions a fact, for which it is still more difficult to account, that the same fever brought to this country in several American ships, attacked those only who had been on board the ships, others remaining uninfected, notwithstanding the freest intercourse with the sick on shore.

* See the observations on the states of body which dispose to infection, towards the end of this section.

The stools, it has been observed, especially if unusually fetid, are most apt to communicate the contagion to the air ; next to these, the patient's breath ; and then the effluvia from his body.

The last of the ways in which a contagious disease may spread, is by *fomites*, or matters impregnated with the contagion. Fomites often retain contagion for a great length of time, and may convey it to any distance. It is a general opinion, that a disease caught from fomites is more dangerous, than when received immediately from a person labouring under it. " It appears to me " probable," Dr. Cullen observes, " that contagions as they arise " from fomites are more powerful, than as they arise immediate- " ly from the human body." In the observations of Sir John Pringle and others, we find striking instances of the virulence of infection from fomites. Fomites are not only said in general to communicate the disease in a worse form, but more readily also, than the sick themselves. Dr. Lind remarks, " I am convinced, " from very extensive experience, that the body of the sick is not " so apt to commmunicate the infection, as the dirty linen, &c. " which has been about him. The sick, Dr. Smith observes, and even the dissection of those who died, were not so apt to communicate the disease, as substances which had been in contact with them.*

Contagion adheres to the furniture and utensils employed about the sick, as well as to all kinds of clothes, woollen, cotton, linen, &c. and even lurks in the walls of the apartments where the sick have lain. Woollen materials and wood are thought more apt to retain contagion than most other substances.

It is a curious and wholly unaccountable fact, relating to this part of the subject, that contagious diseases generally run a certain course, notwithstanding all the means which can be employed to check their progress, and after this cease spontaneously, while the walls of the houses, furniture, &c. must still be supposed to be highly impregnated with the contagion. This observation is made by Russel and others on the plague, and has been made, indeed, on all contagious diseases.

Those who have been near the sick may infect others without having the disease themselves. Nay, those who have only been exposed to putrid effluvia may communicate typhus to others, while they themselves escape.†

---

* It is even said, that contagion may be conveyed in the smeke arising from fomites while burning. Dr. Mead makes this observation with respect to the contagion both of small-pox and typhus. See Mead's Monita et Præcepta Medica. The same observation is also made by Van Swieten and others.

† " The most pernicious infection next to the plague," Lord Bacon observes, " is the smell of the jail, where the prisoners have been long, and close, " and nastily kept, whereof we had in our time experience, twice or thrice,

, The greater the debility is, and the more strongly marked those symptoms are which have been called putrescent petechiæ, fetor of the breath, and perspiration, &c. the more contagious in general is typhus. This, however, is far from being an universal rule; the milder forms of typhus are sometimes as contagious as the more malignant.

. The time during which the contagion is applied before it excites the disease, is different in different cases. Sometimes its effects are almost immediate; in general, however, the infected leave the place, where they receive the contagion, in good health, and feel no symptom of the complaint for one, two, three, or more days, and in some cases, though much more rarely, even for weeks after.

. It sometimes happens, that when those employed about patients labouring under contagious diseases are suddenly taken ill, the illness proves to be different from that under which the sick labour. People have, for instance, on approaching those ill of the small-pox, been suddenly attacked with sickness, head-ach, pain in various parts of the body, and other febrile symptoms, which with the help of proper remedies went off without shewing any of the symptoms peculiar to small-pox.* Dr. Chisholm observes, that those exposed to the contagion of the fever of Grenada, were often immediately seized with nausea and slight rigours, which always proved transitory, the fever not appearing till the 2d or 3d day, or perhaps not appearing at all.†

. It is not only true, that many exposed to the action of contagion escape infection, but it appears from a variety of observations, that many escape infection who have actually received the contagion of typhus into the system, or have it lurk-

" when both the judges, who sat upon the jail, and numbers of those who
" attended the business, sickened upon it and died, therefore it were good
" wisdom, that in such cases the jail were aired before they be brought
" forth. It is probable," Sir John Pringle observes, after quoting this
passage, " that one of the times hinted at, by this noble author, was at
" the fatal assizes held in the year 1577, of which we have a more par-
" ticular account in Stow's Chronicle, in these words. On the 4th, 5th,
" and 6th days of July, were the assizes held at Oxon, where was ar-
" raigned and condemned Rowland Jenkins for a seditious tongue, at
" which time, there arose amidst the people such a damp (an expression
" in the language of those days signifying bad air) that almost all were
" smothered, very few escaped that were not taken, here died in Oxon
" 300 persons, and sickened there, but died in other places 200 and odd."
* Cases of this kind are mentioned by Dr. Lind and others.
† Similar to these observations are those of Sydenham and Rush, respecting the measles. What Sydenham calls the morbillous fever, and Rush the internal measles, are complaints in certain respects resembling, in others differing from, measles; but which frequently attacked those, who were exposed to the contagion of measles. Rush also observes, that he frequently met with a slight feverish complaint, which those who formerly had had the measles were subject to, on approaching patients labouring under this disease.

ing about them for a considerable time, in such a manner, that it may be readily excited to action by slight causes. This observation is sufficiently confirmed by Dr. Lind in his Treatise on Fevers and Infections. He found that those who had been but slightly exposed to the contagion often escaped the disease, if not soon after subjected to the action of debilitating causes; and many recovering from contagious fevers, their bodies not yet being free from the contagion, had the fever renewed by such causes. Dr. Lind remarks, that he has often seen these observations confirmed in sailors, after they had been for some time on shore. The fever, which at first seemed merely the effect of a debauch, or some other cause, soon assumed the precise form of that which raged in the ship they had left. In such cases we find contagion acting merely as the predisposing cause. These observations are farther illustrated by what is said by other authors, particularly by what Dr. Rush says of his own situation while the yellow fever raged at Philadelphia.

In speaking of the means of preventing the progress of contagious diseases, I shall have occasion to mention circumstances favourable to, or tending to prevent, their spreading, which to save needless repetition I omit at present; particularly those states of body which are favourable to, or tend to prevent, infection. It is a remarkable fact. relating to this part of the subject, that although typhus, as has been observed, sometimes arises among brute animals, in the same way as among men, and is communicated from one to another in the same manner, yet brutes cannot communicate the complaint to men, nor men to brutes;* nor can one species of brute animal communicate it to another. Hogs, for instance, cannot communicate typhus to sheep, nor vice versa. It is remarkable that white people cannot communicate certain contagious fevers to blacks. And I have been informed by West Indians, that there are among the negroes many contagious febrile complaints, to which white people are not subject.

I am now to consider the last and most important part of the subject,

The Means of preventing the Generation, and checking the Progress, of Typhus.

With regard to the means of preventing the generation of typhus, all that is necessary to be known was delivered in speaking

---

* Illud præterea notabile est (Waldschmidt observes) venenum pestilentiale, hominibus infestum, non nocere brutis; et e contrario, brutorum pestem non nocere hominibus. See Haller's Disput. ad Morb. Hist. et Cur. pertinentes, vol. v. There are instances, however, of human contagion proving fatal to brute animals. Bocacce says, he saw two hogs eat some pieces of bread thrown from a poor man's house, who had died of the plague, in consequence of which they were seized with convulsions and died in an hour.

of the sources of typhus. If these are avoided, the generation of the complaint will be prevented. It will be necessary to speak at greater length of the means to be employed for checking its progress.

, On what has been said of the different ways in which contagious diseases spread, are founded many of the precautions employed for checking their progress. It is obvious that the first of these, actual contact with the sick, is to be avoided. The means suggested, by our knowledge of the air being a medium through which contagion spreads, are more various.

As the contagious atmosphere extends only for a short distance round the patient, a principal means of avoiding infection is not to approach the sick. But as contagion is carried from place to place by the wind, and as every place where the sick have been, even for a short time, may be supposed to be more or less impregnated with it, it must frequently happen, in close and crowded parts of cities, when the number of sick is great, that the whole atmosphere will become more or less loaded with contagion. And it is difficult for those who inhabit such places to escape infection. It is prudent, therefore, on the breaking out of pestilential distempers, to remove to the less populous parts of the city. Europeans residing at Aleppo, and other places frequently visited by the plague, choose the suburbs for their residence. By this means, and by shutting themselves up in their houses, and avoiding all intercourse with their neighbours, while the distemper rages, they rarely suffer from it. Even the inhabitants of colleges and monasteries in these countries, who live in a great measure secluded from intercourse with their neighbours, frequently escape, while pestilential disorders rage.

For those, however, who are obliged to remain in crowded parts of the city, where the deaths are numerous, it is proper to use some further precautions. When it is probable that the surrounding atmosphere is more or less impregnated with contagion, the first thing that suggests itself is, that the way to exclude the contagion is to exclude the external air. It is impossible, however, to do so entirely ; nor, if possible, could a house be long inhabited without a fresh supply of air. The following observations deserve the attention of those, who may be placed in such circumstances.

Contagion sufficiently diffused becomes inert ; were not this the case, the very purifying of goods impregnated with contagion, (which is generally done by exposing them to the air) would be sufficient to spread the disorder on all sides. Whether it is owing to this circumstance, or the specific gravity of contagion, it is not easy to determine. But it has been observed, that those who reside in the upper parts of houses often escape, while those living on the ground floor are attacked with, pestilential fevers.

The greater purity of the air at some distance above the surface, of the earth, in places where such disorders rage, has been so thoroughly ascertained, in eastern countries, that those who shut up (as it is termed) during the plague, converse with their neighbours from high windows, or if those who live next them are also cut off from intercourse with the infected, the families meet on the house top without dreading the fever which rages below. Dr. Russel* was accustomed to prescribe for a crowd of patients in the plague who daily assembled under his window, and by whom the air to a certain height must have been strongly impregnated with contagion ; yet he neither received the disease himself, nor communicated it to those he lived with.

It should be the endeavour, therefore, of those who live where the deaths are numerous, to be supplied with air from the tops of their houses. A very simple expedient is sufficient for this purpose, and will at the same time promote a free circulation of air in the house. If fires be kindled in several of the apartments, as the air of the house ascends through the heated chimnies, the doors and windows being kept close, the external air can enter only by the chimnies which have not been heated. By similar means miners procure a current of fresh air, when they work at a considerable depth under ground.

A free ventilation is generally kept up in the wards of hospitals, by kindling fires at the ends of the wards and throwing open the upper parts of the windows. It appears, however, that these means are less effectual than at first sight they appear to be. Maret observes, in the Memoires de Dijon for 1788, that in a ward, where the hospital fever raged, he found from several experiments, that the air towards the cieling, on a level with the open windows, was pure enough to preserve the life of birds ; while in the lower parts of the same wards, on a level with the patients beds, they sickened and died. The fact tends to confirm the observations just made ; and shews the necessity of ventilating the wards of hospitals, where contagious fevers rage, by openings near the floor as well as the cieling ; and it is probable, that the former of these modes of ventilation will be found the most effectual.

Such are the simplest means of checking the progress of contagious diseases, suggested by the knowledge of the air being a medium through which they spread.

The same knowledge has suggested another set of means, those which seem to destroy, or correct the noxious properties of, the contagion, while suspended in the air.

It is necessary, however, to premise that it is impossible in every instance to discover whether these means operate by destroying, or correcting the properties of the contagion ; or merely by for-

* See Russel on the Plague.

tifying the body against its action. Many of them may be supposed to act in both ways. I shall arrange under the present head, those which may be supposed to act in the former way ; and under another division, point out the means which act evidently by fortifying the body against the effects of the contagion. There can be no objection to this mode of arrangement, if the hint here suggested be kept in view.

. We may determine whether any particular means possess the power of destroying, or correcting the properties of, contagion, by observing whether they are capable of purifying fomites. What means have, in this way, been proved to possess the power of destroying, or correcting the properties of, contagion, will be pointed out in speaking of the purification of fomites.

. One of the most ancient means employed for destroying, or correcting the properties of, contagion suspended in the air, is caloric. It has been a favourite opinion ever since the days of Hippocrates, that by exposing air impregnated with contagion to the action of fire, the contagion is as it were burned out. And it will appear, when we consider the means employed for purifying fomites, that there is probably a great deal of truth in this opinion. But how shall we apply the temperature sufficient for this purpose, which we shall find is very considerable, to the infected air ? Fires have frequently been made in the streets throughout a whole city, where the plague or other pestilential fevers raged. From this however we should not, a priori, expect much benefit ; and the fact is, that where it has been put in practice it has not proved successful, and seemed often prejudicial. In the year 1721, the plague raged at Toulon with such violence, that in the space of 10 months it destroyed about two thirds of its inhabitants. Many having insisted on fires being made in different parts of the city, the public records were consulted, and it was there found that on a similar occasion the same means had been tried without success. This, however, did not prevent the inhabitants from repeating the experiment. Wood was therefore laid before every house, and at the sound of a bell all the fires were lighted, by which the city was involved in a thick smoke for nearly a whole day. The plague, however, suffered no abatement. The same measure was had recourse to both at Marseilles and London, when the plague raged in these cities, with no better success.

It even appears, upon the whole, that large fires by heating, the atmosphere prove hurtful ; probably in consequence of the relaxation induced by the heat. Dr. Rush observes, that bakers, hatters, and blacksmiths, are more liable than others to contagious diseases. Thus it was perhaps that when fires had been kept burning for three days in London, while the plague raged there, on the night which succeeded these days no less than 4000 died, although not more than 12000 had been destroyed during the preceding three or four weeks.

It appears, I think, upon the whole, that there are two ways in which caloric proves useful in checking the progress of conta- gious diseases, the one by supporting a free circulation of air, in the manner which has been pointed out; the other by destroying, or correcting the properties of, contagion lurking in fomites. The manner in which caloric is employed for this purpose we shall presently have occasion to consider. If fires do not produce one of these effects they seem to do little good, and if they over- heat the atmosphere they do harm. Some have supposed, that caloric is of service in contagious diseases, by drying the air, es- pecially in damp situations. It appears, from what has been said of damp air, that drying the air may be serviceable, by tending to prevent infection.

There is a variety of substances which are supposed, while burning, to have a peculiar power of destroying, or correcting the properties of, contagion, independently of the evolution of caloric, which attends the use of them. Most of these, however, being employed for the purpose of purifying fomites as well as the contagious atmosphere, will be considered with more propri- ety under the next division. The firing of gunpowder, indeed, is chiefly employed with a view to purify the air, and is frequently used in hospitals, on shipboard, &c.

. How this acts has not been certainly ascertained; the agitation of the air, occasioned by the sudden explosion, must diffuse the contagion through a larger tract of air, and may thus render it innocent, or at least milder, and its properties, as some have sus- pected, may be corrected by the elastic fluid disengaged during the conflagration of gunpowder.

It has long been thought, that the carbonic acid gas tends to correct the properties of contagion; and the opinion seems to de- rive some support from its having been observed, that in south- ern climates pestilential fevers generally suffer a check during the vintage. This has been ascribed to the gas evolved from the fermenting vats.

Of whatever service this gas may be, there are many other circumstances during the vintage, which tend to moderate the violence, and check the progress, of contagious disorders: The fresh fruits, the approach of the cold season, and the general cheerfulness which autumn inspires. It would be worth while, however, since this gas may easily be procured, to determine, by more accurate observation, whether it tends to purify air impreg- nated with contagion.

A variety of strong smelling substances seem to destroy, or correct the properties of, contagion, without the assistance of fire. This quality is commonly ascribed to the odour of pitch and tar. When the plague raged in London, few of those em- ployed about the shipping, it is said, were seized with it. We are also informed, that those who work in storehouses of spices are less liable to contagious disorders than others. One of the most celebrated of this class of substances is juniper.* There are none of them, however, on which much dependence can be placed. Camphire, so generally used as a preservative from infection, is supposed to act rather by fortifying against contagion, than by correcting its properties.

A means belonging to this head, which is probably more effectual, is the steam of water, or, what seems to be better, of lime water, which has been recommended for purifying the air in jails and hospitals.† Many have thought, that large tubs filled with cold water, and placed in the apartment of the sick, especially in summer, are serviceable; and some recommend fresh willow and other boughs to be thrown into the water. The fumes of mineral acids have lately been proposed as a means of destroying, or correcting the properties of, contagion, and seem, from the experiments which have been made, to be very effectual.‡

We are now to consider the means of preventing infection through the medium of substances, which have been in contact with, or near, the sick, for fomites may receive the contagion from the air.

It was once a custom to destroy the apparel, and other substances, which had been in contact with the sick; and, if the disease was of a highly contagious nature, even to pull down their houses.

The total destruction of clothes, furniture, &c. however being expensive, various means have been proposed, and practised with success, to preserve the goods, and at the same time destroy the contagion which lurks in them. It is unnecessary to give a detail of all the means which have been employed with this view. It will be sufficient to point out those which have been found most successful in use.

* " Juniper," Dr. Monro observes in a note to his Treatise on Inoculation, " being a plant unsuspected of having any thing poisonous in it, " there could be no harm in making some experiments with it, on ac- " count of the following facts communicated to me. A lady, when the ", small-pox raged in her neighbourhood, bathed all her children daily in " a bath made with juniper, and burned juniper in their rooms. Not " one of eight or nine had the small-pox. On telling this to a gentleman," Dr. Monro observes," he asked me, if this might not possibly be the rea- " son why none of a parish, where juniper grows in great quantity, were " infected by the plague, so destructive to Scotland, about the time of the " Restoration, while the neighbouring parishes suffered greatly, which he " assured me, he had been well informed was a fact."

† See Considerations on Contagion in Maidstone Jail by Mr. Day; and Dr. Alderson's Essay on Contagion.

‡ See Dr. Carmichael Smith's Treatise on the Effect of the Nitrous Vapour in preventing and destroying Contagion, ascertained by a variety of trials, made chiefly by Surgeons of His Majesty's Navy, &c. See also the Report of the Council of Health on purifying the Air in the Military Hospitals of the French Republic.

'The most simple means of purifying houses and goods, is washing and exposing them to the air, and these means are very generally practised with success. It is common to wash, or what is better white-wash the walls of houses, where the sick have lain; and to procure a free circulation of air by opening the windows, and making fires in the house. The clothes, and other articles which have been in contact with the sick, are washed and exposed to the air for a considerable time. And in the different lazarettos of Europe, exposure to the air, for a certain length of time, is generally thought sufficient to purify merchandize, even from cities where the plague rages.

Washing seems to be a less powerful means of purification than exposure to air; and those employed in washing fomites run the risque of infection. Dr. Lind particularly cautions against washing clothes, impregnated with contagion, in warm water, as the steam is dangerous, unless they have been steeped for some time in cold water, or cold soap lees. The same author observes, that the air around fomites is sometimes so impregnated with contagion, that it is capable of communicating the disease.

Fomites, highly impregnated, should be fumigated in the manner about to be pointed out, before they are exposed to the air, both on account of the circumstance just mentioned, and because the purification of substances highly impregnated with contagion, ought not to be trusted to exposure to air alone. This means is generally thought sufficient for the purification of fomites, which have not been in contact with the sick, but received the contagion from a contagious atmosphere.

The means most to be depended on is fumigation. This has been performed in various ways, and with a great variety of materials.

The most simple way is smoking with coals or wood; the latter is preferred by Dr. Lind, and some think charcoal preferable to either. The articles to be purified being inclosed in a convenient place, fires are kindled, and the smoke and caloric confined, which are thus applied to the fomites for a considerable time. If a house or ship is to be purified, the windows and other openings are closed, and fires kindled within.

Much of the good effects of smoking in this way seems to depend on the temperature, which, it is said, should be but little inferior to that for baking bread. And this degree seems capable of destroying contagion in every thing which can be exposed to its action for a sufficient length of time.

But in order to make the purification as complete as possible, different articles have been added to the fire. The chief of these are yellow and white arsenic and sulphur. The last has been known as an antidote against infection since the infancy of medicine. In the same manner are used occasionally tar, pitch, rosin, frankincense, camphire, cascarilla, various spices and aromatics, juniper, pine tops and shavings, turpentine, &c.

It is often adviseable to purify a house or ship, when, from various circumstances, the patients are prevented from leaving it. We must then avoid the use of sulphur, arsenic, or other articles, whose fumes would prove pernicious; we must employ a less degree of temperature; and be cautious not to diminish too much the oxygenous part of the air; and in particular avoid the use of charcoal. The purification, on these accounts, will be much less perfect than when the inhabitants can be removed, but it may still be serviceable. It is even found useful to burn cascarilla, and other aromatics, at the patient's bedside.

When the inhabitants can be removed, and the dwelling smoked as above pointed out, the contagion seems to be, in every instance, wholly eradicated. Dr. Lind observes that he never knew an instance in which a ship, after being smoked, did not become quite healthy.

It is to be observed, under this head, that there should be as little furniture as possible in the bed-rooms of the sick. It is an observation of Dr. Rush, which has not been sufficiently attended to, that every thing around a patient being charged with the contagion, not only renders those about him more liable to infection, but increases the virulence of his complaint. To this circumstance we must in part attribute the benefit derived from removing those labouring under contagious diseases to fresh apartments.

Wood and woollen materials, which, as has been observed, seem particularly apt to retain contagion, should be used by the sick as little as possible. The bedsteads in hospitals should be of iron; and Howard advises the floors to be laid with bricks.

Certain states of body have been observed to be more favourable to infection than others. These, which to avoid repetition I omitted to point out in considering the ways in which typhus spreads, I am now to consider, together with the means of inducing the states of body which are unfavourable, and preventing or correcting those which are favourable, to infection.

When the body is vigorous, and the mind undisturbed, we are least liable to infection. Whatever debilitates and relaxes is favourable to infection. These observations point out most of the means to be employed, and most of the circumstances to be avoided, by those who are exposed to contagion.

The most effectual means of preventing infection is a generous, but temperate diet, and regular exercise. Wine has been long celebrated as a preservative when contagious fevers rage; and it is, upon the whole, the best we are possessed of. This can only be said, however, of the moderate use of wine. The body is at no time more liable to infection than after intoxication. There is sufficient proof of this in the observations of many of the authors whom I have had occasion to mention. Those, Dr. Chisholm observes, who were addicted to the abuse of intoxicating liquors, were most subject to the fever of Grenada. If, however, when the debility subsequent to a debauch in wine commences, it be driven off by again having recourse to wine, the tendency to infection is prevented. Thus it has frequently been observed, that habitual drunkards escape contagious diseases.

Distilled spirits are more apt to be followed by debility, and strengthen the body less than wine. On these accounts they are a less powerful preservative against infection.

Opium and tobacco seem to act in the same way, but are inferior to wine. Tobacco,* whether used as snuff, smoked, or chewed, has long been a celebrated preservative against contagion. Chewing tobacco, in the presence of the sick, has the additional advantage of reminding us not to swallow the saliva, which, in a contagious atmosphere, is believed to be dangerous. It would be difficult to prove, that any advantage is derived from an attention to this circumstance ; yet as it is not improbable, from several facts which I shall presently have occasion to mention, that the first attack of contagion is sometimes on the stomach, and as swallowing the saliva may be the means of conveying it thither, a precaution so easy should not be neglected. For similar reasons we are advised to stand with the back towards the patient.

To this head belong those remedies which have been termed tonic. The Peruvian bark, when it neither oppresses the stomach nor otherwise deranges the system, may be ranked next to wine, as a preservative against infection, and should be used along with it when the danger is great. Pure bitters are also used, but their effects are more doubtful. To these might be added, an endless variety of articles of less note, most of which do not deserve to be mentioned. Vinegar is used in various ways ; frequently washing the mouth and hands with vinegar, or dossils of lint dipt in it, or in a mixture of vinegar and spirits of rosemary, and put into the nostrils, are precautions little to be relied on. Some place confidence in chewing lemon peel and other aromatics. The opinion, that mercury tends to prevent infection, has in some places gained ground. Whatever be the truth of this opinion, quicksilver worn in a quill, which is sometimes done even by medical men, can be regarded as nothing better than an amulet ; a great variety of these are in use among the vulgar in every country.†

We have reason to believe, from the observations of Dr. Currie in a treatise which I shall have occasion to mention more par-

---

* See Van Swieten's Comment. in Aph. Boerhaavii.

† What truth there is in the observation, that those who have issues in any part of the body are less subject to infection than others, it is difficulty to say. See Dr. Smith's Treatise on the Jail Fever of Winchester.

ticularly in considering the treatment of fever, that the cold bath will be found a better preventive against infection, than most of the means wich have been employed for this purpose.

There is one powerful means of fortifying the body against infection, which on many accounts deserves attention, namely, frequent exposure to contagion. It is well ascertained, that those who are frequently exposed to contagion become at length, in some measure, hardened sgainst its effects, just as those who are accustomed to drink much wine are less readily intoxicated by it, than others. Thus nurses and physicians often escape even the plague itself, although freely exposed to its contagion.

Few things are better preservatives against infection than fortitude and equanimity. Nothing we are informed, by those who voluntarily exposed themselves to the contagion of the most pestilential fevers was found an equal preservative against its effects with a steady adherence to what they believed their duty, banishing from their minds, as much as possible, all thoughts of danger, and avoiding every kind of passion, particularly the depressing passions. Every body knows, how much fear disposes to infection ; on this account it is of consequence to strengthen the faith of the ignorant in the efficacy of any thing they believe capable of preserving against infection.

Not only fear, and the other depressing passions, but every thing else that debilitates, disposes to infection. "The yellow "fever," Dr. Lining remarks, " was most fatal to those deprived " of fresh air, those from cold climates, those who had most " dread of it, those who overheated themselves by exercise in the " sunshine, or by intoxicating liquors." And Dr. Chisholm observes, that convalescents, and those labouring under chronic disorders, were remarkably subject to the fevers of Grenada ; visiting the sick with an empty stomach, he adds, or when perspiring was dangerous.

In short, every cause of debility, whether of mind or body, predisposes to infection ; immoderate evacuations ; the depressing passions, or the debilitating effects of the exciting ; a poor and scanty diet, or excess in eating and drinking ; much heat, or a cold and damp air ; long continued vigilance, and even sleep, in which the circulation is more languid than while we are awake, and which has been very generally observed to be favourable to the action of contagion.

It is remarkable, that so slight a debilitating cause as a disagreeable odour may have the same effect. Every kind of soap, Van Swieten observes, has a nauseous smell, but particularly the coarser kinds, which are made of impure alkaline matters and quick lime mixed with train oil. Diemerbroeck observes, that in his hospital, three women who had been washing linen were next morning seized with the plague, and were all of them persuaded they had taken it from the fetid smell of the soap.

In checking the progress of contagious diseases, it is of great importance, as much as possible, to separate the sick from the healthy. No more attendants should be employed than are absolutely necessary; and on the breaking out of a contagious fever, a proper house should be prepared for the reception of the poor, who are attacked with the disease.

.The proper choice of nurses and other attendants, is also a matter of consequence. As those employed about the sick are unavoidably exposed to infection, it is of importance to choose such as are least liable to it. The attendants on the sick in particular should be made acquainted with the circumstances which dispose to, or tend to prevent, infection; and when, as frequently happens, there is any set of people in the place, who from having formerly had the disease, from having been frequently exposed to contagion, or from any other cause, are less liable to infection than others, they should be induced to undertake the office of attendants.

All the exanthemata, and even the yellow fever of sultry climates, are less apt to attack those who have formerly laboured under them. It was observed, that negroes are not subject to the yellow and some other fevers. This is true, however, only of those negroes who have come immediately from the coast of Africa, or have been born and bred in the West Indies. It appears from the observations of Dr. Jackson, that negroes who have been in Europe, or the higher latitudes of America, are subject to the yellow fever. It was probably owing to this circumstance, that Dr. Rush having assured the black inhabitants of Philadelphia that they were in no danger from the fever which lately raged there, many of them perished in consequence of attending the sick.

It has been said, that people of different shades between white and black are as subject to the fevers of white people as those themselves are. Dr. Chisholm remarks, of the fever of Grenada, however, that although people of all colours were subject to it, mulattoes and mustees were less subject to it than whites, and negroes least of all.

The habit of mind and body, as well as other circumstances which dispose to infection, have just been pointed out. An attention to these, it is evident, is proper in choosing attendants for the sick. People labouring under certain disorders are less liable to infection than others. It has been observed, for instance, that scorbutic patients are less subject to typhus than people in health. But from the diseased we cannot choose attendants.

While such as are least subject to infection, are chosen for attendants, care should be taken to prevent those from approaching the sick, who from any peculiarity in their situation are particularly liable to it.

It is observed, in cities where pestilential distempers rage, that those lately from the country are particularly apt to be attacked by them, and that the fevers of warm climates are most apt to seize on those from cold latitudes. It often happens in the West India islands, that fevers are kept up for years, wholly in consequence of a constant supply of fresh troops from Europe. Dr. Jackson observes, that it is uncommon for people to have the yellow fever a second time, unless between the first and second attack they have been for some time in a cold climate.

Such are the circumstances relating to the contagion of typhus, which deserve attention. Concerning the manner in which this contagion acts, or on what parts of the system it makes its first attack, nothing satisfactory has been determined. It is a common opinion, that it makes its first attack upon the stomach. This is far from being ascertained; although some probable arguments may be adduced in support of the opinion. A disagreeable sensation in the stomach, and other disorders of this organ, are often the first symptoms of contagious fevers. Dr. Lind even observes, that an uneasy sensation in the stomach is sometimes perceived the instant the patient is infected. " Many have " been sensible of a disagreeable sensation at the moment they " received the infection, and being questioned, said it was a dis- " agreeable smell reaching down to their stomach, not cadave- " rous, but like the smell of a newly opened grave." It is also in favour of this opinion, that dyspeptic affections often occasion irregular chills, resembling the cold stage of contagious fevers; and that fevers are sometimes cut short at their commencement, by the operation of an emetic; and sometimes though more rarely, by diarrhœa. But when we reflect on the sympathy which subsists between the stomach and other parts of the system, the inference from these facts is rendered very doubtful. It has been observed, that contagious fevers are particularly apt to derange any part of the system which has been debilitated, and consequently rendered more sensible to injury, by former disease or any other cause. From which it does not appear improbable, that the superior sensibility of the stomach is the only cause of its being particularly affected at the commencement of fevers.

It is remarkable that contagious diseases seem (to use the language of medical authors) to change others into their own nature; so that while a contagious fever rages very generally, few other complaints make their appearance, and those which do, commonly partake of the symptoms of the epidemic. The observation has often been made of typhus, and still more frequently of the plague. This curious subject is considered at some length in Dr. Rush's work on the Fever of Philadelphia.

CHAP. III.

Of the Proximate Cause of Fever.

OF the various hypotheses which have prevailed respecting the proximate cause of fever, there are only two which at present deserve attention, that of Dr. Cullen and that of Dr. Brown. With the former it is necessary to be acquainted, because it is blended with the writings of many of the best and latest medical authors; with the latter, both for this reason, and because in part it is founded on observation. Of Dr. Cullen's hypothesis it will only be necessary to give the reader a short account, that he may not find himself at a loss when he sees it alluded to; Dr. Brown's it will be proper to consider at greater length.

SECT. I.

Of Cullen's Hypothesis.

I cannot give a shorter account of this hypothesis than its author gives in the 46th paragraph of his First Lines. "Upon the "whole," he observes, "our doctrine of fever is explicitly this: "The remote causes are certain sedative powers, applied to the "nervous system, which diminishing the energy of the brain, "thereby produce a debility in the whole of the functions, and "particularly in the action of the extreme vessels. Such how- "ever is, at the same time, the nature of the animal œconomy, "that this debility proves an indirect stimulus to the sanguiferous "system; whence by the intervention of the cold stage, and "spasm connected with it, the action of the heart and larger ar- "teries is increased, and continues so, till it has had the effect of "restoring the energy of the brain, of extending this energy to "the extreme vessels, of restoring therefore their action, and "thereby especially overcoming the spasm affecting them; upon "the removing of which the excretion of sweat and other marks "of the relaxation of excretories, take place."

How the debility of the functions proves an indirect stimulus to the sanguiferous system; how this stimulus acts in exciting the cold stage and spasm; how through the intervention of these the action of the heart and larger arteries is increased; how the energy of the brain is restored, and how this energy is extended to the extreme vessels; Dr. Cullen attempts not to explain. Whatever rests on these points, therefore, is confessedly hypothetical; but if what rests on these is excluded from the account of his hypothesis, what remains will be found nothing more than a short recapitulation of the symptoms of fever. It is to be remembered, that a reference to the *Vis Medicatrix Naturæ* in reasoning, respecting the proximate cause of diseases, always amounts to a confession of ignorance. See a more detailed account of Dr. Cullen's hypothesis, from the 33d to the 46th paragraph of his First Lines.

SECT. II.

Of the Brunonian Doctrine.

OF the medical systems which have been proposed to the world, Brown's alone is in a great measure founded on observation. Many parts of it are simple deductions from facts, which must be admitted independently of all hypothesis. In a more advanced state of science, when the systems of Stahl, Hoffman, Boerhaave, and Cullen are forgotten, there will still remain enough of the Brunonian doctrines to preserve the memory of their author.

Dr. Brown alone has made several steps towards a true system of medicine. But in taking a few right steps, he has, (as indeed might have been expected from the state in which he found the subject) taken many wrong ones. It has proved unfortunate for medicine, that those who have attempted to construct systems have never been contented with advancing as far as they found themselves conducted by observation; but when this guide forsook them, have groped their way without assistance, determined, whatever might be the faults of the system, to give it the appearance of a complete system.

It is an attempt, worthy the pains it will cost, to separate the true from the false parts of the Brunonian doctrines ; to point out, and detach from the rest, what is really valuable in them. This attempt I shall make in the present section, and in the next, endeavour to advance a few steps in addition to those which Dr. Brown has taken, towards a true system of medicine.

The present section may be divided into two parts ; the one, comprehending an account of the Brunonian system,; the other, the observations I shall make upon it.

That power, by which the phenomena peculiar to the living state are produced, is termed, by Dr. Brown, excitability. Under this term he includes both the nervous and muscular power,[*] and seems in some places to suppose, that it includes a power different from either of these.[†] He considers every agent capable of producing any change on the living body, as an exciting power ;[‡] that

---

[*] In the following notes the numbers refer to the paragraphs of Dr. Brown's Principia Medicinæ, and the Greek letters to the sections of the paragraphs. "For the sense in which Dr. Brown uses the term excitability, see X, XI, XII, XIV, &c.

[†] See CLXVII.

[‡] See XIX, &c.

is, a power capable of exciting the action of the living solid.
These powers he terms stimuli,* and their effect on the living
solid he terms excitement†. The application of every agent to a
living body, therefore produces excitement‡, and in proportion
as it has this effect, it exhausts the excitability ; that is, it renders
the living body less capable of being excited by stimuli.§ Dr.
Brown does not admit that there is any agent capable of producing
a sedative effect ; but maintains, that when the excitement, unless
it is from an excess of stimuli, is diminished, (that is when the
sedative effect takes place) it is always in consequence of the abstraction of stimuli.¶

The excitability produces no effect, and according to the
Brunonian system has no existence, except when acted upon by

* Dr. Brown supposes the action of all stimuli the same, differing
only in degree ; he, however, divides them in different parts of his work,
in three different ways, into universal and local ; diffusible and natural or
durable ; and direct and indirect. "The effects common to all the exciting
"powers are sense, motion, mental exertion, and passion. Now these
"effects being the same, it must be granted, that the operation of all the
"powers is the same." See XV. "Stimuli are either universal or local.
"The universal stimuli are exciting powers, so acting upon the excitabili-
"ty as always to produce some excitement over the whole system. The
"appellation of universal is convenient, to distinguish them from the
"local. The local stimuli act only on the part to which they are applied,
"and do not, without previously occasioning some change in it, affect the
"rest of the body." See XVII, a, 6, γ. Dr. Brown uses the
terms natural or durable stimuli, in contradistinction to diffusible, by
which he means the stronger stimuli ; such as distilled spirits, musk, vol.
alkali, ether, opium, &c. See CIV, CV, CVI, CXXVI, CXXX, φ, and
CCXC.
"The stimulus of the articles of diet, not exclusive of the diffusible
"stimuli, should be denominated direct, because it acts directly and im-
"mediately on the excitability of the part to which it is applied. Direct
"stimulus, at least in so far as it regards the food, is assisted by another
"stimulus, depending upon a distension of the muscular fibres, on which
"account, for the sake of distinction, the latter should be called indirect.
"The latter is owing to the bulk of animal and vegetable food ; the
"former is produced by a relation or affinity of the stimulus to the ex-
"citability. The indirect acts upon the living solids, in so far as they are
"to be considered as simple ; the direct acts upon them as living only."
See CXXXVII, see also CCLXVIII, &c.

† "The effect of the exciting powers, acting upon the excitability, may
"be denominated excitement."

‡ See XIX, and a variety of other passages, in Brown's Elements of
Medicine.

§ See XXIV, and a variety of other passages.

¶ "The sedative affections as they are called, are only a less degree
"of the exciting ones ; thus fear and grief are only diminutions or
"lower degrees of confidence and joy, not passions different in kind.
"The subject of the passions admits of the same reasoning in every
"respect as that of heat ; and in the same manner all the bodies in na-
"ture that seem to be sedative are debilitating, that is, weakly stimula-
"ting, inducing debility by a degree of stimulus inferior to the proper
"one." XXI, η.

stimuli.* By the total abstraction of stimuli it is as effectually destroyed, as by their excessive application, ; it is on this account that Dr. Brown terms life a forced state.

He does not consider the excitability as a property residing in and depending upon the mechanism of particular parts, but as an uniform, undivided property, pervading the whole system, which cannot be affected in any one without being affected in a similar way in every other part.† Upon the whole, according to the Brunonian system, the excitability (the power on which the phenomena of life depend) is an uniform undivided property, residing in every living body whether animal or vegetable, to whose existence the constant application of stimuli is necessary, which excitement tends constantly to exhaust, which may be destroyed by the excessive application of stimuli, and which accumulates in consequence of their partial abstraction.‡

1. With respect to the powers to which we are to attribute the accumulation of excitability, Dr. Brown leaves us wholly in the dark. The powers in question, it may be said, are those of digestion and assimilation. But how shall we reconcile this with a favourite hypothesis of Dr. Brown—That a certain quantity of excitability to last through life is bestowed on every living body

* " If the property which distinguishes living from dead matter, or " the operation of either of the two sets of powers," (that is, either the external agents, or those which exist in the body itself) " be with- " drawn, life ceases ; nothing else than the presence of these is ne- " cessary to life." XIII.

† " Whether the excitement has been increased or diminished in a " particular part, and whether its diminution has been owing to direct or " indirect debility, and in either way the asthenic diathesis has been pro- " duced, all the rest of the body soon follows the kind of change which " has taken place, because the excitability is an uniform, undivided, uni- " versal property of the system." CLXVII. " And must we, giving up " our fundamental principle, after so compleat an establishment of it, " allow that the excitability is not the same uniform, undivided property " over all the system," &c. CCXXXII. See also a note belonging to this paragraph. Dr. Brown however admits, that although the excitability is always affected in the same way in all parts of the system, yet it is affected in a greater degree in that part on which the stimulus acts than in any other. He maintained another opinion respecting the excitability, that a certain quantity is bestowed on every animal at its first existence, which determines the natural duration of its life. But this opinion, for reasons which will afterwards appear, I shall not at present regard as forming any part of the Brunonian system, with the other parts of which it is impossible to reconcile it.

‡ See XVIII, XXIV, XXXIX. In one of these paragraphs he observes, " this mutual relation obtains between the excitability and excitement, " that the more weakly the powers have acted, or the less the stimulus " has been applied, the more abundant the excitability becomes. The " more powerful the stimulus, the more abundant the excitability becomes the more exhaust- " ed." In XXXIX he observes, " in this case the excitability becomes " abundant ; because in consequence of the stimuli being withheld, it is " not exhausted," &c. See what is said of sleep in CCXXXIX.

at its first existence ? This is a part of the subject on which Dr. Brown did not choose to enter.*

Between the healthy state, in which the excitability and stimuli applied are in due proportion ; and death, in which the excitability is extinguished, either by an excess, or too great an abstraction of stimuli ; the Brunonian system supposes all possible gradations. These are evidently to be divided into two classes ; those in which the excitability is to a certain degree exhausted by too great an application of stimuli ; and those in which a morbid accumulation is supposed to take place in consequence of too great an abstraction of stimuli. In the latter of these, the body is said to be in a state of direct,† and in the former of indirect‡ debility. These are supposed its morbid states.

It is evident however, that there is a state of body different from either of these, and different also from the healthy state. When stimuli are too much abstracted, debility is supposed immediately to insue ; but debility is not the immediate consequence of too great an application of stimuli ; the immediate consequence of this is increased excitement. Dr. Brown therefore, although he maintains, that in the greater number of diseases the system is in a state of debility ;§ yet admits, that there are many, in which it is in a state of increased excitement.¶ The diseases of excitement he terms Sthenic ; those of debility, Asthenic. Which two classes include all general diseases.

These principles Dr. Brown regarded as fully demonstrated, and with a want of caution altogether inexcusable, founded on them his modes of practice.

* See Dr. Beddoes's Observations on this part of the Brunonian system, in the introduction to his edition of Dr. Brown's Elements of Medicine.

† " The debility arising from defect of stimulus may be called *direct*, " because it is not produced by any positive noxious power, but by a sub- " duction of the things necessary to support life." XLV. For an account of this species of debility, see various parts of the Principia Medicinæ, particularly the XXXVIIIth and eight following paragraphs.

‡ " The excitability thus exhausted by stimulus constitutes debility, " which may be denominated *indirect*, because it does not arise from de- " fect, but excess of stimulus." XXXV. For an account of this species of debility, see a variety of passages in the Principia Medicinæ, particularly the XXVIIth and ten following paragraphs.

§ See an account of the diseases of debility, from DIII to DCXCV.

¶ See CCLI. In CCCXXVIII, Dr. Brown observes, " to every sthe- " nia, to all sthenic diseases, increased excitement over the whole sys- " tem is a common circumstance ; it appears during the predisposition, in " an increase of the functions of body and mind ; and after the arrival of " disease, in an increase of some of the functions, a disturbance of others, " and a diminution of others, in such sort that the two latter phenomena " are easily perceived to arise from the noxious powers that produce the " former, and to depend upon their cause." See an account of diseases of excitement from CCCXXVIII to CCCCLIII.

As he allows excess of excitement to be a morbid condition of the body which we frequently meet with, he admits that an abstraction of stimuli is in some cases requisite;* but what he chiefly depends on for the cure of diseases is the addition of stimuli. On this, his plan of treatment in the diseases both of direct and indirect debility is founded. In the former, we are taught, that the morbid accumulation of excitability is to be reduced by a cautious application of more stimuli.† In the other, in which the excitability has been morbidly diminished by too great an application of stimuli, the only mode of cure is, to begin by a stimulus but a little weaker than that which produced the disease, and bring the system to the healthy state by gradually diminishing the quantity of stimulus employed; giving time for the excitability to be sufficiently restored for the functions of the system to go on, in consequence of the application of the natural stimuli alone.‡

Such is the Brunonian system; or rather the system which may be collected from Dr. Brown's Elements of Medicine; for as delivered in that work, it is clogged with so many contradictions, that in order to give the reader a distinct view of the author's doctrines, I have been obliged to separate the system always aimed at, and often clearly expressed in the writings of Dr. Brown, from many of his opinions, which have introduced much confusion into, and often directly contradict the fundamental principles of, his system. It is owing partly to this, and partly to Dr. Brown's never having given any concise view of his doctrines, but left the reader to collect them from his Elements of Medicine, that there are scarcely two people, who, if questioned, would give the same account of them.

Although the opinions here alluded to are not to be regarded as any part of the Brunonian system, since they are incompatible

* See CVI, &c. and the mode of treatment in sthenic diseases from CCCCLIII to DIII.

† In DCLXXXVIII, Dr. Brown observes, "In direct debility, where "the redundancy of excitability does not admit of much stimulus at a "time, ten or twelve drops of laudanum every quarter of an hour, till the "patient, if, as is usually the case in such a high degree of debility, has "wanted sleep long, falls asleep. Afterwards when some vigour is pro- "duced both by that and the medicine, and some of the excessive excita- "bility worn off, a double quantity of the diffusible stimulus should be ad- "ded, and in that way gradually increased, till the healthy state can "be supported by stimuli, less in degree, more in number, and more "natural."

‡ In DCLXXXVII, Dr. Brown observes, "When indirect debility has "had more concern in the case, as in agues or more continued fevers, oc- "casioned by drunkenness; and in the confluent small-pox; the same "remedies are to be employed, but in an inverted proportion of dose. "We should consequently set out here in the cure with the largest doses, "such as are next in effect to that degree of stimulus which produced "the disease; then recourse should be had to less stimuli, and a greater "number of them, till, as was said just now, the strength can be supported "by the accustomary and natural stimuli."

with it; it is necessary to say something of them, that my account of this system may not appear defective.

One of the most striking inconsistencies in the writings of Dr. Brown is his supposition, that every living body at the commencement of its existence, receives a certain quantity of excitability, which if not extinguished by violent stimuli, or by too great an abstraction of stimuli, will last for a certain length of time. The quantity received (he supposes) determines the natural duration of life, it being impossible to protract it after that quantity is exhausted. "We know not," he observes, " what " excitability is, or in what manner it is affected by the exciting " powers. But whatever it be, whether a quality or a substance, " a certain portion is assigned to every being upon the com- " mencement of its living state. The quantity or energy is dif- " ferent, in different animals, and in the same animal at different " times. It is partly owing to the uncertain nature of the sub- " ject, partly to the poverty of language, and partly to the no- " velty of this doctrine, that the phrases of the excitability being " abundant, increased, accumulated, superflous, weak, not well " enough sustained, not well enough exercised, or deficient in " energy, when enough of stimulus has not been employed ; ti- " red, fatigued, worn out, languid, exhausted, or consumed, when " the stimulus has operated in a violent degree ; at other times " in vigour, or reduced to one half, when the stimulus has nei- " ther been applied in excess, or defect, will be employed in dif- " ferent parts of this work."*

It is almost unnecessary to observe, that the different parts of the foregoing quotation are perfectly irreconcileable. The confusion, which Dr. Brown here attributes to the poverty of language and the novelty of the subject, arises from the most evident contradictions in his hypothesis. Dr. Beddoes justly observes, that " he who assumes that a certain portion of excitability is origi- " nally assigned to every living system, by his very assumption " denies its continual production, subsequent diffusion, and ex- " penditure, at a rate equal to the supply, or greater or less.",

An inconsistency in the Brunonian doctrines, if possible, still more remarkable than this, is the supposition, that both the above species of debility may exist in the same body at the same time. In CCXL, he observes, " as debility therefore, whether direct or " indirect, or both conjoined," &c. and after pointing out the doses of medicine suited to his two species of debility, he observes, in DCXCI, " when the affection is more a mixture of " both sorts of debility, these proportions of the doses must be " blended together." If direct debility be that state in which the excitability is morbidly accumulated ; and indirect debility, that in which a morbid exhaustion of the excitability has taken place, in what state shall we suppose the system to be, when both species of debility are conjoined? For when the excitability and

* See XVIII.

stimuli applied are in due proportion, according to the Brunonian
hypothesis, it is in a state of health. Nay, in some places, he
seems to maintain, that the same agent 'may at the same time
induce both species of debility. In CXXXVII he observes, " the
" same thing is to be said of excess in venery, which is partly an
" indirect, partly a direct, always a great debilitating power."

Is it possible to suppose that sleep should ever be the consequence of what Dr. Brown calls direct debility, of that state of
the system in which every agent produces a greater degree of
excitement than in the healthy state? Yet in a variety of passages
direct debility is regarded as capable of producing sleep.*

Although he maintains, that the mode of action of every agent
on the living body is the same, (CCCXV, CCCXVI, CCCXVII,
&c.) yet he is constantly obliged to admit, that there is a difference
in the effects of different agents. (CCCI, CCCIX, &c.) Towards the end of the latter of these paragraphs he observes,
" when the excitability is worn out, by any one stimulus, any new
" stimulus finds excitability and draws it forth, and thereby pro-
" duces a farther variation of the effect." If the operation of all
stimuli is the same, a new stimulus can produce no effect which
may not be produced by changing the quantity of that first applied.

Are not the supposed states of direct and indirect debility opposite conditions of body? Can we suppose them to produce
precisely the same train of symptoms? Yet Dr. Brown is constantly forced into this inconsistency. (CLXI, CC, CCXXXIV,
&c.) In CC he observes, " Epilepsy depends likewise on debi-
" lity, and the same scantiness of fluids, only here the debility is
" commonly of the direct kind. Fevers may arise from indirect
" debility, as in the confluent small-pox, or where drunkenness
" has been the principal exciting noxious power applied, but at
" the same time the most frequent cause of fever is direct
" debility."

A variety of similar inconsistencies in the writings of Dr.
Brown might be pointed out. In stating and commenting upon
his system, we must regard the spirit of his writings, and overlook the passages which cannot be reconciled to the doctrines in
general maintained in them.

When we consider the comprehensive nature and simplicity
of the Brunonian system, and that many of the facts on which it

* See CCL, &c. If it be said, that the Brunonian system does not suppose that stimuli necessarily occasion a greater degree of excitement when
the system is in a state of direct debility than in health, what shall we
understand by the excitability being accumulated in the former case? Is
there any other test of the excitability being accumulated but the greater
degree of excitement produced by the same stimuli? It is true, indeed,
Dr. Brown often loses sight of this, one of the fundamental principles of his
system.

CONTINUED FEVERS.

rests are such as we every day experience in our own bodies, can
we be surprised that it laid hold of the minds of all who were not
wedded to former systems? Dazzled by its lustre, it required
some time for the observer to discover its defects. These, however, are not less than its excellencies.

I shall adopt the same mode of arrangement in the following
observations on Dr. Brown's system, which has been followed in
giving an account of it.

All agents, according to the Brunonian system, are stimuli.
Every thing, capable of producing any change in the living body,
excites the action of the muscular or nervous system or both;
and in proportion as it produces excitement the excitability is
diminished. According to this system then, there is no agent
capable of diminishing the excitability without occasioning previous excitement. Let us consider if this be a fact.

It seems indeed to be a law of the living solid, that every agent
applied to it in a certain degree, acts as a stimulus, that is, produces more or less excitement; and if its action be on the nervous system, the subsequent exhaustion is always proportioned
to that excitement. Applied in other degrees, however, the
same agent acts no longer as a stimulus. Distilled spirits received into the stomach occasion excitement, and to a certain
extent the greater the quantity the greater the excitement. But
the immediate effect of a large quantity of distilled spirits suddenly received into the stomach has often been instant death.
Is this excitement?

The same is true of those agents whose first operation is on
the mind. The passions within a certain degree of intensity act
as stimuli, but beyond this they sometimes instantly extinguish
life; that is, destroy the excitability without previous excitement.
It is needless to multiply illustrations; every one's reflection will
supply him with many.

These agents act on the nervous; let us see how far the Brunonian doctrine applies to those whose action is confined to or
chiefly exerted on the muscular system.

A small quantity of opium applied to the heart occasions increased excitement. A large quantity does not excite in it violent contractions, followed by the loss of excitability, but instant
paralysis without any previous excitement.

The first instance then, in which the Brunonian system departs
from truth, is, in supposing that every thing, capable of acting on
the living body, is a stimulus, and that there is no agent which
directly destroys the excitability.

It appears also, that excitement may take place in the muscular
fibre, without being followed by a corresponding exhaustion of

its excitability; a circumstance of which Dr. Brown was not aware, and which strikes at the fundamental principles of his system. The influence discovered by Galvani, it is said, is so far from tending to exhaust, while it produces excitement, that it preserves the excitability of the muscular fibre in circumstances where it would otherwise have been lost.

The excitability we have seen according to the Brunonian doctrine is an uniform, undivided property of the system, which cannot be increased or diminished in any one part, without being affected in the same way, although in a less degree, in every other.

This is true of the excitability when the term is confined to that of the nervous system. As sensation and voluntary motion, in every part of the body, depend on the sensorium commune; and the excitability of this organ may be diminished by stimuli applied to any part of the system, every part is affected in consequence of the excitement of any one.

If we fatigue one limb by violent exertions, we find that we have, though in a less degree,* diminished the power of every other. Dr. Brown laid hold of this and some analogous facts, and (as in many other instances) his excessive fondness for generalisation made him overlook a distinction of great importance.

The excitability of the nervous system may be said to be indivisible, the nervous excitability every where depending on the state of one particular organ. But the muscular excitability exists in every muscle independently of its existence in any other.

If we apply a strong solution of opium, for instance, to the denuded muscles of a limb, they are instantly deprived of their excitability. But the excitability of every other muscle of the body remains as entire as it was before the application of the opium. If an animal be killed by destroying the excitability of the heart, that of every other muscle remains after death, gradually becoming less in consequence of the powers of assimilation being suspended.†

The excitability of the muscular and that of the nervous system obey laws wholly different from each other; a circumstance which Dr. Brown either overlooked, or could not prevail on himself so far to encroach on the simplicity of his system (which

* The exercised limb is more debilitated than other parts of the body, because it not only suffers in common with these from the debilitated state induced on the sensorium, but the excitability of its muscles is also impaired in consequence of the contractions excited in them. It is proved, in an experimental essay on opium, alluded to when speaking of the modus operandi of this medicine, that contractions excited in the muscles of voluntary motion, through the medium of the nervous system, impair the excitability of the muscles in which the contractions are excited without affecting that of any other.

† See the experiments with opium above alluded to.

he considered its chief excellence) as to acknowledge. No man
will make any considerable advancement in science, whose mind
is not prone to generalise, but of all its propensities this requires
to be watched with most care; it is that which is most apt to lead,
to error. Dr. Brown seized on the great outlines of his subject
with an impetuosity that would not permit him to examine its
parts in detail.

Another opinion, respecting the excitability which makes part,
of the Brunonian system,* is, that the constant application of,
stimuli is necessary to its preservation, and that life consequently
may be regarded as a forced state; an opinion which seems also
to have arisen from a general and very inaccurate view of the
subject.

Upon a cursory view of the animal machine, the position appears to be just. If we deprive the heart and arteries of their
proper stimulus, (the blood) the excitability in every part of the
system is soon extinguished. That the excitability is extinguished
in consequence of the abstraction of the stimulus, is the inference
which Dr. Brown draws from this fact; for I think it could easily
be shewn, that it is this fact alone which he keeps in view, although he speaks as if his inference were drawn from a great
variety of observations, which however are not specified.

Is there any other way of explaining this fact? If there be,
Dr. Brown's inference is rendered doubtful. If it can be shewn,
that this explanation is not supported by a solitary fact only, but
by a variety of facts, which are inconsistent with the Brunonian
opinion, it must then be admitted that Dr. Brown's inference is
false.

As there is a constant waste, there must be a constant supply
of excitability. What the excitability is, and how it is supplied,
have not been determined. We have reason perhaps to believe,
that it is a property of the nervous matter and muscular fibre,
depending on their mechanism; that the different degrees of
exhaustion depend on this mechanism being more or less deranged; and that the supply is to be attributed to the restoration of the proper mechanism by the powers of assimilation.

Whatever be said of the rest of these positions, this we are
well assured of, that a constant supply of excitability is necessary;
and that this supply somehow or other depends on the powers of,
assimilation. It follows then, that these powers being destroyed,
excitability must cease. When therefore we observe the excitability lost soon after the stimulus of the blood is withdrawn,
we are not to infer that the presence of this stimulus is necessary

* I say, which makes part of the Brunonian system, because I regard
the opinion of a certain quantity of excitability being bestowed on every
living body at the commencement of its existence, and some other opinions which have been mentioned, as making no part of that system, because they are inconsistent with it.

to the existence of excitability ; for we cannot deprive the heart
and arteries of the stimulus of the blood, without at the same time
destroying the powers of assimilation on which the supply of
excitability constantly depends. Dr. Brown's inference therefore
is doubtful.

But we may go a step farther. If this inference be just, the
excitability must either be, as Dr. Brown supposes it, an uniform,
undivided property of the system, so that we may suppose its existence maintained in every part, by the action of stimuli on any
one ; or every part of the system must be subjected to the uninterrupted application of stimuli.

That the former of these positions is unfounded has just been
shewn ; and the latter has not I believe been maintained. Stimuli applied to any part of the living body produce excitement.
Does excitement take place in the muscles of voluntary motion
during sleep? Yet their excitability remains. Dr. Brown's inference therefore is false.*

We are now to consider the two great hinges on which the
Brunonian system turns, the states of direct and indirect debility.

It was observed above, that between the healthy state, in which
the excitability and stimuli applied are in due proportion ; and
death, in which the excitability is extinguished, either by an excess or too great an abstraction of stimuli ; Dr. Brown supposes
all possible gradations. These are to be divided into two classes ;
those states of body in which the excitability is to a certain
degree exhausted by too great an application of stimuli ; and
those in which a morbid accumulation takes place in consequence
of too great an abstraction of stimuli. The body in the latter of
these classes is said to be in a state of direct, and in the former of
indirect, debility. In the first place—of indirect debility.

According to the Brunonian system a state of indirect debility is that in which the excitability is more or less exhausted ;
and consequently the same stimuli produce a less degree of excitement than in the healthy state.

We need only reflect on what we have a thousand times observed in our own bodies, to be convinced of the truth of the
following position ; that in proportion as we have been subjected
to the action of stimuli, we become less capable of being excited
by them ; and if their application is continued, the strongest
fail to rouse the system to any further exertion, till a state of

* As the stimulus of the blood is necessary to the existence of the powers of assimilation, and as the existence of excitability in every part of
the system depends on these powers, the constant stimulus of the blood
is indirectly necessary to the existence of excitability. In this sense, but
as far as I can judge in no other, can life be said to be a forced state.
The loss of the excitability is not the immediate effect of the abstraction of the blood, but of the suspension of the powers of assimilation in
consequence of its abstraction.

sleep (during which, if it be sound, there is the greatest abstraction of stimuli which is consistent with health) has to a certain degree renewed its excitability. We read of men in long continued sieges sleeping at the breech of a cannon. And we know that the most violent tortures produce sleep in the hardy savage, who can bear a long application of such powerful stimuli without having life extinguished.

The moderate application of the ordinary stimuli of life renders sleep during a certain portion of the day necessary to our existence. We may delay sleep by constantly applying a stronger stimulus than that which preceded it ; but in proportion as it is thus delayed, it becomes the more irresistible, and the longer its continuance must be in order to restore the due degree of excitability.

This part of the subject Dr. Brown has illustrated at length. His doctrine of indirect debility is, (with two exceptions afterwards to be pointed out) a fair deduction from a numerous train of facts, which he has arranged in a more systematic manner than any preceding author.

The same observation will not apply to his doctrine of direct debility. This according to Dr. Brown is a state of debility, in which the excitability is accumulated, and consequently every stimulus produces a greater degree of excitement, than in that condition of the system which alone he allows to be the healthy state.

The first question which here presents itself is, what is that condition of body which the Brunonian system admits to be the healthy state ? How shall we define that state in which it supposes the excitability and stimuli applied to be in due proportion ?

In the morning the quantity of excitability is proportionably great, in the evening it is small, and between these there are infinite gradations. Which of these states does Dr. Brown consider that of perfect health ?

From a review of his system it appears, that wherever there is any addition made to the stimuli necessary for preserving the body in a state of health, a morbid degree of excitement takes place, and a morbid exhaustion of the excitability follows.* However trifling the degree of morbidity may be, according to the Brunonian system it is a morbid state. According to this system then we are only in a state of perfect health on waking after a sound sleep.

But what will support the doctrine of direct debility, if it

* Admitting the Brunonian system, this is the only state of health which can be defined : When an addition is made to the stimuli necessary for preserving the body in health according to this system, a condition of body differing only in degree from the most morbid, must be the consequence.

can be shewn, that this is that state of the system in which stim-- uli of every kind produce the greatest degree of excitement ; that in which the excitability is accumulated in a greater degree than in any other ? If it can be shewn, that the definition which Dr. Brown gives of direct debility, applies, and applies only, to that state which, according to his system, is the only state of perfect health ?

We come now to that part of the Brunonian system where truth for the first time wholly forsakes us. In other parts, if errors have appeared, they are the errors of rash induction ; that, we are about to consider, is, as far as I am capable of judging, altogether unfounded. I mean the application of the Brunonian doctrine of excitability to explain the phænomena and treatment of general diseases ; which turns wholly on the supposition, that in all diseases of the whole system, except those of increased excitement, (concerning the general nature of which there is no dispute) the body is in one of those states which Dr. Brown terms direct and indirect debility. Let us in the first place take a view of the diseases of direct debility.

.. On reviewing all that Dr. Brown says of the hypothesis of direct debility, I can find but one fact on which it is founded ; and that a fact which, although at first view it seems favourable to this doctrine, if fairly examined will not be found to afford any argument in support of it ; namely, that the living body is strongly affected by the application of certain agents, food and caloric, when they have not for a considerable time been applied in the usual degree. The mildest food will often destroy life in animals who have fasted for several days ; and a moderate temperature will produce violent effects on those who have been exposed to a great degree of cold. .

Of these states of body, supposing them in the extreme, it may be observed in the first place, that neither heat in the one case, nor food in the other, occasion excitement, which were the excitability accumulated, as the Brunonian system supposes, they ought to do.

But admitting that the effects of these agents in such states of the body, are what they ought to be, according to the doctrine of direct debility, they will go but a short way towards establishing this hypothesis. A state of direct debility is that, in which all agents occasion a greater degree of excitement than in health. Do all agents produce a greater than ordinary excitement in an animal that has been exposed to hunger or cold ? Instead of applying caloric to the animal that has been exposed to cold, and giving food to that which has fasted ; to the former give food, and let caloric be applied to the latter. According to the Brunonian system violent excitement should still in both cases be the consequence. In both the excitability is supposed to be accumulated, and to both according to this system powerful stimuli are applied.

. But so much the reverse of this is the fact, that caloric in those who have fasted, and are still deprived of food ; and food in those who have been exposed to cold, and are still deprived of caloric, occasion a much less degree of excitement than in health. The truth is, that in animals under the operation of hunger or cold, every agent, except that whose application in the usual degree has been interrupted, produces less powerful effects than in ordinary states of the system.

The effects of every agent are proportioned to the change it induces on the body. It is not difficult therefore to account for the effects of a temperature of 100°, being more remarkable in an animal which has been exposed to that of 10°, than in one that has been exposed to a temperature of 60° ; or for a hearty meal producing more powerful effects on him who has fasted for several days, than on one who has fasted for a few hours, although exposure both to hunger and cold tends to exhaust the excitability ; which we know to be the case, from the effects of other agents. It is a well known fact, that such a quantity of fermented liquor as proves a strong stimulus in the temperature of 50°, may be taken while the body is exposed to the temperature of 15° without producing any marks of excitement ; yet in the latter case, according to the Brunonian system, an accumulation of excitability has taken place.

According to this system, sensation is one of the effects of stimuli. Are there any sensations more acute than the pains of hunger and cold ? The sensation of cold, it is true, is occasioned by the abstraction of caloric, that of hunger by the want of food ; but these sensations nevertheless are followed by the same exhaustion which succeeds powerful sensations from any other cause.

The few facts on which the doctrine of direct debility is founded, are referable to a law of the animal œconomy, by which the body is rendered more sensible to the action of those agents whose constant or frequent application is necessary to health, by their being for some time withdrawn or not applied in the usual degree. Exercise is another agent of this kind. A person who has long indulged in indolence is overcome by the slightest exertion ; but a high temperature or a full meal occasions no greater excitement in him than in those accustomed to exercise.

We have instances of the same kind in the various natural agents which excite the different organs of sense—light, noise, sapid and odoriferous bodies. An animal which has lived long in the dark, is strongly affected by light ; one which has been long accustomed to quietness, is disturbed by the least noise. The palate that has been habituated to insipid articles of diet, is strongly affected by animal food ; and he that is accustomed to a pure atmosphere, is sensible of odours, which are not perceived by the inhabitants of a large city. But in none of these instances is the body rendered more sensible 'to any other agent than that whose application in the usual degree has been interrupted.

The doctrine of direct debility supposes that the abstraction of any one of these agents renders the system m_{ore} sensible to every agent, and that the effect of all is at all times excitement. *The facts* are, that the abstraction of any one of these agents, only renders the body more sensible to the action of that agent, and that the effect of that agent is not always excitement; but either excitement, or the reverse, according to the degree in which it is applied and the state of the body at the time, that is, according to the change it induces.

If the change is moderate, it proves a stimulus, and within a certain range the greater the change is, the greater is the excitement. Beyond this, it occasions debility, and when excessive, death. Food in an animal that has fasted 12 or 14 hours, occasions excitement; and a full meal occasions a greater degree of excitement, than a scanty one. In an animal that has fasted three or four days, even a small quantity suddenly received into the stomach occasions debility; a larger quantity, death.

The same is true of every other agent, whether natural or artificial, of every thing capable of producing any change on the living body. While the change induced is moderate, while it is consistent with the health of the parts, on which the agent acts, excitement is always the consequence; but wherever the change induced is sufficient to derange the mechanism of the living solid, (if I may use the expression) to induce a morbid state, its immediate effects are debility or death. It ceases to produce any degree of excitement. Thus, with regard to the diffusible, that is the artificial, stimuli, a small quantity of opium or tobacco, applied either to the nervous system or muscular fibre, occasions excitement; and within a certain range, the more we apply, the greater the excitement; but beyond this, their effect is not excitement, but a direct diminution or destruction of the powers of life. These facts will be stated at greater length in the next section; it is sufficient here to shew, that they are incompatible with the Brunonian doctrine of debility.

The morbid states we have been considering, namely, those in which the animal body is exposed to the effects of cold and hunger, are the supposed states of direct debility, of which Dr. Brown speaks with most precision. It is unnecessary to consider particularly any of the others, because one observation applies to all of them; there is none in which many agents do not produce as little or less excitement than in health; therefore there is none in which the excitability is accumulated.

With regard to the diseases in which Dr. Brown supposes the system to be in a state of diminished excitability, a similar observation applies to them; there is no general disease in which the

system is rendered less sensible to the action of all agents. In
typhus, it is less sensible to that of opium and wine ; but a degree
of exercise or heat which would not incommode us in health, is
in this complaint often capable of destroying life.

Upon the whole, the following, as far as I am capable of judging, are the facts which Dr. Brown overlooked in framing his
hypotheses of direct and indirect debility.

Every agent is capable of producing either excitement, or debility, without previous excitement, (which may be termed
atony*) according to the degree in which it is applied.

In health, the degree in which any agent produces moderate
excitement,† and that in which it produces excessive excitement‡
or atony, are in a certain ratio to each other ; and this ratio is
such, that the natural agents applied in the usual degree, viz. a
certain temperature, a certain quantity of blood, a certain quantity of exercise, &c. always occasion moderate excitement, never
excessive excitement or atony.

In general diseases the laws of excitability are changed. The
same degree of temperature, the same quantity of blood, the same
quantity of exercise, &c. either stimulate in excess, as in the diseases of excitement ; or produce atony, as in those of debility.

This change in the laws of excitability Dr. Brown overlooks,
and constantly supposes them the same in health and disease,
that is, he supposes the effect of agents in all cases either of health
or disease to be excitement, and this excitement always to be followed by exhaustion ; so that when he observes, that any agent in
a diseased state of the system does not occasion so powerful an
effect, or occasions a more powerful effect, than usual ; he supposes the body to be rendered in the same degree more or less
sensible to the action of all other agents ; because in health it is
found that when those parts of the system on which the animal
functions depend become more or less sensible to the action of
any one agent, they are at the same time rendered more or less
sensible to that of every other.   The facts here alluded to will be
considered at length in the next section.   1 ras

It must appear to every one who attentively considers the Brunonian system, that its author, in speaking of diseases, has constantly in view the healthy state of the animal body, and attempts
in vain to apply to its morbid states those laws which by fair induction he has demonstrated regulate the excitability of certain parts
of the system in health.   For if we confine the application of the
Brunonian theory to the organs on which the animal functions

---

* See the definition of atony, in the next sect. (III.)
† See the definition of moderate excitement, in the next sect. (VIII),
‡ See the definition of excessive excitement, in the next sect. (X.)

depend* in a state of health, in which all agents are stimuli, (atony being always a morbid state) and suppose the condition of these organs in the morning that of accumulated, and their condition in the evening that of exhausted excitability, we shall find this theory (with a few exceptions relating to the nature of excitability) equally simple and just.

SECT. III.†

Facts relating to the Laws of the Excitability of the Animal System in a State of Health and Disease.

L

Excitability is that quality of the living solid which distinguishes living from dead matter.

In the title of this section I use the term living system, instead of living solid, because I do not speak of particular parts of a living system, but of the living system as a whole, capable of being generally affected by certain causes, which may therefore be termed general, in contradistinction to those whose action is confined to particular parts of the system, and which only affect the excitability of those parts.

Dr. Brown, it has been observed, maintained, that there is no cause which partially affects the excitability of a living system; but facts have been adduced to prove this opinion erroneous; of such causes however I am not to speak, but of those affecting the excitability more generally.

How it happens that certain causes applied to a part affect the excitability of the whole, or a great part of the system, it is not necessary to enquire; it is sufficient to be assured of the fact. I have already had occasion to remark, that this seems to depend on the nervous matter being diffused through every part of the system, and its state every where depending on that of one organ, the brain, which in its turn is affected by every cause acting on any part of the nervous matter.

It is to be recollected then, that in the following observations an attempt is made to trace the laws of the general, not the local, affections of the system; our knowledge of the latter being extremely imperfect. Every occurrence in life is an experiment on the animal system as a whole; consequently on this part of the subject our observations are as extensive as perhaps they ever

* It will appear, as far as I can judge from what is said in the next section, that it is to these organs alone, that the Brunonian doctrine of excitability is at all applicable.

† About six years ago, the rude outlines of the following section were read before the Royal Medical Society of Edinburgh, and inserted in the Books of the Society.

can be. When an animal is exposed to the action of agents, exercise, food, caloric, &c. it is easy to observe their effects upon it as a whole ; but it would require a train of minute experiments and a far more extensive knowledge of the animal œconomy than we possess, to determine the manner in which they act on each particular part of the system. A full meal we know produces in a healthy animal general activity; but in the production of this effect, what part is to be attributed to the action of the food on the stomach and bowels, what to the effects of the increased flow of chyle into the mass of blood, what to the change induced on the brain, what in short to that induced on the nervous or muscular matter in each particular part of the system ? To trace the laws of the local affections of the system, we must make experiments for the purpose ; and the results of the best conducted experiments of this kind must ever be fallacious till we know how far and in what manner one part of the system depends on another. If we wish for example to trace the laws of the muscular fibre exclusively of other parts of the system, on the very outset our progress is checked, by a doubt which the united labour of physiologists has not yet been able to solve—Do agents applied to the muscular fibre act directly on that fibre, or through the intervention of nervous matter ?

I confine the following observations to the animal system, because we are not possessed of a sufficient number of facts to trace the laws of the living vegetable system.

II.

Excitement is a state of activity.

By excitement is not necessarily implied contraction ; because the term is not confined to the muscular system ; the nervous system may be excited without occasioning any contraction in the muscular. I do not adopt Dr. Brown's definition of excitement, that it is the effect of agents on the living solid ; because they often produce a state very different from excitement.

III.

Atony is a state of inactivity, that is, of debility, in which every part of the system is preternaturally sensible to the action of some agents, and preternaturally insensible to that of others ; and watchfulness is the consequence.

IV.

Agent is any thing capable of occasioning a change in the state of the living solid.

In the Brunonian doctrine it is supposed, that every agent produces excitement, that is, is a stimulus. The term agent is therefore rejected by Dr. Brown, and that of stimulus used in its stead. But it appears from the foregoing observations on that system, that the effects of agents on the living solid are either excitement or

atony, according to the degree in which the agents are applied.
When an agent occasions excitement, it is a stimulus; when it
occasions atony, it must have some other appellation expressive
of this effect.

V.

Agents are either *Stimuli* or *Atonics*.

VI.

Stimuli are those agents which produce excitement. (II.)

VII.

Excitement is either *moderate* or *excessive*.

VIII.

i *Moderate excitement* is that which is followed by *exhaustion*.

IX.

Exhaustion is a state of inactivity, that is, of debility, in which
those parts of the system, on which the animal functions depend,
become uniformly less sensible to the action of all agents; and
sleep, that is, a suspension of the animal functions, is the consequence.

This state is always the effect, and the degree of it is proportioned to that of the preceding excitement.

This is the only state either healthy or morbid, to which Dr.
Brown's definition of indirect debility will at all apply; and here
it applies only to those organs on which the animal functions depend; for those on which the vital and natural functions depend
are never in a state of exhaustion.

During sleep these organs suffer no diminution of vigour* but
what is the consequence of the suspension of the animal functions. This is another distinction of importance which Dr. Brown
overlooks.

The state of the heart and blood vessels after each systole is
not that of exhaustion, as exhaustion is defined by Dr. Brown, nor
does he indeed suppose it to be so. That it is not a state of exhaustion might be demonstrated in various ways. It is sufficient
however to observe, that the exhausted excitability can never be
restored while the stimulus which exhausted it continues to act.
A man will never recover from the fatigue of a long walk while
he continues walking; nor will the retina ever recover its sensibility while exposed to the same degree of light which impaired
it. But the contractions of the heart continue to recur, although
it is exposed to the uninterrupted action of the agent which excites them; for, as I have frequently observed in frogs, if a ligature be thrown round the aorta so that the heart continues uniform-

* Dr. Darwin even alleges that the vital functions are most vigorous
during sleep.

ly gorged with blood, its fibres are still alternately contracted and relaxed, and for the space of four or five minutes with the same frequency as before the ligature was applied. Thus, if we sprinkle salt on a muscle, we do not produce permanent contraction followed by exhaustion, but alternate relaxations and contractions followed by exhaustion. But the state of the $mu_{sc}l_e$ in the relaxation which intervenes between the contractions, is essentially different from its condition in that relaxation which succeeds them, because in the former case the same agent, although its application has not been interrupted, is still capable of exciting the muscle to action.*

The vital and natural functions are the powers of assimilation, by which the excitability of those parts of the system which suffer exhaustion is renewed. If these powers also suffer exhaustion, to what powers in the animal machine shall we attribute the renewal of their excitability ? It is impossible that any exertion of these powers themselves can renew it ; because every thing capable of exciting their action must increase the exhaustion, that is, still further diminish the excitability.† Besides, it is impossible that the excitability of the parts on which the vital and natural functions depend, could be renewed while the same agents which occasion its exhaustion continue to be applied. If the organs on which the vital and natural functions depend were subject to the same exhaustion with those concerned in the animal functions, no animal could exist above a few hours.

The excitability of the organs on which the animal functions depend, is renewed during sleep, because the stimuli which occasioned the exhaustion are withdrawn ; and the powers of assimilation, that is, the powers of life, remain. But if the natural stimuli occasioned exhaustion in the organs on which these powers depend, as the stimuli are never withdrawn, would not their uninterrupted application, a fortiori, prevent any renewal of the excitability, which they had been the only means of impairing.‡

* See what is said of the nature of exhaustion in the last paragraph of this division.

† It is this objection to the Brunonian system which forced its author into the supposition, that a quantity of excitability, which is to last through life, is bestowed on every animal at the commencement of its existence. In forming his system he could not but perceive, that admitting every part of the body to be in a state of exhaustion, there is no power inherent in it capable of restoring its excitability. This formidable objection he found it necessary to get rid of, although at the expense of introducing into his system the most palpable inconsistencies.

‡ There is one set of the organs indeed, on which the vital functions depend, which are subject to exhaustion, the intercostal muscles and diaphragm. These are muscles of voluntary motion ; we can interrupt, renew, increase, and diminish their action at pleasure, and like other muscles of voluntary motion they are subject to exhaustion. But the slight degree of exhaustion which takes place after each of the moderate contractions of these muscles in ordinary respiration, is sufficiently restored

ı In diseased states indeed the organs on which the vital and natural functions depend are often debilitated. But this debility we shall find to be of a nature so different from exhaustion, that excitement, instead of increasing, is the only means of removing it.

By the addition of stimuli, we may rouse to action the organs on which the animal functions depend while they are in a state of exhaustion. A powerful affection of the mind, for example, will excite these organs while under the influence of fatigue, but it will leave them in a state of still greater exhaustion. What Dr. Brown says of the action of stimuli in removing this state is wholly unfounded ; the excitability of those parts of the system on which the animal functions depend, the only parts subject to exhaustion, is most speedily and effectually restored during the total absence of every stimulus capable of affecting them. It may be assumed as an axiom, that that debility which can be removed by the operation of stimuli, is not exhaustion.

X.

Excessive excitement (VIL) is that which is followed by atony. (III.)

If we except cases of local disease, *atony* and its effects are the only species of debility to which those organs, on which the vital and natural functions depend, are subject. And to these, they are subject in common with the other living solids, those on which the animal functions depend.

In exhaustion, (IX.) there is but *one set of organs* debilitated : those concerned in the animal functions ; and these are rendered uniformly less sensible to the operation of all agents, till at length they cease to be excited, and sleep is the consequence.

· In atony (III.) *every part of the system* is debilitated, and becomes preternaturally sensible to the action of some agents, namely, the natural agents, food, caloric, exercise, &c. (XI.) which in this state of the system, instead of acting as stimuli are atonics ; and preternaturally insensible to that of others, namely, those which still act as stimuli, termed by Dr. Brown diffusible or artificial ; and watchfulness is the consequence.

ꝛ·It must be recollected, that what is here said, is said of general, uninfluenced by local, affections. Local affections are so various and their nature so obscure, that it is impossible in the present state of our knowledge, to trace their laws. It will appear, as far as I am capable of judging, from the following observations, that

by the interval of rest which intervenes between these contractions, during which the stimulus which produced them is removed ; there is no muscle of the body which could not during the whole life of the animal undergo such moderate contractions with the same interval of rest, were there a stimulus fitted to excite them both in our sleeping and waking hours, as in the case of the muscles of inspiration.

it is owing to pathologists not having properly distinguished the local and general affections, that so much difficulty has occurred in tracing the laws of the latter, which seem to be very simple.

XL.

Atonics are those agents (V.) which produce atony.

It has been observed, that every agent may produce either excitement or atony, according to the degree in which it is applied. Atony is always produced by a greater degree, than that which produces excitement. A certain quantity of those agents, whose first impression is on the body, such as opium, tobacco, &c. as well as a certain degree of those agents whose first impression is on the mind, occasions excitement. (IL.) A greater quantity both of the one and the other produces atony. (III.)

The degree of excitement which any agent is capable of producing, is not in any particular ratio to the degree of atony which a greater quantity of the same agent will produce. Thus, tobacco will not occasion the same degree of excitement that opium or distilled spirits do ; but it is better fitted to produce atony. The exhibition of opium or distilled spirits will not be immediately followed by atony, unless given in doses very great, compared with those which produce moderate excitement ; (VIII.) but a dose of tobacco, very little greater that which produces moderate excitement, will produce atony.

The same is true of those agents whose first impression is on the mind ; grief, fear, hatred, disgust, are ill calculated to occasion excitement ; although when present only in a small degree, they have this effect ; but they are chiefly calculated to produce atony.* Love and joy, on the contrary, produce much excitement ; and only occasion atony when in excess.

With respect to what Dr. Brown says of the depressing passions, as it makes a part of his doctrine of direct debility, it must fall with that doctrine. Unless we allow that grief, fear, hatred, &c. occasion an accumulation of excitability, there is nothing which Dr. Brown† says on this subject that can be admitted. His assertion, that grief is only a less degree of joy, and fear nothing more than a diminution of confidence, is quite gratuitous. He might with equal reason assert, that confidence is a diminution of fear, and joy a less degree of grief. The one set of passions are as positive agents as the other ; and if the one tend more to excite, and the other to depress, it is only what is true of agents of every other species. A negative passion implies an

---

* It is to be recollected, that when these agents are present to such a degree as to occasion derangement of the brain, the general laws of excitability no longer apply.

† Those under the operation of grief are rendered more sensible to joy ; those under the operation of fear, to confidence ; but they are rendered less sensible to the operation of every other agent.

absurdity. Every agent then is either a stimulus, or an atonic, according to the degree in which it is applied.

It appears from what has been said, that atony is either the immediate consequence of the action of atonics, that is, of agents applied in a greater degree than that which produces excitement; or it is the consequence of excessive excitement. (X.)

That exhaustion is never the immediate consequence of the action of agents applied in any degree ; but always the consequence of moderate excitement.* (VIII.)

XII.

The system in general is either in a state of *health* or *disease*. Predisposition to general disease is a state that cannot be defined.

There is perhaps no part of the writings of Dr. Brown more exceptionable than his observations on predisposition to disease. These however, as they do not properly form any part of his system, it did not appear necessary to consider here.

XIII.

Health is either a state of moderate excitement, (VIII.) or exhaustion. (IX.)

That excitement which is followed by exhaustion is always healthy. The debility it occasions affects no parts of the system but those on which the animal functions depend, and in them only occasions debility by diminishing their excitability ; in consequence of which they cease for some time to be excited, and the animal functions are suspended, that is, sleep takes place ; during which the excitability of the organs concerned in these functions gradually increasing, they become sufficiently sensible to be again roused to action by the usual stimuli. The same stimuli again in a short time impair their excitability, which is again in like manner restored ; hence the constant alternation of vigilance and sleep. During neither of these states are the powers of life at all impaired, the system is in as perfect health in a state of exhaustion, as in that of moderate excitement. The powers by which the body is preserved do not partake of this alternation, it is confined to those powers, by which the animal is connected with the external world, by which he perceives and acts.

The latter set of powers cannot exist independently of the former, but the former may without the latter. We have reason to believe, that this is the case in the less perfect animals, which seem to possess no powers but those on which their existence depends, and which may be regarded as the link that connects the more perfect animal with the vegetable world.

* When a state resembling exhaustion occurs without previous excitement, or when the exhaustion is not proportioned to the previous excitement, there is then present a morbid affection of the brain.

We have ample proof than even in the most perfect animals, the vital and natural functions may be in a state of perfect vigour, where the powers on which the animal functions depend never existed: Human and other fœtuses have been born without the head, in other respects well formed and of the full size. Such a fœtus dies as soon as a ligature is thrown round the umbilical chord, because the blood no longer undergoes that change, which is caused by the vicinity of the maternal blood in the placenta, and which is effected after birth by respiration ; a function which, depending on the nervous system, cannot be performed by an animal without the brain. Could such a fœtus after birth be made to respire, and supplied with nourishment, we have every reason to believe, from what we know of the animal œconomy, that it would live and increase in size after birth as it does before it ; but it would certainly experience no alternation corresponding to that of vigilance and sleep in the more perfect animal.

The states then of moderate excitement and exhaustion, that is, of vigilance and sleep, are equally states of health. In both, the powers of life are unimpaired ; and the greater the excitement is, provided it occasions no degree of atony, and the more complete the exhaustion which follows it, the more perfect is the healthy state. We are now to take a view of the states of general disease.

XIV.

General disease is either a state of excessive excitement, (X.) or atony. (III.)

That excitement only is morbid which is followed by atony. This degree is always sufficient to derange some of the functions, and therefore properly termed excessive.

Atony is a state of general debility, and is always a morbid state. In health the powers on which the vital and natural functions depend are never debilitated.

The circumstance which distinguishes a state of general disease from that of health, is a change in the laws of excitability.

The natural agents no longer produce moderate excitement, followed by exhaustion, proportioned to that excitement; but either excessive excitement or atony. The healthy alternation of vigilance and sleep therefore is disturbed, and uninterrupted watchfulness is the consequence. I must again observe, that I am speaking of general disease, strictly so called, that is, disease which neither is in any degree caused, nor influenced, by any local affection. It is true, that sleep occurs in typhus, which is a general disease ; but it is either a morbid sleep, a degree of apoplexy depending on a local affection of the brain, which is apt to supervene in this fever ; or the sleep is natural, and then the degree of fever is slight, there not being present a sufficient degree of atony wholly to counteract the natural alternation of vigilance

aud sleep; thus it is, that in fevers natural sleep is almost a certain indication of recovery.

In a state of general disease, the artificial, or as they have been
termed diffusible stimuli, produce either a greater or less degree
of excitement than in health. In that state which is characterised
by excessive excitement, the smallest quantity of opium or fermented liquors has violent effects. In atony, large quantities of
such stimuli are required to produce the degree of excitement
consistent with health.

XV.

Atony is to be removed by inducing moderate excitement.

As in atony all the natural agents, food, caloric, exercise, &c.
are atonics, we are obliged to have recourse to stimuli, which in
the healthy state occasion excessive excitement, but in the atonic
are the only means by which we can induce moderate excitement. In proportion as we succeed in maintaining this degree
of excitement, we relieve the morbid state ; and in proportion as
this happens, the laws of excitability are changed to those which
prevail in health ; the natural stimuli begin to produce excitement, and we find it necessary to diminish the quantity of the
artificial, till by degrees the healthy laws of excitability are restored, and the artificial stimuli laid aside.

XVI.

Excessive excitement is to be removed by changing excessive
into moderate excitement.

As excessive excitement in general disease is occasioned by the
presence of the natural agents, the only means we have of diminishing the excitement are, diminishing the quantity of some of
these, namely, of caloric, of the blood, and other fluids, and entirely
preventing the application of others, food, noise, light, exercise,
&c.

In atony where our object is to increase excitement, we employ
stimuli ; but in excessive excitement, where our object is to diminish excitement, we do not, employ atonics, because the state
which they induce is always a morbid one.

XVII.

General disease includes infinite varieties, from the greatest excess of excitement, to the extreme of debility.

Between any two of these varieties however no other line of
distinction can be drawn, but that which divides them into those
in which the excitement is above, and those in which it is below
the healthy, that is, moderate excitement. (VIII.)

XVIII.

Simple fever is the only general disease, and may be defined, an excessive excitement or debility of all the functions, without any local affection.*

When fever is in any degree occasioned by a local affection, such as inflammation, hæmorrhagy, &c. or has itself occasioned any local affection, it is no longer a simple fever. Then the general derangement is influenced by the local affection, the preceding observations will not apply to it, and the indications of cure in general diseases are not sufficient to restore the healthy state.

It was shewn in the Introduction that we cannot give a definition of fevers by any enumeration of their symptoms; for the catalogue of symptoms will either be defective, and then will not apply to every case of fever; or too long to serve the purpose of a definition. The above definition is sufficiently concise, and it will be found to include every case of fever, at the same time excluding every other disease.

XIX.

All other diseases are either local, or general and local.

The only diseases which can be mistaken for simple general diseases, are affections of the heart and brain. A local affection of the brain is known by the presence of delirium, coma, or convulsions; a local affection of the heart, by the presence of palpitation or syncope. When these symptoms occur in fever, the case is complicated; it is a case of general and local disease combined; and the preceding observations will not apply to it.

XX.

The laws of excitability are changed in fever. This change is sufficient to account for the phænomena essential to fever, without supposing any change induced on the fluids.

We know that the laws of excitability in fevers are different from those which prevail in health, because the same external agents, the same degree of exercise, the same degree of temperature, the same quantity of food, of light, of sound, &c. which in health occasion moderate excitement, followed by exhaustion; in fever produce excessive excitement or atony. The state of the living solids being thus changed, there must be a corresponding change in the effects of the internal agents, the circulating and other fluids; hence the phænomena of fever.

XXI.

The proximate cause of fever therefore is a change in the laws of excitability; in consequence of which the same agents no longer produce the same effects.

How the remote causes of fever act in inducing this change, and on what change in the living solid this change in the laws of

* That is, without any part of the system being more particularly affected than every other.

excitability depends, we neither can, nor ever shall perhaps be able to determine. This part of the subject is involved, in the, utmost obscurity. From the facts which have been stated, it is certain that the causes of fever do effect this change, and it is evident that such a change in the living solid must occasion the phænomena of fever.

We could have told, a priori, that if the natural agents either stimulate in excess, or become atonics, the phænomena of fever would be the consequence.

Some of these phænomena may be explained, by supposing that the principal natural agent, the blood, is so changed as to produce effects on the living solid, different from those consistent with health. There is a species of fever evidently produced by this cause. When opium or fermented liquors are received into the mass of blood, they so change the properties of this fluid, that it stimulates the heart and blood-vessels to more frequent and powerful contractions than usual. But if a quantity of these agents has not been received into the body sufficient to effect a change in the laws of excitability, the other symptoms of fever do not appear ; and this always proves temporary, the excitability of the heart and blood-vessels being affected by the blood in the usual way, as soon as this fluid has regained its usual properties, in consequence of the expulsion of the offending matter by the excretories.

It required but a very imperfect knowledge of the animal œconomy to suggest that some of the phænomena of fever may be occasioned by the blood's acquiring morbid properties ; and till the time of Stahl, Hoffman, and Boerhaave, physicians laboured in vain to shew that the blood is so changed in fevers as to account for all their phænomena, on the supposition of the solids remaining in the same state as in health. The chimerical hypothesis of Stahl was ill calculated to effect any favourable change on the systems which preceded it. Hoffman was the first who pointed out the insufficiency of what has been termed the humoral pathology, and directed the attention of physicians to the solids. " Porro " etiam omnes, quæ morbus gignunt, causæ," he observes, in recapitulating the outlines of his doctrine,* " operationem suam " pottissimum perficiunt in partes motu ct sensu præditas, et ca- " nales ex his coagmentatos, corum motum, et cum hoc fluido- " rum cursum, pervertendo ; ita tamen, ut sicuti variæ indolis " sunt, sic etiam varie in nerveas partes agunt, iisdemque noxam " afferunt. Demum omnia quoque eximiæ virtutis medicamenta " non tam in partes fluidas, carum crasin ac intemperiem corri- " gendo, quam potius in solidas et nervosas, earundem motus al- " terando ac moderando, suam edunt operationem : de quibus " tamen omnibus, in vulgari usque eo recepta morborum doctrina, " altum est silentium."

* See the 3d vol. of the Medicina Rationalis Systematica of Hoffman.

Boerhaave was sensible of the important change which the observations of Hoffman had affected in medical systems ; but in modeling, he did not improve his doctrines. Boerhaave attempted to explain the symptoms of diseases by attending almost solely to the state of the simple solid. His error was detected by succeeding writers ; and Dr. Cullen at length attempted a new, system more nearly allied to that of Hoffman, and pointed out the properties of the living solid, as those by which we are to explain the phænomena both of health and disease. But it was Dr. Brown who first taught the proper mode of investigating these properties.

In the foregoing observations, I have attempted to add something to what he has done, by which as far as I can judge the laws of excitability and in particular the state of the living solid in fevers are better ascertained. The following observation however must be kept in view ; the properties of the living solid cannot be altered without producing some corresponding change in the fluids, so that although it is certain that most diseases are the consequence of a change in the living solid, yet some of their phænomena must in a certain degree depend on changes induced on the fluids.

XXII.

In simple fever then there are only two indications of cure ; the one to moderate excitement, the other to remove atony. (XV, XVI.)

The means of fulfilling each of these indications have been pointed out in general. (XV. XVI.) We are presently to consider them in detail.

RECAPITULATION.

I.

Excitability is that quality of the living solid which distinguishes living from dead matter.

II.

Excitement is a state of activity.

III.

Atony is a state of inactivity, that is, of debility, in which every part of the system is preternaturally sensible to the action of some agents, and preternaturally insensible to that of others ; and watchfulness is the consequence.

IV.

Agent is any thing capable of occasioning a change in the state of the living solid.

V.

Agents are either *Stimuli* or *Atonics.*

VI.

Stimuli are those agents which produce excitement.

VII.

Excitement is either *moderate* or *excessive.*

VIII.

Moderate excitement is that which is followed by *exhaustion.*

IX.

Exhaustion is a state of inactivity, that is, of debility, in which those parts of the system, on which the animal functions depend, become uniformly less sensible to the action of all agents ; and sleep, that is, a suspension of the animal functions, is the consequence.*

X.

Excessive excitement (VIL) is that which is followed by atony. (III.)

XI.

Atonics are those agents (V.) which produce atony.

XII.

The system in general is either in a state of *health* or *disease.* Predisposition to general disease is a state that cannot be defined.

XIII.

Health is either a state of moderate excitement, (VIII.) or exhaustion. (IX.)

XIV.

General disease is either a state of excessive excitement, (X.) or atony. (III.)

XV.

Atony is to be removed by inducing moderate excitement.

XVI.

Excessive excitement is to be removed by changing excessive into moderate excitement.

XVII.

General disease includes infinite varieties, from the greatest excess of excitement, to the extreme of debility.

XVIII.

Simple fever is the only general disease, and may be defined ; Excessive excitement or debility of all the functions, without any local affection.

XIX.

All other diseases are either local, or general and local.

* The sleep which is not the effect of, and proportioned to, the preceding excitement, is not natural, and is the consequence of a morbid affection of the brain. It is a local disease produced by compression, by various substances applied to the brain, such as opium, tobacco, &c.

XX.

The laws of excitability are changed in fever. This change is sufficient to account for the phænomena essential to fever, without supposing any change induced on the fluids.

XXI.

The proximate cause of fever therefore is a change in the laws of excitability ; in consequence of which the same agents no longer produce the same effects.

XXII.

In simple fever then there are only two indications of cure ; the one to moderate excitement, the other to remove atony. (XV. XVI.)

CHAP. IV.

Of the Treatment of Continued Fever.

W E may observe, in perusing the works of medical writers, that there are two general principles, on the one or other of which the treatment of fevers has been conducted.

In speaking of the modus·operandi of the medicines employed during the paroxysm of an ague, it was observed, that such is the constitution of the animal system, that any extraneous body introduced into, and injuring any part of it, excites certain motions which tend to expel the offending cause ; and facts illustrating this observation were adduced. This property has been termed the *Vis Medicatrix Naturæ.*

It has long been a favourite opinion among physicians, and perhaps it is a just one, that fever arises from this property, that it is an effort of the system to expel some offending cause or restore the vigour of some debilitated part, that is, that the causes of fever in consequence of the peculiar mechanism of the animal machine excite motions calculated to expel them from the body, or repair the injury they have done.

This opinion led physicians to mark with care the phænomena of fever, when left to run its natural course ; and in their plans of cure to attempt nothing more but to regulate and promote the salutary efforts of nature.

Others observing, that fevers, left to run their natural course, often terminated fatally ; and being aware, that the operations of nature are but ill understood, have constructed their plan of treatment on a different principle. Their attention has been directed to ascertain the symptoms which denote danger, and paying little attention to the operation of the Vis Medicatrix, they have endeavoured to obviate these symptoms.

Both modes of practice have occasionally been found successful; and from both we are to extract what experience has proved to be valuable. In the one, our practice is wholly empirical. We observe, for instance, that spontaneous sweating frequently attends the change from fever to health; we therefore endeavour to induce this symptom; but are wholly ignorant of the manner in which it acts in removing the disease. The other mode of practice is founded on our knowledge of the animal œconomy. If, for instance, the action of the heart and arteries is so violent as to threaten danger, that knowledge teaches us that their action may be moderated by diminishing the quantity of the stimulus which supports it. It is only in the latter mode of treatment therefore that we can properly lay down indications. All that can be said of the former, is simply to relate what parts of it have proved serviceable.

This I shall do before entering on what may be called the general plan of cure, in which our endeavours are directed to obviate the symptoms indicating danger, because confounding the other with this mode of treatment, which is better understood, tends to involve the whole in obscurity.

When speaking of the crises of fevers, I had occasion to consider an opinion, very prevalent among those who attempt to promote the operations of nature, that the peculiar symptoms termed critical, are always the cause of the relief which attends their appearance. From which they inferred, that a principal part of the treatment of fevers, consists in inducing these symptoms. Let us endeavour to determine to what extent this inference is just.

SECT. I.

Of the Means of stopping a Fever at its Commencement, by inducing a Crisis.

IT is only at the commencement of fever, we shall find, that we can attempt to induce a crisis, or at least that the attempt ever proves wholly successful. It was formerly observed, that it is only at an early period that spontaneous crises occur. A fever seldom terminates spontaneously by a crisis after the 10th or 12th day; and a crisis is rarely induced by art after the 3d or 4th. The nearer to the commencement of the fever the attempt is made, the better is the chance of success.

It appears from what was said of the crises of fever, that the symptoms most frequently critical are, the furfuraceous or lateritious sediments of the urine, sweat, vomiting, diarrhœa, hemorrhagy, eruptions, swelling and suppuration of glandular and other parts, and cold chills followed by the other symptoms of the paroxysm of an intermittent. We are now to enquire what advantage has arisen from inducing these symptoms by art, and what means are to be employed for this purpose.

We can only induce the critical sediments of the urine by re-moving the fever, or inducing sweat, so that of this symptom there is nothing to be said here.

The propriety of inducing sweat, a point of much importance in the treatment of fevers, Dr. Cullen has considered at some length. I shall quote his observations, making the additional re-marks which the experience of others has supplied.

" A third means, " he observes, " of determining to the sur-" face of the body, and taking off the spasm subsisting there, is " by the use of sudorific medicines and of sweating.

" The propriety of this remedy has been much disputed, and " specious arguments may be adduced both for, and against the " practice.

" In favour of the practice it may be said,

" 1. That in healthy persons, in every case of increased action " of the heart and arteries, a sweating takes place, and is seeming-" ly the means of preventing the bad effects of such increased ac-" tion.

" 2. That in fevers their most usual solution and termination " is by spontaneous sweating.

" 3. That even when excited by art, it has been found mani-" festly useful at certain periods and in certain species of fever.

" Upon the other hand, it may be urged against the practice of " sweating,

" 1. That as in fevers a spontaneous sweating does not imme-" diately come on, so there must be in these some circumstances " different from those in the state of health, and which may " therefore render it doubtful whether the sweating can be safely " excited by art.

" 2. That in many cases the practice has been attended with " bad consequences. The means commonly employed have a " tendency to produce an inflammatory diathesis'; which if not " taken off by the sweat following their use, must be increased " with much danger. Thus, sweating employed to prevent the " accessions of intermitting fevers, has often changed them into " a continued form, which is always dangerous..

" 3. The utility of the practice is farther doubtful, because " sweating, when it happens, does not always give a final deter-" mination, as must be manifest in the case of intermittents, as well " as in many continued fevers, which are sometimes at the begin-" ning attended with sweatings, which do not prove final, but on " the contrary, whether spontaneous or excited by art, seem of-" ten to aggravate the disease.

" From these considerations, it is extremely doubtful if the

" practice of sweating can be admitted very generally; but at
" the same time, it is also doubtful if the failure of the practice or
" the mischiefs said to have arisen from it, have not been owing
" to the improper conduct of the practitioner.

" With respect to this last, it is almost agreed among physi-
" cians,

" 1. That sweating has been generally hurtful when excited by
" stimulant, heating, and inflammatory medicines.

" 2. That it has been hurtful when excited by much external
" heat, and continued with a great increase of the heat of the bo-
" dy.

" 3. That it is always hurtful when it does not soon relieve, but
" rather increases the frequency and hardness of the pulse, the
" anxiety and difficulty of breathing, the head-ach and delirium.

" 4. That it is always hurtful if it be urged when the sweat is
" not fluid, and when it is partial and on the superior parts of the
" body only.

" In these cases it is probable, that either an inflammatory dia-
" thesis is produced, which increases the spasm on the extreme
" vessels, or that from other causes the spasm is too much con-
" firmed to yield easily to the increased action of the heart and ar-
" teries ; and upon either supposition it must be obvious, that ur-
" ging the sweat, as ready to produce a hurtful determination to
" some of the internal parts, may be attended with very great dan-
" ger.

" Though the doubts stated above are to be attended to, and al-
" though the practices above mentioned having been found hurt-
" ful are therefore to be rejected, it still remains true,

" 1. That sweating has certainly been often useful in pre-
" venting the accession of fevers when the times of this have been
" certainly foreseen, and a proper conduct employed.

" 2. That even after fevers have in some measure come on,
" sweating when properly employed, either at the very beginning
" of the disease or during its approach and gradual formation, has
" often prevented their further progress.

" 3. That even after pyrexiæ have continued for some time,
" sweating has been successfully employed in curing them, as
" particularly in the case of rheumatism.

" 4. That certain fevers produced by a very powerful sedative
" contagion, have been generally treated, so far as we yet know,
" most successfully by sweating."

If we compare the last observation with other parts of the quotation, we shall find that it is to be understood in a very limited

sense. Where there is a tendency to a general sweat, which is
accompanied with an abatement of the symptoms, it should be
encouraged ; or even where no such tendency appears, if by the
means about to be pointed out we succeed in bringing out a sweat
which is thin and generally diffused, it seldom fails to bring relief.
There are no other circumstances in which a sweat proves serviceable in continued fever.

If it be brought out by much warmth and heating medicines,
or if it be partial and clammy, it will do no good. Even when
spontaneous, profuse, and general, if not soon attended with an
abatement of the symptoms, it will generally be found to have
no other effect than that of reducing the patient's strength. When
the sweat is partial and clammy, it is needless to encourage it.
When it is profuse without bringing relief, we must always endeavour to check it, by cautiously removing part of the bed clothes,
cooling the air of the room, and allowing the patient to take cool
drink ; while at the same time we endeavour by proper medicines
to remove the debility which is the cause of such sweats. It is
only in the more alarming forms of typhus that these sweats are
apt to appear. Nothing is to be apprehended from checking
them, but the worst consequences to be feared from their continuance.

. It sometimes happens in this fever that very debilitating sweats
occur, which yet relieve the febrile symptoms. In such cases
we can only attempt to moderate the sweating, and obviate its
hurtful effects, by employing the means which tend to restore the
vigour of the system ; which will be considered at length in the
general plan of treatment.

. " These instances," Dr. Cullen continues, " are in favour of
" sweating, but give no general rule, and it must be left to fur-
" ther experience to determine how far any general rule can be
" established in this matter. In the mean time, if the practice
" of sweating is to be attempted, we can venture to lay down the
" following rules for the conduct of it.

" 1. That it should be excited without the use of stimulant,
" inflammatory medicines.

" 2. That it should be excited with as little external heat and
" with as little increase of the heat of the body as possible.

" 3. That when excited, it should be continued for a due length
" of time, not less than twelve hours, and sometimes for twenty-
" four or forty-eight hours ; always however providing that it pro-
" ceeds without the circumstances mentioned ;" that is, provided
it relieves the symptoms, and is not partial and clammy.

" 4. That for some part of the time, and as long as the person
" can easily bear, it should be carried on without admitting of
" sleep.

"5. That it should be rendered universal over the whole body; "and therefore particularly that care be taken to bring the sweat"ing to the lower extremities.

"6. That the practice should be rendered safer by moderate "purging excited at the same time." The propriety of this regulation seems very doubtful. It appears, from a variety of observations, that the only purpose for which we ought to move the body while we are endeavouring to promote sweat, is the regular expulsion of the fæces; and clysters in these cases are preferable to cathartics, because they are less apt to check the perspiration.

"7. That it should not be suddenly checked by cold any how "applied to the body.

"When attention is to be given to these rules, the sweating "may be excited, 1. By warm bathing, or a fomentation of the "lower extremities. 2. By frequent draughts of tepid liquors, "chiefly water rendered more grateful by the addition of a light "aromatic, or more powerful by that of a small quantity of wine. "3. By giving some doses of neutral salts; most effectually and "perhaps most safely by a large dose of an opiate, joined with a "portion of neutral salts, and of an emetic.

"In what cases may cold water, thrown into the stomach in "large quantities, be employed to excite sweating? See Celsus, "lib. iii. chap. viii.—ix."

These means it will be necessary to consider at greater length.

The employment of wine and opium in fevers will be considered in the general plan of treatment. Practitioners have now very generally abandoned the practice of giving wine with a view to promote sweat in fevers; and opium is rarely employed with this view except in intermittents,* or in small doses to aid other medicines.

Nauseating doses of emetics are more frequently employed for the purpose of promoting sweat in continued fever. The following are the circumstances to be attended to in their exhibition.

1. Both because a fever is seldom terminated critically after it has lasted for a considerable time; and because nauseating doses of emetics are debilitating either by promoting sweat† or catharsis; they have been found most useful at an early period.

2. They may often be employed with advantage at later periods if given about the commencement of the exacerbations, when these are distinctly marked.

* See the treatment of an intermittent during the paroxysm, in book i. of this vol.

† They are most apt to promote sweat when given with small doses of opium. When given alone however they generally have more or less of this effect, which should be promoted by the use of mild tepid liquors.

3. When much debility is expected, and they do not soon relieve the symptoms, we should not persevere in exhibiting them.

Ipecacuanha and the preparations of antimony are the medicines usually employed. The latter are preferable, both because they more powerfully promote the action of the skin, and because small doses of ipecacuanha are more apt to excite vomiting. James's powder and tartar emetic are the preparations of antimony at present generally used in fevers. Most practitioners prefer James's powder. How far this preference is well founded it is difficult to say ; tartar emetic has the advantage of our being able with more certainty to regulate its dose.

The power of neutral salts in promoting diaphoresis is seldom considerable, although almost all of them seem to possess this property in a greater or less degree. The salts composed of an acid and ammonia, particularly the saline mixture, prepared with ammonia and given in a state of effervescence, or the aqua ammoniæ acctatæ, (the spiritus mindereri) seem to possess this property in a greater degree than others.

But the means of promoting diaphoresis in fevers which chiefly demand attention, is the external and internal use of cold and warm water ; which from the observations which have lately been made on it, promises to form an important part of the treatment in these diseases.

The external and internal use of water, both cold and warm, is employed in fevers for other purposes besides that of promoting sweat. I shall therefore have occasion to mention it in other parts of the treatment. It will be the most distinct plan however to give at once view the result of the observations which have been made on it, and when I have occasion to mention it afterwards to refer to what I am to say here.

I. Of the employment of *cold* water in fevers.

Both the external and internal use of cold water in fevers was known to the ancients ; but among the moderns, it is only lately that the former has demanded much attention. Washing the body with cold water is said to have been first practised in fevers, in modern times, at Breslaw in Silesia ;* and it appears that the practice was followed in some of the neighbouring countries. The external use of cold water in fevers however has never been prevalent in Europe, perhaps as Dr. Currie supposes from the manner in which it should be regulated not having been understood.

Several late practitioners in sultry climates, particularly in the West Indies, have employed it freely ; and in 1786, Dr. Wm.

---

* See a Dissertation entitled, Epidémia Verna quæ Wratislaviam anno 1737 afflixit, in Act. Nat. Curios. vol. X.

Wright, who had practised for many years in the island of Jamaica, gave an account of some cases of fever successfully treated by the affusion of cold water, in the London Medical Journal. Dr. Wright has since published some additional observations on the same subject, in a letter to Dr. Garthshore, in the 7th vol. of the Medical Facts and Observations, in which he gives an account of Dr. Gregory's manner of employing this remedy, and the success which attended its use in the Royal Infirmary of Edinburgh; and in the 2d vol. of Annals of Medicine, he again gives a favourable testimony of its effects in the fevers of the West Indies. Dr. Jackson* and others also employed this remedy. Even the alternation of the warm bath and affusion of cold water has been practised in thess fevers, and it is said with the best effects. But no other writer has bestowed so much attention on the use of cold water in fevers, and so accurately observed its effects, as Dr. Currie of Liverpool.†

1. The manner of using cold water externally in fever.

The most effectual way of employing cold water externally in fever is by affusion. The patient is stripped naked, and a bucket of cold water is thrown over him. The temperature of the water should be from 40° to 60°; the quantity from three to five gallons.

Dr. Wright used sea water; Dr. Currie at first used fresh water, afterwards fresh water and vinegar, lastly a saturated solution of common salt. " I was led," the latter author observes, " to prefer salt water to fresh on account of the stimulating effect " of sea salt on the vessels of the skin, by which I apprehend the " debilitating action of cold is prevented. Salt water, either for " the purpose of immersion or affusion, is more grateful to the " patient than fresh water; and it is well known that it may be " applied to the surface for a length of time with much less hazard. " Persons immersed in sea water, and especially in saturated brine, " for some time together, preserve the lustre of the eye and the " ruddiness of the cheek longer than those in fresh water of an " equal temperature; and such persons exhibit the vital reaction " stronger when removed from it."

Dr. Currie used a saturated brine in preference to vinegar and water, on account of the greater expense of the latter; but thinks that vinegar and water of a proper strength will probably be found preferable to brine. He observes however, that no bad consequences ensued from performing the affusion without the addition of either salt or vinegar.

2. The period of the disease proper for the external use of cold water.

* See Dr. Jackson's Treatise on the Fevers of Jamaica.
† See Dr. Currie's Treatise entitled, Medical Reports on the effects of water cold and warm as a remedy in fever and other diseases.

The proper period of the disease for the employment of the cold affusion is the commencement of the hot stage. It cannot be employed too early, provided the chills are over, and the hot stage completely formed. On the first or second day,* it often puts a stop to the progress of the fever. It rarely has this effect when employed on the third or fourth day, and never at a later period. Still however, during the first eight or ten days, it is found to moderate the symptoms, and shorten the disease. Dr. Currie says he has seen it of service on the eleventh, twelfth, or thirteenth day. At an advanced period however, he observes, the water should not be more than fifteen or twenty degrees below the heat of the body; and in most cases he thinks that after the ninth or tenth day, or earlier if the patient be much debilitated, washing the body with tepid vinegar and water answers better than the cold affusion. He also observes, that injury is done by continuing the employment of the cold affusion during the period of convalescence; an application of cold, safe in the violence of fever, often proving hurtful after the fever is removed.

Dr. Currie frequently employed the cold affusion twice in the day, at noon and in the evening. When it was only employed once in the day, the evening was found the properest time. " The safest and most advantageous time," he observes, " for " using the aspersion or affusion of cold water, is when the ex- " acerbation is at its height, or immediately after its declination " is begun; and this has led us almost always to direct it to be " employed from six to nine o'clock in the evening."

3. The effects of the external use of cold water in fever.

The immediate effects of the cold affusion are a diminution of the temperature and frequency of the pulse, which are soon followed by diaphoresis and sleep.

In the following quotation Dr. Currie enumerates the cautions to be e in view, in having recourse to this remedy.

" lk If the aspersion of cold water," he observes, " on the " surface of the body be used during the cold stage of the parox- " ysm of fever, the respiration is nearly suspended; the pulse " becomes fluttering, feeble, and of an incalculable frequency; " the surface and extremities become doubly cold and shrivelled, " and the patient seems to struggle with the pangs of instant dis- " solution. I have no doubt from what I have observed, that in " such circumstances the repeated affusion of a few buckets of " cold water would extinguish life. This remedy therefore should " never be used when any considerable sense of chilliness is pre- " sent, even although the thermometer applied to the trunk of the " body should indicate a degree of heat greater than usual." In the 37th and 38th pages of his Treatise, Dr. Currie relates a stri-

* That is, if the cold chills have ceased, and the hot fit is completely formed at so early a period.

king instance of the bad effects of the cold affusion employed during the chills.

" Neither ought it to be used when the heat measured by the
" thermometer is less than, or even only equal to, the natural heat,
" though the patient should feel no degree of chilliness. This is
" sometimes the case towards the last stages of fever, when the
" powers of life are too weak to sustain so powerful a stimulus.

" It is also necessary to abstain from the use of this remedy
" when the body is under profuse perspiration ; and this caution
" is more important in proportion to the continuance of this per-
" spiration. In the commencement of perspiration, especially
" if it has been brought on by violent exercise, the affusion of
" cold water on the naked body, or even immersion in the cold
" bath, may be hazarded with little risk, and sometimes may be
" resorted to with great benefit." The justness of this observation is doubtful, at least not fully established. Dr. Currie relates
a case (p. 40 and 41) in which the cold affusion was employed at
the commencement of perspiration, and although the event proved favourable, yet it suddenly produced a degree of cold in the
extremities that was alarming, and had not the temperature at the
time of affusion been very high, (106°) it is probable that it would
have had worse effects. " After the perspiration has continued
" for some time and flowed freely, especially if the body has re-
" mained at rest, either the affusion or immersion* is attended
" with danger, even though the heat of the body at the moment
" of using them be greater than natural. Perspiration is always
" a cooling process in itself, but in bed it is often prolonged by
" artificial means, and the body is prevented from cooling under
" it to the natural degree, by the load of heated clothes.
" When the heat has been thus artificially kept up, a practitioner,
" judging by the information of his thermometer only, may be
" led into error. In this situation however I have observed that
" the heat sinks rapidly on the exposure of the surface of the body
" even to the external air ; and that the application of cold water
" either by affusion or immersion is accompanied by a loss of heat
" and a deficiency of reaction, which are altogether inconsistent
" with safety."

* * *

" When employed in the advanced stages of fever, where the
" heat is reduced and the debility great, some cordial should be
" given immediately after it, and the best is warm wine."

Almost all the trials which have been made with the cold affusion have been in contagious fevers,† that is, in those fevers in

* The immersion is more troublesome and less beneficial than the affusion. The former was the manner in which the ancients used this remedy in fevers.

† The cold affusion has also been employed in intermitting fever ; and

which more or less of the synocha is succeeded by a greater degree of the typhus, which forms the chief part of the complaint. It is while the symptoms of synocha last, however, as appears from the foregoing observations, that the cold affusion is most beneficial. How far it is proper in the fevers arising from cold, &c. in which the synocha prevails through the greater part of the complaint, still remains to be determined.

Dr. Currie relates many striking proofs of the good effects of the cold affusion in contagious fevers; one of the most remarkble is, that, of seventeen soldiers attacked with a fever of this kind, all of whom were immediately subjected to the cold affusion once or twice a day, in fifteen the fever was cut short, in two it went through its ordinary course.

What Dr. Currie calls the cool affusion, is a milder form of the cold; the temperature of the water employed in the cool affusion is from 75° to 87°. This is recommended where from the debility of the patient, or continuance of the disease, the cold affusion is judged to be hazardous.

Washing the body with cold water, or cold water and vinegar, is also a milder, though less effectual, way of using this remedy, and may be employed with advantage when the patient refuses to submit to the affusion. The same cautions however are still to be attended to, whether we recommend affusion, immersion, or simply washing the body. When there is a sense of burning in the palms and soles of the feet, keeping them moistened with vinegar is often very beneficial, and always safe and refreshing.*

With respect to the internal use of cold water, Dr. Currie's conclusions correspond with those which have been made by others, and indeed by most practitioners in the course of their own practice. Cold water is not to be used as a drink in the cold stage. It increases the chills and other symptoms of this period. After the hot stage is completely formed, and especially when the heat is considerably above the healthy degree, there are few things either more grateful or more beneficial than large draughts of cold water. They produce the same effects as the cold affusion, but in a less degree, diminishing the heat and frequency of the pulse, and disposing to sensible perspiration and sleep.

After the sweat has become general, cold water is inadmissible. " At this time," Dr. Currie observes, " I have perceived in more " than one instance, an inconsiderate draught of cold water pro- " duce a sudden chilliness both on the surface and at the stomach,

from what is said in the 31st and following pages of Dr. Currie's Treatise, it is probable that it will be found an effectual means of shortening the hot fit. On the effects of the cold affusion in intermittents, however, observations are still wanting. Dr. Currie also used the cold affusion with success as a means of preventing the accession of the paroxysm, when the strength was sufficient to bear this remedy in the absence of the fever.

* See Dr. Currie's Treatise, p. 71.

" with great sense of debility and much oppression and irregula-
" rity of respiration. At such times, on applying the thermome-
" ter to the surface, the heat has been found suddenly and greatly
" reduced. The proper remedy is to apply a bladder filled with
" water heated from 110°, to 120° to the scrobiculus cordis, and
" to administer small and frequent doses of tincture of opium, as
" recommended by Dr. Rush. By these means the heat is spee-
" dily restored."

Dr. Currie remarks however, that at the commencement of the
sweat, before it flows freely and where the heat is considerable,
a draught of cold water will often reduce the temperature to the
degree at which perspiration flows more freely, and thus bring the
fever to a speedier issue.

From the foregoing observations it appears, that the action of
cold drink in fevers, is in every respect similar to, but less powerful than, that of the cold affusion, and that the same cautions are
necessary in the exhibition of both.

II. Of the use of warm water in fevers.

The tepid affusion is performed in the same way as the cold.
There is no addition made to the water, and the proper temperature is from 87° to 97°. When the water is applied by immersion it should be some degrees colder.

It may appear at first view, that the tepid affusion would be a
means of raising the temperature of the body; that it should be
employed where the cold affusion is improper; and avoided in
cases where the latter is found beneficial. All this is contradicted
however by the trials which have been made with it. " At first,"
the author just mentioned observes, " I imagined that the tepid
" affusion might be beneficial in cases where the heat of the body
" is below the degree necessary to render the cold affusion safe.
" I employed it therefore in those stages of fever where the heat
" did not exceed the temperature of health. A little experience
" however convinced me that this practice was not without hazard,
" for I found that in many cases at least the heat of the human
" body is lowered as speedily by the affusion of tepid water, as by
" the affusion of water that is cold. If I mistake not, the heat is
" lowered more speedily by the tepid water."

It appears from Dr. Currie's observations, that the tepid affusion is beneficial in all those cases of fever, and in those only, in
which the cold affusion has been found so; but that the effects of
the former are much less permanent. He never saw the tepid
affusion stop the progress of fever.

The effects of immersion in tepid water however do not correspond with those of the tepid affusion. The tepid bath is always
improper where the temperature is considerable, and often serviceable when it has fallen too low.

The same may be said of the internal use of warm water in fover. During the cold fit, or in a more advanced stage, when the temperature has fallen below the healthy degree, warm drink is proper; and where the temperature is not much above this degree, tepid drink assists the operation of other sudorifics. The drink should also be tepid after the sweating has commenced, by whatever means induced, except in those debilitating sweats which occur in typhus, and reduce the strength without bringing relief, the means of checking which have been pointed out. With these exceptions, cold drink is more beneficial in fevers.

It will be necessary afterwards to make some additional observations on the internal use of water as a means of diminishing excitement.

Such are the means of promoting sweat in fevers,* and the circumstances in which this ought to be attempted.

The crises we are next to consider, are vomiting and diarhœa, concerning which a very few words will be sufficient.

Spontaneous vomiting at an early period is often serviceable; and excited by art on the first or second day it seems sometimes to cut short the disease.† At a more advanced period however it is rarely beneficial, and when there is much debility always hurtful.

* To these means may be added the use of mercury, which is very generally recommended by the practitioners of sultry climates, and whose good effects seem in part, but not chiefly, to depend on its diaphoretic property. " By calomel," Dr. Wright observes, " the pores of the " skin were opened, a resolution of the fever was brought about, and the " patient happily recovered." In another place he observes, " And we " recollect no instance, where mercury had been freely given, and " persevered in till it shewed itself in the mouth, which was not attended " with the happiest consequence." . ,

Dr. Chisholm gave mercury to a very great extent, endeavouring as soon as possible to excite a salivation. He sometimes gave ten grains every three hours till this effect was produced, by which means he observes he has succeeded in cases which seemed desperate.

It is probable however that these observations will not be found to apply to the fevers of this country. I have already had occasion to remark, that the fevers of sultry latitudes are generally accompanied with some local affection. For many of these, mercury is found a powerful remedy.

Dr. Chisholm is one of the few practitioners who have given us any account of the appearances on dissection after death in the fevers of sultry latitudes. From his dissections it appears that, besides other local affections, the liver, as indeed might be inferred from the symptoms of most of the fevers of the West-Indies, was almost always diseased. The benefit derived from mercury in affections of this organ has been well ascertained by the observations of a variety of authors on the hepatitis. It is owing to the local affections which attend the fevers of sultry latitudes, that their treatment is so difficult, and that that which succeeds in one epidemic is often hurtful in another.

† See Dr. Lind on Fevers and Infections.

Diarhœa we have seen sometimes proves critical in fevers ; it is a crisis however which we never attempt to induce. We often indeed excite a moderate catharsis with another view, which will be pointed out in the general plan of treatment.

We shall there also consider at length the cases of fever in which venesection ought to be employed. Venesection, that is, artificial hemorrhagy, seldom perhaps never proves a crisis in fever. Its only effect appears to be that of diminishing excitement. It is therefore unnecessary to say any thing here of hemorrhagy.

With respect to eruptions and glandular swellings, these are symptoms which we have it not in our power to induce. There is a succedaneum for them however, if I may be allowed the expression, which is sometimes serviceable ; I mean blisters and rubefacients.

The first observation to be made on the use of blisters is, that they are improper both in the well marked synocha, and in the worst forms of typhus. In the former their irritation increases the excitement ; in the latter, which is generally attended with a disposition to gangrene, they are often the means of inducing it.* The species of continued fever therefore in which blisters are chiefly employed is the typhus mitior, or what is commonly called the nervous fever. And respecting the propriety of employing them even in this fever, unattended by any local affection, there is much difference of opinion.

No author has given so favourable a testimony of the effects of blisters in the typhus mitior as Dr. Lind. He recommends their application at an early period, and observes, that " In a " moderate infectious fever, where the source of infection is not " very violent, if twenty patients be blistered, sixteen will next " morning be entirely free from head-ach, heat, pain, and fe- " ver." Dr. Cullen was also a strong advocate for the use of blisters in fever ; but thought that they are employed with most advantage at an advanced period of the disease. " It appears to " me that blistering may be employed at any period of continued " fever ; but that it will be of most advantage in the advanced " state of such fevers, when the reaction being weaker, all ambi- " guity from the stimulant power of blistering is removed."

When we compare these with the observations of other authors, however, we cannot help suspecting that both Dr. Cullen and Dr. Lind formed too favourable an opinion of this remedy. " Whether exciting inflammation," says Dr. Fordyce, " has or " has not the same effect in a regular continued fever, which it

---

* See the observations of Sir John Pringle, Mr. Clark, and others. A thick tough matter, like leather, covering blistered parts, shews a tendency to gangrene. " If under this," Dr. Lind observes, " white or ruddy " specks appear, it is a favourable symptom ; if pale or dark, a very " bad one."

" has in health, can only be known by making these applications
" to the body of a person affected with regular continued fever.
" As far as the author's experience goes, when any stimulus has
" been employed so as to produce inflammation, when a patient
" has become weak towards the end of a regular continued fe-
" ver, the only difference which has occurred has been, that
" phlegmonous inflammation has not produced hardness, fulness,
" and strength of the pulse ; but both phlegmonous inflamma-
" tion and inflammation of the skin have occasioned greater fre-
" quency of the pulse, have rendered it weaker and smaller, and
" as in health have prevented sleep, and the patient taking the
" same quantity of nourishment, and have depressed and deranged
" the whole system."*

Sir John Pringle observes, that blisters were only of service
in the jail fever when the patient was threatened with an inflammatory affection of the brain. " Blisters before *useless* became
" then of service."† He also remarks of the inflammatory fever,
that at first he used to employ blisters at an advanced period of
the disease, when he thought the patient could not bear any further loss of blood, but afterwards confined their use to those cases
where the head-ach was considerable, which they seldom failed
to relieve.

" Notwithstanding my having watched the effects of blisters,"
Dr. Moore‡ observes, " with all the attention I am capable of,
" and formerly with a strong prepossession in their favour, I can-
" not assert that I ever knew vesications of any use in this dis-
" ease," the typhus mitior, " but I have frequently seen the pa-
" tient teazed by their irritating quality without their seeming to
" have any other effect."

Upon the whole, although it is probable that the observations of
Dr. Cullen and Dr. Lind are not wholly without foundation, those
of the majority of writers tend to prove that little is to be expected from blisters in fevers unaccompanied by local affections. For
the removal of many of these, they are among the most powerful remedies we possess. They are often employed with advantage in fevers for the removal of coma or delirium. When used
with this view, the head should be shaved, and the blister applied
over it. For like other local remedies, blisters are the more
powerful in relieving local affections, the nearer they are applied
to the part affected.||

* Dr. Fordyce's third Dissertation on Fever.

† Observations on the Diseases of the A: my.

‡ Medical Sketches.

|| Blisters sometimes occasion a degree of strangury from the absorption
of the cantharides ; this effect may generally be prevented or removed
by small doses of camphire or merely by dilution. Some anoint the part
to be blistered by camphorated oil. It is difficult to say, whether the
small quantity of camphire which may be absorbed in this way is of any
service.

With respect to rubefacients, they are still more improper than blisters in the synocha, because they occasion an equal or greater degree of irritation, and are unattended by any discharge. In the worst forms of typhus indeed they are safer than blisters; even rubefacients however may be the means of inducing gangrene, where there is much tendency to it, and it does not appear, that in any kind of typhus, unattended by local affections, rubefacients have been found serviceable. Mustard poultices applied to the feet are often employed with advantage when coma supervenes on the typhus mitior.*

Such are the circumstances respecting the artificial inflammation of the skin in fevers which deserve attention; a practice probably suggested by the relief which sometimes attends spontaneous eruptions in these complaints.

With regard to the last symptom mentioned among the crises of fevers, shivering followed by the other symptoms of the paroxysm of an intermittent, as we have no means capable of inducing it, there is nothing to be said of it here.

SECT. II.

Of the Treatment of Continued Fever when we fail to induce a Crisis at its Commencement.†

When we fail to induce a crisis at the commencement of continued fever by some of the means which have been pointed out, which very frequently happens, we are then from our knowledge of the animal œconomy, assisted by the experience we have had of the effects of a variety of remedies which have been employed in fever, to endeavour to moderate or remove the symptoms which indicate danger; nor is this part of the treatment to be neglected while we are attempting to induce a crisis, if such symptoms shew themselves, which they seldom do at the commencement of the fevers of this country.

For conducting this, the most important part of the treatment

* It is the custom in such cases to apply rubefacients to the feet. This practice originated from the doctrine of derivation; according to which a congestion of blood in any part of the system is best relieved by occasioning a determination of blood to the part most distant from that affected. We have every reason to believe, that in the case mentioned in the text, rubefacients like other local means would be found most useful applied to the head, that is, as near the part affected as possible. The same prejudice once influenced the employment of blood-letting, and it was the practice in affections of the head to let blood from the feet.

† With respect to the modus operandi of the medicines employed in continued fevers, I shall as we proceed, in considering the treatment of these complaints, make such observations as the state of our knowledge permits, in addition to what was said on this part of the subject when speaking of intermittents. It is unnecessary to make a separate section for the few observations which remain to be made on this head.

of continued fever, there are two indications, which were pointed out in the last chapter, namely,

1. In the synocha, to change excessive into moderate excitement.

2. In the typhus, to change atony into moderate excitement.

The first of these indications is answered by avoiding the application of some of the natural agents, and diminishing the quantity applied, or stimulating power of others.

The second is answered,

1. By removing as far as can be done with safety, the natural agents which now act as atonics.

2. By applying those agents which still act as stimuli.

I. *Of the Treatment of Synocha.*

The indication of cure in synocha, it has just been observed, is to change the state of excessive into that of moderate excitement; which is effected by avoiding the application of some of the natural agents, and diminishing the quantity applied, or stimulating power of others. Such is the simple outline of the treatment in synocha, and the principle on which our practice in all idiopathic fevers, where the symptoms of synocha prevail, is conducted.

The natural agents which are to be wholly removed in exquisitely formed synocha, and the total removal of which is more or less necessary according as the symptoms are more or less violent, are,

1. All exercise either of body or mind.

2. Every thing which makes an impression on the external senses.

3. All kinds of aliment, and the presence of feculent or other matter in the alimentary canal.

1. Every kind of motion is to be avoided, and that posture preferred which requires least exertion of the muscles, the horizontal. The bed should be soft, that the patient may be as little as possible oppressed with his own weight, and the covering should be light. Speaking, Dr. Cullen justly observes, as it accelerates the respiration, is particularly to be refrained from.

With respect to the mind, whatever excites the attention, whether business or amusement, is hurtful ; and whatever excites the passions, still more so. Every cause of anxiety must be carefully avoided. There are no causes of anxiety more frequent in fever than thirst and a noxious atmosphere.

. The former is to be removed by permitting the patient to drink as freely as he pleases.

A noxious atmosphere is to be avoided by proper ventilation, by permitting only one attendant to remain in the patient's room, by the speedy removal of all excremental matters; and as it is necessary that the patient should not only respire a pure air, but that his body should not be long immersed in its own effluvia,* he should have frequent changes of linen, than which there is nothing more refreshing to febrile patients. The linen should not be warmed; it is sufficient that it is dry. In all kinds of fever, except where the temperature is below the healthy degree, the cooler it is the better. Even while the symptoms of synocha remain distinctly marked, if the disease has arisen from contagion, the body of the patient is found to generate it. In such cases therefore, to the foregoing means of preserving the purity of the air, should be added occasionally some of those for destroying or correcting the properties of contagion, pointed out when speaking of the causes of continued fever. When synocha arises from cold, or the other causes which more particularly belong to this fever, this set of means are unnecessary till the symptoms of typhus shew themselves.

2. All impressions on the external senses are prejudicial. The patient must be kept quiet, and the light excluded, which is the more necessary as the eyes are generally inflamed when the symptoms of synocha run high. " With respect to avoiding im- " pressions of all kinds," Dr. Cullen observes, " an exception is " to be made in the case of a delirium coming on, when the pre- " senting of accustomed objects may have the effect of interrupt- " ing and diverting the irregular train of ideas then arising in the " mind." This observation however is less applicable to synocha than typhus, both because delirium is a less frequent symptom in synocha, and because when the symptoms run high in synocha, the only case in which delirium is apt to supervene, impressions made on the external senses are most hurtful, and in this fever indeed seem often to induce the delirium.

3. With respect to the agents whose immediate action is on the stomach and intestines, food of every kind is hurtful while the symptoms of synocha run high. But after we have succeeded in moderating the excitement, the patient should be induced to take some of the lighter kinds of aliment; for in the treatment of synocha we must keep in view the state of debility which constantly succeeds. With respect to the drink in synocha, every thing stimulating should be avoided. The best drink in this fever is water, of the use of which I have already had occasion to speak. The diet in continued fever will be considered more particularly when speaking of typhus. It is in that fever that it demands most attention.

* There is reason to believe, that the application of fresh air to the surface is also useful in another way; it has been found, that the air is vitiated by the skin in the same manner as by the lungs, although less rapidly.

While the symptoms of synocha are considerable, we must not only avoid the introduction of aliment, but be careful to free the primæ viæ both of that and any feculent matter which they happen to contain. It has already been observed, that an emetic is often serviceable at the commencement of all kinds of fever. This ought to be followed by a cathartic,* which, when the synocha is well marked, should be repeated till we are assured that the primæ viæ are cleared. It is also proper to employ means for correcting the irritating properties of any part of their contents which may still remain, when such means are known. Thus, acids are found useful when there is much bile in the alimentary canal, and absorbents when there is much acid. It is also useful in most cases of fever, to defend the stomach and bowels against the irritation of their contents, by mixing some mucilaginous matter with the drink. On this account water gruel or barley water is generally preferable to plain water, especially at an early period ; in a more advanced stage the contents of the alimentary canal are for the most part inconsiderable.

The natural agents, the constant presence of which is necessary to existence, and which cannot therefore be wholly removed, are the circulating fluids and caloric. The quantity of these is to be diminished in synocha.

Of the means of diminishing the temperature of the body in synocha.

This is to be done by cool air, cold drink, and the external use of cold or tepid water.

It was observed, when considering cold as a cause of fever, that the temperature of the human body is not diminished by so rare a medium as the air, unless its temperature be under 62° ; nor in air at this temperature is the caloric disengaged by the human body permitted to accumulate so as to become unpleasant; the rapidity with which it is abstracted is duly proportioned to the quantity evolved. But if the body disengage more caloric than in health, a lower temperature will be required for its due abstraction.

This happens both in synocha, and in most cases of typhus.† In these therefore the temperature of the surrounding air should

---

* Calomel, which has already been mentioned as often serviceable in another way in the fevers of warm latitudes, is generally regarded as the best cathartic in these fevers, and many practitioners prefer it to others in the fevers of this country. See the observations of Drs. Wright, Rush, Chisholm, &c.

† We have reason to believe, from a variety of experiments, (see the different works on animal temperature) that, wherever the temperature of the body is increased, the blood in a given space of time passes through the lungs more frequently than in health, and consequently that the rapidity of the circulation is increased. That this should happen in synocha cannot appear surprising ; but in typhus, where the powers supporting

always be below 62°. How much below this, will be determined by the temperature of the patient. In synocha ·the temperature is higher than in typhus. In the former therefore, when there is no tendency to local inflammation, a freer application of cold is proper. In well marked synocha the temperature of the patient's bed-room, when the state of the weather permit us sufficiently to diminish it, should never perhaps exceed 35° or 40°, and may often with advantage be still more diminished.

It is not meant that it would be proper constantly to expose the body to air of this temperature, but it is better that the proper temperature of the body be preserved by covering, that the patient may enjoy the refreshing effects of breathing a cool atmosphere.

' When the temperature of the surrounding air is too low, there are many evident ways of raising it. The only circumstances to be attended to in raising the temperature of the air in the patient's bed-room are,

1. That it shall be as uniformly raised as possible.

2. That the patient shall not be exposed to a current of air; and

3. That the proper proportion of oxygen gas in the air shall not be diminished.

For the last purpose we have only to take care that no part of the vapour arising from the burning fuel shall be permitted to remain in the room, and that the external air shall have free access.

For heating the patient's bed-room, a stove is preferable perhaps to an open fire, because by it the air may be more uniformly heated, and it is less apt to occasion currents of air. It is not to be overlooked however that a current of air passing through the room, provided the patient is not exposed to it, may for reasons formerly pointed out, be of service in contagious fevers.

It is much to be regretted that we are not possessed of means for lowering equally efficacious with those for raising the temperature of the air.

the circulation are weakened, we should expect to find the circulation less rapid than in health, and consequently a less quantity of caloric disengaged; and this is the case in exquisitely formed typhus, in which the temperature of the body falls below the healthy degree. But in other cases of ·this fever, the increased frequency of contraction in the heart and blood vessels, more than compensating for its feebleness, the rapidity of the circulation is increased, and thus a greater quantity of caloric disengaged.

In determining the temperature in typhus, we should always use the thermometer; if we judge by the feeling, the acrid secretion by the skin which occurs in this fever will generally make the temperature seem higher than it really is. This circumstance is particularly to be attended to in the application of cool air, and the external use of cold and tepid water, in typhus. In the 35th and 36th pages of Dr. Currie's Treatise, above mentioned, he describes the thermometer, and the manner of using it, which he found most convenient.

When from the state of the weather the temperature of the patient's bed-room is too high, which it always is in well marked synocha if it exceed 45°, we have no means capable of diminishing it many degrees; and this seems to be the chief reason of the great fatality of the fevers of warm countries. The hotter the weather, the more fatal the fevers of sultry latitudes are always observed to be; and it is even said of the yellow fever of the West Indies, that the weather becoming very warm or cool while a person labours under it, is often sufficient to save or destroy him.

The only means we have of lowering the temperature of the patient's bed-room in warm weather, is as much as possible to exclude the light, and frequently sprinkle the floor and other parts of the room with cold water.

As in warm countries we cannot diminish the temperature of the air of the bed-room many degrees, other means have been proposed for diminishing that of the patient's body. "Whenever the "patient is in a climate, whose heat is less than 97 degrees of Fa-"renheit's thermometer, which is nearly the heat of the body of "the patient, removing the air which is in immediate contact, "by means of putting the atmosphere in motion by any kind of "fan, renders that which is in immediate contact with the body "much colder than it would otherwise be. Such means in case "of too warm an atmosphere seem to be very proper to be em-"ployed."[*] "When the object is to diminish heat, that may be "obtained with great certainty by the repeated use of the tepid "affusion, suffering the surface of the body to be exposed in the "interval to the external air; and if the beams of the sun are ex-"cluded, and a stream of wind blows over it, the heat may thus "be reduced, where cold water cannot be procured, even in the "warmest regions of the earth—on the plains of Bengal or the "sands of Arabia."[†] Dr. Wright practised a still more effectual method of reducing the febrile heat, but one whose employment requires much caution. "Some lucky expedients, however, "have been practised, which success alone can justify; thus when "the most urgent symptoms had been subdued, the patients were "wrapt up in a wet blanket, a profuse sweat was brought on, and "an immediate recovery was the consequence."[‡]

For farther observations on the external and internal use of water, as means of diminishing the temperature in fever, the reader is referred to what was said when considering the means of inducing sweat.

The most important part of the treatment in synocha still re-

* See Dr. Fordyce's third Dissertation on Fever.

† Dr. Currie's Treatise on the Use of Warm and Cold Water in Fevers, &c.

‡ See Annals of Medicine, vol. ii.

mains to be considered; I mean diminishing the quantity of the circulating fluids.

As the increased excitement of the heart and blood-vessels supports that of every other part of the system; and as it appears, from the observations made when speaking of blood-letting in intermittents and the modus operandi of this remedy, that diminishing the quantity of the blood is the most powerful means of diminishing the action of the heart and blood-vessels; it is not surprising that blood-letting has been found the most effectual remedy in synocha.

It is true indeed, that the mass of circulating fluids may be diminished by other evacuations, by promoting a discharge from the skin, kidneys, or intestines. The two former we have it not always in our power to command, and although we had, there would still remain the same objection to these as to the last, the discharge by the intestines. This objection has already been considered at some length, namely, that in proportion as the evacuation is made more slowly than in blood-letting, it must be carried to a greater extent, in order to produce the same diminution of excitement. On this account it was observed, that purging is to be regarded as a means of diminishing excitement in no other way than by removing from the alimentary canal any cause of irritation, or at most that very mild cathartics are to be employed to aid the more powerful remedy.

" But it is to be observed, that as the fluid drawn from the ex-
" cretories opening into the intestines, is not all drawn imme-
" diately from the arteries, as a part of it is drawn from the mu-
" cous follicles only ; and as what is more immediately drawn
" from the arteries, is drawn off slowly, so the evacuation will
" not, in proportion to its quantity, occasion such a sudden de-
" pletion of the red vessels as blood-letting does, and therefore
" cannot operate so powerfully in taking off the phlogistic diathe-
" sis of the system.

" At the same time as this evacuation may induce a conside-
" rable degree of debility, so in those cases where a dangerous
" state of debility is likely to occur, purging is to be employed
" with a great deal of caution ; and more especially as the due
" measure of the evacuation is more difficult to be applied than in
" the case of blood-letting.

" As we shall presently have occasion to observe, that it is of
" great importance in the cure of fevers to restore the determina-
" tion of the blood to the surface of the body ; so purging, as in
" some measure taking off that determination, seems to be an
" evacuation not well adapted to the cure of fevers."*

Mild cases of synocha indeed often yield to this remedy, to-. gether with the other means just pointed out ; it being only ne-

* See Cullen's First Lines.

cessary in such cases to remove every cause of irritation, wheth- er from without or existing within the body, and the evacuation which the cathartic occasions doubtless promotes recovery. But in more urgent cases, where it is necessary to diminish the vol- ume of blood, this is always best done by venesection.

There are many circumstances to be attended to in the em- ployment of blood-letting in synocha. For the same reason that blood-letting is the most powerful of all remedies in this fever, it is dangerous to employ it needlessly, or in any case to push it too far. If venesection be the most powerful means of dimin- ishing excitement, it is consequently the most apt to induce de- bility ; and this caution is particularly necessary in the synocha, which, if the patient is not carried off, or the fever terminated by a crisis at an early period, is constantly succeeded by a disease of debility.

" When the violence of re-action," Dr. Cullen observes, " and " its constant attendant a phlogistic diathesis, are sufficiently man- " ifest ; when these constitute the principal part of the disease, " and may be expected to continue throughout the whole of it, " as in the cases of synocha ; then blood-letting is the principal " remedy, and may he employed as far as the symptoms of the " disease seem to require, and the constitution of the patient will " bear. It is however to be attended to, that a greater evacuation " than is necessary, may occasion a slower recovery, may ren- " der the person more liable to a relapse, or may bring on other " diseases.

" In the case of synocha* therefore, there is little doubt about " the propriety of blood-letting ; but there are other species of " fevers, as the synochus, in which a violent re-action and phlo- " gistic diathesis appear, and prevail during some part of the " course of the disease, while at the same time these circumstan- " ces do not constitute the principal part of the disease, nor are " to be expected to continue through the whole course of it ; and " it is well known, that in many cases the state of violent re-ac- " tion is to be succeeded, sooner or later, by a state of debility, " from the excess of which the danger of the disease is chiefly " to arise. It is therefore necessary, that in many cases, " blood-letting should be avoided ; and, even although during " the inflammatory state of the disease it may be proper, it will " be necessary to take care, that the evacuation be not so large " as to increase the state of debility which is to follow.

" From all this it must appear, that the employment of blood- " letting in certain fevers requires much discernment and skill, and

* It was formerly observed, that the pure synocha is a fever which we never meet with. At least the term synocha cannot be applied to any fever of this country which lasts above a few days, and those which ter- minate favourably in so short a time are generally very mild ; which seems to be the reason that the state of debility towards their termination either does not supervene, or is inconsiderable.

" It is to be governed by the consideration of the following circum-
" stances:

" 1. The nature of the prevailing epidemic.
" 2. The nature of the remote cause.
" 3. The season and climate in which the disease occurs.
" 4. The degree of phlogistic diathesis present.
" 5. The period of the disease.
" 6. The age, vigour, and phlethoric state of the patient.
" 7. The patient's former diseases and habits of blood-letting.
" 8. The appearance of the blood drawn out.
" 9. The effects of the blood-letting that may have been al-
" ready practised."

In the treatment of fever, it is not always sufficient to study
the symptoms of the case for which we prescribe. If the complaint be epidemic, we must acquire a knowledge of the general
course of the disease, that we may know what symptoms to expect ; for our conduct in the treatment of fever is often regulated
as much by what the state of our patient will be, as by what it is.
If much debility is expected, we must be cautious in recommending evacuations. An attention to the prevailing epidemie, therefore, is mentioned by Dr. Cullen as the first circumstance to be attended to in considering the propriety of blood-letting in fevers.

We are next to attend to the nature of the remote cause.

It appears from what was said of the causes of fever, that an
atmosphere loaded with putrid effluvia is one of the most common,
and that a fever thus produced is afterwards communicated by its
peculiar contagion. All fevers, it was observed, arising from putrid effluvia or contagion, whatever be the state of the patient at
the time he is attacked, or the nature of the symptoms at an early
period, will soon assume the form of typhus. In such cases
therefore blood-letting is seldom admissible, even although the
excitement at the commencement be considerable.

When, on the contrary, the fever has arisen from cold, from
strong passions, violent exercise, &c. although we know, that if
it be protracted for many days, the symptoms of synocha will be
succeeded by those of typhus, yet we have reason to believe, that
the synocha will form the principal part of the complaint, and that
if the excitement be not permitted to run high at the commencement, the debility towards the termination will not be considerable.
In these fevers therefore blood-letting is more frequently proper.

The season, climate, and even situation, are not to be overlooked in prescribing blood-letting in fevers.

On this part of the subject some observations were made when
speaking of the employment of blood-letting in intermittents.

This remedy is most to be dreaded in those circumstances in which the fever is apt suddenly to assume the form of typhus; both because in these cases the symptoms of debility are generally more alarming than where the change is more gradual; and because the typhus supervening soon after the blood-letting, is often attended with fatal consequences.

The changes of fevers are more sudden in sultry than in cold and temperate climates, and in large cities than in the country; in autumn than in spring. In sultry climates it is often difficult to determine what is best to be done. At the commencement, the symptoms are sometimes so violent as to endanger life; and yet we have no means of diminishing the excitement without the risque of involving the patient in dangers no less alarming.

In perusing the works of those who have practised in warm climates, we find them much divided in their opinion respecting the employment of blood-letting in fevers. Some advising the liberal use of the lancet; and others, having frequently experienced its dangerous consequences, almost binding themselves by a solemn engagement never to recommend it again in idiopathic fevers within the tropics.

In this, as in most other cases, extremes are to be avoided. And there is reason to believe, that we give the patient the best chance of recovery, if we never in such climates recommend blood-letting in idiopathic fever, except when the violence of the excitement threatens to prove fatal, either by carrying off the patient in the height of the synocha, or by the debility which always follows violent excitement, and then only push it to that extent which the urgency of the symptoms absolutely requires. What the symptoms are which mark this degree of excitement, I shall presently endeavour to point out.

Although the changes of fever are more sudden, and consequently blood-letting more dangerous, in large cities than in the country, even in temperate climates; yet this case never proves as perplexing as the former. In the populous cities of temperate climates, the excitement at the commencement of fevers is generally moderate, and there is no occasion for the copious evacuations which some employ.

In most of these fevers venesection is improper. All that is necessary in general is to moderate the excitement at their commencement, by clearing the primæ viæ, and other gentle means, till the fever has assumed the form of typhus, and then we must treat it as such. Whether blood-letting is ever proper in typhus, will be considered in laying down the treatment of that species of fever. The same observation applies to the autumnal fevers of temperate climates; the excitement is rarely such as warrants the use of blood-letting.

The next circumstance which demands attention in recommending blood-letting in idiopathic fever, is the degree of excitement present.

In determining the degree of excitement which warrants blood-letting, we are influenced by the observations just made ; for the same degree of excitement which would induce us to recommend this remedy when the epidemic partakes much of the synocha, does not warrant its employment when the prevalent symptoms are those of typhus.

The same degree of excitement which indicates blood-letting when the fever has arisen from cold, from rage, or violent exercise, does not indicate it in fevers from putrid effluvia or contagion. In the latter case, although the excitement at an early period be considerable, we know that the nature of the fever will soon overcome it. In the other, if the excitement is not diminished at the commencement, there is reason to believe that it will increase, while at the same time we know that the debilitating effects of blood-letting in this case are less to be dreaded.

Let the nature of the fever be what it may, however, the following observation is to be kept in view : That violent excitement is itself a highly debilitating cause, and often debilitates more than a well-timed blood-letting which relieves it.

Lastly, the degree of excitement which warrants blood-letting in the cold and temperate climates and in the country, does not warrant it in sultry climates and large cities, because in the latter cases we in general dread more the diminution than the excess of excitement.

From these observations it is evident, that no general rule can be laid down respecting the degree of excitement in fevers which demands blood-letting. The determination of this question, unless the violence of excitement be extreme, depends as much on the consideration of the circumstances just mentioned, as the symptoms present.

When the excitement is such as to be accompanied with delirium, which when it arises from violent excitement is of the furious kind, or when coma, which more rarely happens, appears in well marked synocha, we must always have recourse to blood-letting.

In temperate climates the symptoms of synocha seldom run so high, and almost never in any of those circumstances which render blood-letting dangerous. In sultry climates they often do, and then as the affection of the brain either in the furious delirium or coma seems to increase the general excitement, (as most local affections allied to inflammation do) it may often be adviseable to try the effects of local means, particularly leeches applied to the head or scarification of the temples, before we have recourse to general blood-letting.

Delirium is mentioned as a symptom denoting a degree of excitement which renders blood-letting necessary in all cases of synocha ; But in general it is indicated by a much less degree. If the face be flushed, the pulse full and strong, and the heat considerable, this remedy to a greater or less extent is usually employed with advantage.*

There are other circumstances to be considered in the employment of blood-letting in fever. Among these is the period of the disease. What was said on this head when speaking of intermitting is nearly applicable to continued fevers. As soon as the symptoms of synocha begin to decline, the proper period for blood-letting is past. Even Huxham, prejudiced as he and most of his cotemporaries were in favour of this remedy, admits in his treatise on fevers, that " bleeding, unless in the beginning, seldom did " service."

· The age, vigour, and plethoric state of the patient are also to be attended to. Young people, it has already been observed, and people in the vigour of life, bear evacuations of all kinds better than those advanced in age. The same may be said of people of a full habit, compared with such as are naturally infirm or reduced by disease or other causes.

The patient's former diseases and habits of blood-letting are also to be considered ; if he has been subject to inflammatory complaints, these are apt to be renewed on slight occasions ; and consequently symptoms indicating their approach must often be removed by more vigorous means than are necessary for the removal of the same symptoms in those who have not been subject to such complaints. If the patient has been in the habit of losing blood, it is often proper to employ this remedy where it would not otherwise have been necessary. Habitual blood-letting produces habitual plethora, which constantly demands a repetition of the same remedy.

We must attend to the appearance of the blood drawn, in order to determine the propriety of repeating the blood-letting.

There are three morbid states of the blood which have particularly demanded the attention of physicians.

1. Where there is much of the inflammatory diathesis, the blood is either more fluid or coagulates more slowly than natural, so that the red globules in part subside before the coagulum is formed. Hence there are no red globules on the upper part of the coagulum, which on this account appears of a buff colour, and has been termed the buffy coat. In different cases it is thicker

* Blood-letting in infants, Vogel observes, is not necessary in the synocha ; nor is it necessary in adults, unless the face be red, the head much pained, the pulse very full, or blood bursts from the nose, except when the mind is deranged, or the fever has arisen from the abuse of spirituous liquors. Prælect. Acad. de Cog. et Cur. Morb.

or thinner, according as the blood has remained fluid for a longer or shorter time. The thicker the buffy coat is, it generally indicates the greater degree of inflammatory diathesis. The buffy coat however, though for the most part, does not universally indicate the presence of this diathesis, nor does it universally appear when the diathesis is present. I shall afterwards have occasion to observe more particularly, that the buffy coat is sometimes, though rarely, absent even in cases of actual inflammation, and now and then it appears when the system is in a state very opposite to the inflammatory diathesis.

The buffy coat may also appear thicker or thinner, or its appearance may be wholly prevented, by the circumstances of the blood-letting. If the blood flows slowly, and is permitted to trickle down the arm, the coagulation will begin before it reaches the vessel, and consequently the red globules, if they subside at all, will subside more slowly. If the blood is received into a broad shallow vessel, it will coagulate more quickly than if received into a narrow deep vessel, and the buffy coat consequently will be thinner in the former case. These circumstances therefore are to be attended to in forming our judgment from the buffy coat.

When this coat appears, the crassamentum is generally firm, and that part which forms this coat being free from red globules, is firmer than the crassamentum of healthy blood, which is every where crowded with globules that diminish its cohesion, in the same way as any other powder would do.

, 2. There is a light kind of blood in which there are comparatively few red globules, and the proportion of water is too great. Such is the state of the blood in many diseases of debility, in the typhus mitior, the different kinds of dropsy, &c.

3. The last kind of blood is found in the vessels of those labouring under typhus gravior and scurvy. It has a dissolved appearance, does not coagulate so readily as healthy blood, the serum is of a redder colour than natural, and the crassamentum of a looser consistence.*

If the blood drawn in fever be of the first kind, if after standing some hours it be covered with the buffy coat, this gives encouragement for repeating the blood-letting, should the symptoms seem to require it.

If, on the contrary, the blood be of the second or last kind, we have committed a serious error in recommending venesection, a repetition of which might destroy the patient.

In determining the propriety of repeating the blood-letting, we must also attend to the effects it has produced. If the symp-

* The different appearances which this kind of blood assumes are well described in a quotation from Dr. Fordyce's third Dissertation on Fever, given when enumerating the symptoms of continued fever.

toms are alleviated, if the pulse from being strong and full becomes nearly natural, and the heat is diminished, there is no occasion for repeating the blood-letting. If the strength is much reduced, if the complaint begins to assume the form of typhus, which sometimes very suddenly happens after an ill-timed or excessive blood-letting, the repetition of this evacuation would be attended with the worst consequences. If, on the other hand, the symptoms continue unabated, the operation must be repeated to at least the same extent. Lastly, if the symptoms still continue, but with a considerable abatement, it will be proper to repeat the blood-letting as soon as they begin to suffer an exacerbation, which very often happens, till the operation has been performed several times.*

It appears from what was said of the modus operandi of blood-letting, that it is the more effectual, the more suddenly the blood is abstracted. On this account it was once the practice to let blood from both the arms at the same time. It is enough however to make the orifice pretty large, a circumstance not always sufficiently attended to by surgeons.

For the same reason that we abstract the blood suddenly, namely, that the action of the powers supporting circulation may be diminished with as little loss of blood as possible ; some have recommended, in those cases where much is to be feared from a considerable loss of blood, to keep the patient more or less in the erect posture during the blood-letting, in order to induce a degree of syncope by a small loss of blood. This in idiopathic fevers is not to be attempted. In certain circumstances, hereafter to be pointed out, I have known it practised in the phlegmasiæ with success, but it requires much caution and discernment to practise it with safety.

In general the horizontal posture is preferred, that we may not be prevented by a tendency to syncope from taking away the proper quantity of blood. In this posture many can bear the loss of 16 or 18 ounces with ease, who could not in the erect posture lose half the qantity without falling into syncope. Every cause which diminishes the flow of blood to the brain tends to induce, and every cause that increases it to prevent, syncope. It is in

---

* It sometimes, though rarely, happens in fevers, that the excitement, instead of being diminished, increases after blood-letting ; a circumstance which might disconcert a practitioner not aware of it. In very plethoric habits the quantity of blood seems sometimes to oppress the powers supporting circulation, so that it is not moved with the rapidity which is necessary to occasion the symptoms of violent excitement. Although (says Van Swieten) the most necessary and only remedy in violent fever is blood-letting, yet it sometimes happens in plethoric people, that after venesection the fever from being low becomes very violent. He relates two cases of this kind, one from Sydenham's works, and another which Boerhaave used to relate in his lectures on fevers. Similar cases are to be found in the works of Dr. Rush and others.

In such cases the blood-letting is to be repeated as in other cases of synocha, till the excitement is sufficiently diminished.

this way that the horizontal posture, by which the flow of blood towards the brain is increased, and its return rendered less rapid, is serviceable in blood-letting.

In general blood-letting, that is, when our only view in letting blood is to relieve a state of general excitement, it is of no consequence from what part of the body the blood is taken. The most convenient place therefore, the arm, is generally chosen. But when there is present any local affection which may be relieved by blood-letting, by abstracting the blood from the part affected or its neigbourhood, the same operation may answer the purpose both of general and local blood-letting. Thus when delirium or coma supervenes in synocha, it is better to take the blood from the jugular vein, if this can be readily made to swell, than from the arm. The following caution is to be attended to in bleeding from the jugular in affections' of the head : to compress that vein alone from which the blood is about to be taken. A ligature thrown round the neck in such cases, though not very tight, may be attended with dangerous consequences.

There is perhaps no case which warrants our carrying blood-letting so far as many of the ancients recommend. Copious and early blood-letting, Hoffman observes, is in no fever more requisite than in the synocha. But we are not to follow the advice of some of the ancients, of letting the blood flow till the patient faints ; it is better to repeat the operation than to take away too much at once. ·'

It is generally regarded as an undoubted maxim in the treatment of fevers, that we are not to let blood, give cathartics, or in any manner disturb the system by medicines, when an eruption, or any other of those symptoms which are esteemed critical, makes its appearance. A question of some consequence, says Hasenhorl, may be considered here, whether it is proper to let blood in fevers when an eruption appears upon the skin. Every one believes, he adds, that we are not by any efforts of art, such as blood-letting, catharsis, vomiting, sweating, to disturb the operations of nature, when there is reason to expect a crisis. He justly observes, however, of this maxim, that " juxta illud vulgare nulla regula sine exceptione," and gives the case of pleurisy as an exception to it. He might have added, not only all cases of visceral inflammation, but those also where an eruption or other critical symptom appears in the synocha without relieving the symptoms.

When the state of the symptoms requires both blood-letting and the exhibition of an emetic, the blood-letting should always precede the emetic. One thing, Sydenham observes, is not be overlooked ; if the condition of the sick be such as to require both vomiting and blood-letting, let the blood-letting precede the emetic ; for I could mention several cases, he continues, in which the efforts of vomiting produced such a flow of blood to the head that a rupture of some of the vessels of the encephalon and a fatal apoplexy were the consequence.

A similar observation applies to blistering, when it is judged necessary at the same time with blood-letting. The blister should be delayed till after the blood-letting, because its irritation will be less hurtful when the excitement has been diminished.

Such are the circumstances to be attended to in the employment of blood-letting in synocha.

Evacuations, however, are not the only means of diminishing the quantity of blood. The quantity of this fluid depends on that of the ingesta, and it may be so diminished by abstinence as in a short time to endanger life.

When the excitement runs very high we recommend both evacuations and abstinence; but when it becomes more moderate, or in cases where it has never been considerable, we recommend neither. It is then sufficient to employ those means which diminish the stimulating power of the blood and ingesta; these I am now to point out.

The last means of fulfilling the indication in synocha are those which diminish the stimulating power of such of the natural agents as cannot be wholly removed. These are, caloric, the circulating fluids, and if the synocha be of considerable duration, food.

We have no means of diminishing the stimulating power of caloric; it is only to the circulating fluids therefore, and food, that this indication applies.

As the quantity of blood cannot be much diminished without debilitating every function of the system, it is of consequence where the symptoms run high, to lessen as much as we can its stimulating power, that the excitement may be diminished with as little evacuation as possible.

The means of diminishing the stimulating power of the blood are,

1. Dilution, and

2. The medicines which have been termed refrigerant.

There is a large proportion of water in the blood, to which it owes its fluidity; and the stimulating power of the blood, its quantity being the same, is inversely as the degree in which its saline and other stimulating parts are diluted. Dilution therefore is the most successful means of diminishing its stimulating power, and that which nature by an increase of thirst points out in all cases of excessive excitement. In typhus there is often little or no thirst; but in synocha it is generally insatiable. Every person in this fever, Van Swieten remarks, unless his intellects be deranged, is led by instinct to demand water and watery liquids.

this instinct best points out the quantity of such liquids which ♦ necessary. We are neither, as was once a practice, and there could not be a more improper one, to prevent the patient from satisfying his thirst, nor to run into the extreme of the Dieta Aquea of the Spanish and Italian physicians, and force the patient to take every day eight or nine pounds of water.[*]

When the excitement is considerable, diluting liquids should also be injected per anum. Sydenham made much use of clysters composed of a mild vegetable decoction and sugar, or of milk and water heated to the proper temperature; and so powerful did he find these means in allaying excitement, that he cautions against the immoderate use of them, least the excitement be brought too low. Celsus has justly observed, that clysters are proper where blood-letting is indicated, but the weakness of the patient prevents us employing it, and in those cases where the period proper for blood-letting is past.

Dilution is also the chief means of diminishing the stimulus of the food. The food of a patient in synocha, when food is judged to be proper in this fever, should consist wholly of mild decoctions, thick barley water, or water gruel, or water thickened with sago.

Fresh acidulous fruits make an excellent addition to this diet. These belong to the head of refrigerants, the last set of medicines in the treatment of synocha.

The chief of this class of medicines are acids and neutral salts. They act by diminishing the stimulating power of the food and blood.

If the contents of the stomach and bowels stimulate more than they ought to do, the frequency of the pulse and heat are increased, and temporary fever is the consequence, which may be relieved, and often wholly removed, by receiving into the stomach a quantity of acid or some neutral salt. Thus people drink lemon juice, or cream of tartar, with distilled spirits, to moderate their stimulus.[†]

Refrigerants also, although in a less degree, allay the atonic power of agents[‡], and on this account many of them, particular-

[*] See an account of the Dieta Aquea, in the 36th volume of the Philosophical Transactions.

[†] It may here be alleged, that refrigerants do not diminish the excitement by diminishing the stimulating power of the blood and food, but by diminishing the excitability of the living solid; and it must be confessed, that it is difficult to determine in which of these ways they act.

[‡] A similar objection may be started here. We cannot determine, and it would be of no consequence in the treatment of fever although we could, whether refrigerants diminish the atonic power of agents, or the atonic state of the living solid. We have reason to believe that they act in the former way, because whatever else tends to correct the atonic state of the living solid, increases excitement, which refrigerants tend to diminish

ly acids, are serviceable in typhus as well as synocha, especially in warm climates. We shall find, however, that in the former, from their tendency to diminish excitement, they must be em-, ployed with caution.

The best refrigerants were pointed out when considering the treatment in the paroxysm of an intermittent. " Some metallic " salts," Dr. Cullen observes, " have been employed as refrige- " rants in fevers, and particularly the sugar of lead. But the " refrigerant powers of this are not well ascertained, and its de- " leterious qualities are too well known to admit of its being " freely used."

Of the Treatment in Typhus.

The indication in typhus, it has been observed, is to change the state of atony into that of moderate excitement ; which is to be effected,

1. By removing as far as can be done with safety the natural agents which now act as atonics ; and

2. By applying those agents which still act as stimuli.

In removing or diminishing the quantity of the natural agents in typhus, one caution is ever to be kept in view ; that we do not weaken the action of the powers necessary to life, whose action in typhus is already weaker than it ought to be. Although therefore we are here, as in synocha, to avoid the application of those agents which excite the animal functions, we must be cautious in diminishing the quantity of those on which the vital functions depend. · It is true indeed that these, like the other natural agents, excite a morbid action in typhus ; but this action is capable of sustaining life for a certain length of time, and we can only re- move it with safety by substituting a more healthy action in its stead.

The agents which excite the mind and organs of sense are not necessary to our existence ; they may all be withdrawn without diminishing the powers of life ; and as they excite a morbid ac- tion in all kinds of fever, they must be avoided in the typhus as well as in the synocha. But with respect to the agents that sup- port those powers on which life depends, the indication in synocha and typhus is different. In the former, as they occasion too powerful an action, the indication is to diminish the quantity ap- plied. In the latter, in which the action of the vital powers is too weak, we must abstract with caution the agents which support it, and only guard against their excessive application.

The principal of these agents is the blood. The excessive ap- plication of this agent in typhus is not to be feared, since its quan- tity must always be less than in health ; the quantity of chyle formed being greatly less. It is even necessary, we shall find,

In typhus to use every means in our power to increase the quantity of blood.

The only agent necessary to the existence of the vital functions, which is often applied in excess in typhus, is caloric; but in removing the excess of caloric evolved in this fever, we must be cautious not to diminish the temperature below the healthy degree ; and where, as frequently happens, the powers of life so far fail, that the temperature falls below this degree, we must endeavour to raise it by artificial means.

The agents which excite the natural functions, are neither of such immediate importance to the preservation of life as those on which the vital functions depend, nor are they so little essential to it as those which support the animal functions ; and in the treatment of typhus, we shall find, that although the constant application of these agents in the due degree is not so necessary as that of those which support the vital functions, yet they are never, like the agents that excite the animal functions, to be wholly abstracted in this fever.

While we thus manage the application of the various natural agents, we are at the same time to employ those agents, which more directly tend to remove the morbid condition of the living solid; the cause of the disease. Experience has informed us, that if we succeed in supporting a certain degree of excitement, this morbid state will be removed. This fact is neither the less certain nor the less valuable, because we are unable to explain it. We shall find, that with the exception of the proper management of the natural agents and the crises of fevers, it suggests every thing that has been found serviceable in typhus.

, Such is the outline of the treatment in typhus, and the principles which conduct our practice in all idiopathic fevers in which the symptoms of typhus prevail. We are now to take a more detailed view of the subject.

I. Of the management of the natural agents in typhus.

Of the agents on which the animal and natural functions depend.

Of the agents which excite the animal functions there is little to be added to what has already been said. Wherever the symptoms of typhus are considerable, they must be avoided, with the exception pointed out by Dr. Cullen, which I have already had occasion to notice. In the typhus mitior however, which is often protracted for a great length of time, and in which the febrile symptoms are mild, a moderate application of these agents is often beneficial, particularly the exertion of sitting up a few hours during the day, or, if the weather be mild, of being carried into the open air.* Much caution, however, is requisite in exciting the mind and organs of sense in fever.

* Sydenham observes of this fever, that much benefit is derived from

The agents on which the natural functions depend, demand more attention in typhus than in synocha, both on account of the debility which attends the former, and because it is a complaint of longer continuance.

As the powers of digestion in all fevers are much debilitated, every thing apt to derange these powers is to be avoided. Both for this reason, and because the presence of much food in the stomach is hurtful in all kinds of fever, the quantity taken at one time should be small; but in well marked typhus it ought to be repeated as often as the patient can take it without oppression. It is our view in typhus to restore the vigour of the system, and one means of effecting this, is to procure as considerable a supply of chyle as the state of the digestive organs admits of.

It is doubtful if the irritation of animal food is proper in any kind of fever, when the symptoms run high. In the typhus mitior, especially when of long continuance, the lighter kinds of animal food, chicken, veal broth, or calf's foot jelly, are perhaps the best kind of nourishment; in other cases farinaceous matter, combined with water and coagulated by caloric, seems preferable. It is neither acescent nor flatulent, it is easy of digestion and gives little irritation. We shall find, that in typhus it is proper to combine it with wine; but of wine. I shall afterwards have occasion to speak at greater length.

Fresh fruits are proper articles of diet in all kinds of fevers, especially those that contain a considerable quantity of acid;* and where it is our view to nourish as much as possible, the more farinaceous kinds, such as peaches, are useful. Many fruits are rendered less acescent and more nourishing by being boiled or baked. Roasted and boiled apples are good articles of diet in fevers, but are less nourishing than the farinaceous vegetables.

Farinaceous matter may also be mixed with the patient's drink. Barley water or water gruel, acidulated with lemon juice and mixed with a proper quantity of wine, is the best drink in typhus; and by varying the proportion of the ingredients, the patient can

raising the patient from his bed and making him sit up for a short time. " There are instances," says Dr. Moore, " of patients in the nervous fe- " ver, who while lying in bed thought their strength so much exhausted " that they could not sit in an erect posture even for a few minutes, yet on " being carried on a couch into the open air and remaining there for two " or three hours have been so much refreshed, and have required such an " accession of strength or spirits, as not only to sit up, but even stand, or " walk a little."

*Oranges and lemons are very generally recommended in typhus, and the Asiatics in those countries where malignant fevers are prevalent, consider the juice of lemons as among the most powerful remedies in such complaints. It may seem to imply a contradiction to forbid the use of acescent food and recommend that of acids. Acescent food, however, at the same time that it produces an acid, occasions flatulence, and otherwise impedes digestion; whereas an acid received into the stomach is often found to promote it.

be made to relish it perhaps longer than any other. All kinds of sweets and aromatics soon become disgustful to febrile patients; and for common drink there is no better substitute for that just mentioned, than small beer or butter milk, which are generally very grateful to them. Any of these drinks, are preferable to plain water in typhus.

In all fevers the peristaltic motion of the intestines is lessened, so that artificial means become necessary for the regular expulsion of the fæces, or any other irritating matter which the intestines may contain; the only purpose for which we ought to move the bowels in typhus.

In this fever those cathartics should be preferred which occasion the least evacuation, rhubarb, aloes,* &c. and neutral salts in particular should be avoided, not only because they generally occasion a more copious evacuation, but because refrigerants, if we except acids, are usually hurtful in typhus. When several laxatives are mixed together, Dr. Fordyce observes, they occasion sickness and pain, and are more certain in their operation than when taken singly.

It is only however in the earlier stages of the disease, when the contents of the alimentary canal may be considerable, that cathartics of any kind are well suited to typhus.† When the disease has lasted for some time, and from the diminution of the ingesta there is little matter in the intestines, it is better, because it is less debilitating, to procure the regular expulsion of the fæces by clysters;‡ and it is proper to use the clyster in the evening, that as few causes as possible may conspire to prevent sleep, one of the most favourable symptoms of fever.

Besides removing as far as possible the agents which tend to prevent sleep, most practitioners diminish the sensibility to those still applied by opium in all cases of fever where the excitement is not considerable.

* " Vomitoria et purgantia nunquam admittenda sunt, nisi adsit certitudo, quod alimentum vitiosum adsumtum, ut poma vel pruna immatura " et frigore corrupta, febri malignæ ansam dederint, vires adhuc sufficiant, " nec aliud contraindicans adsit; sed a vomitorio fortiori, vel a purgante " drastico abstinendum " See a Paper on Typhus by Hilscher, in the 5th vol. of Haller's Disp. ad Morb. Hist. et Cur. Pertin.

† It has long been a prevalent opinion, (see the works of Hoffman and others) that purging should be induced in the decline of all fevers, in order, as we are informed, to purge off the dregs of the disease. When we speak of the exanthemata, we shall see the source from which this prejudice took its rise. It is sufficient at present to observe, that in fevers properly so called, the practice is universally pernicious.

‡ From the prejudicial effects of diarrhœa in the plague, the popular dread of all kinds of cathartics in Eastern countries is such, that the natives in that complaint often refuse to submit to any means of evacuating the fæces, which are frequently retained for many days, and sometimes for weeks, and what is remarkable, seemingly without increasing the symptoms of the fever.

Some have opposed this practice, but not on sufficient grounds, and I believe there is no physician who has given it a fair trial, that will not confess he has often found it of much service In exhibiting opium, with a view to procure sleep,* however, some attention to the state of the symptoms is requisite.

When the skin is soft, and the increase of temperature and other symptoms during the exacerbation are not considerable, a moderate use of opium may be given alone; it should then be given at bed-time. But when the skin is parched, and the temperature rises considerably during the exacerbation, we must either delay the opiate till the symptoms begin to suffer some remission, and particularly till the hot parched skin begins to be relaxed, or give a few grains of James's powder or some other antimonial along with it. If this fails to induce a degree of relaxation in the skin, and prevent the opium increasing the heat and restlessness, the latter must in future be delayed, while the exacerbations continue considerable, till towards their decline.

Dr. Currie proposes accompanying the exhibition of opium for the purpose of procuring sleep with that of the cold or tepid affusion. " Even in intermittent fever opium, when given in the " hot stage, will be much promoted in its diaphoretic and salutary " effects by moderate draughts of tepid, or if the heat be great, of " cold, liquids. In continued fever where the heat is great, and " the skin dry, it is proper to lower the temperature of the sur- " face, and if possible to excite sensible perspiration before " opium is administered, if we wish to insure its diaphoretic and " soporific effects ; but even after opium has been exhibited, when " the inordinate heat prevents its salutary operation, it will be " found safe and salutary to use the tepid or cold affusion, and " when the heat is by this means reduced, repose and sleep will " follow. Tepid or cold drink will produce, though in a weaker " degree, similar benefit. These methods of promoting the di- " aphoretic effects of opium seem more certain and advantageous " in fever than the practice of combining it with ipecacuanha, or " the preparations of antimony ; but where opium is to be used " in inflammatory diseases or dysentery, doubtless this last method " is to be preferred. These remarks must be considered, as ap- " plying to opium in its ordinary doses, that is, from half a grain " to two or three grains of the extract, or from ten to sixty drops " of the tincture. Perhaps it has been too much the practice of " late to give this medicine in large doses, and to overlook its ef- " fects in smaller quantities. Experience has convinced us, that " considerable effects are produced on the system by a very few " drops of the tincture properly administered, and that it is always " unwise to employ it in doses larger than necessary to produce " the desired effect."

* Opium produces sleep partly in consequence of the excitement it occasions, but chiefly in consequence of its local action on the brain.

Of the agents on which the vital functions depend.

Of the means of diminishing the temperature of the body in fever I have already had occasion to speak at considerable length, and have nothing to add here to what has been said respecting it. In typhus, and particularly the advanced stages of it, much caution is requisite, we have seen, in employing the means which diminish the temperature of the body, that it may not sink below the healthy degree, which is often followed by fatal consequences.

With respect to the circulating fluids it appears, from the general view of the treatment of typhus which has been given, that no means tending to diminish the quantity of these, are proper in this fever.

Till lately it was an opinion almost universally received among physicians, that the cure of typhus as well as synocha was to be attempted by venesection; and this opinion is still so prevalent in many places, that it will be proper at some length to consider the foundation on which it rests. It is the more necessary to do so, as the arguments adduced in support of it may mislead those who are only entering on the practice of medicine, and because this evacuation is recommended to a greater or less extent in typhus by the majority of those authors whose opinions respecting the treatment of fevers are in most instances chiefly to be relied on.

Blood-letting in typhus has been a prevalent practice from a very early period. Galen particularly recommends it. Celsus looked upon blood-letting as one of the most valuable remedies in pestilential fevers. And Prosper Alpinus informs us, that the Egyptians let blood in all putrid disorders. We know with what freedom Sydenham used the lancet. "Ac proinde," he observes of the continued fevers of 1669, 71, and 72, which were for the most part of the nature of typhus, "eadem ipsa methodo tum " quoad venæsectionem tum repetitas purgationes febrem hanc " aggressus sum, quam in dysenteriæ curatione supra fusius di- " duximus."*

The same practice has been followed by later writers. Huxham recommended blood-letting in all kinds of typhus; "and " here first let me note," says he, " that though malignant and " pestilential fevers at the very onset greatly sink the spirits and " cause surprising and sudden weakness, especially when from " contagion, yet bleeding to some degree is commonly requisite, " nay necessary in the strong and plethoric, not only to lessen the " moles movenda and give a freer play to the oscillating vessels, " but also to prevent any inflammatory obstructions, which may " form in the very beginning, and likewise to moderate the fric-.

* The freedom with which Sydenham employed blood-letting in fevers is conspicuous in almost every part of his writings, and particularly in his mode of practice in the epidemics of the years 1665 and 66, during which time the plague infested London.

" tion and heat, which are often very considerable in the first
" days of the disease, and which more and more exalt the salts
" and sulphors of the blood, increasing the acrimony and putre-
" scent state of the humors, and greatly favour the action of the
" morbific matter." In the former part of this quotation, we
see the practice of Huxham ; and in the latter part of it, the the-
oretical foundation on which it rested.

In the petechial fever, Hoffman observes, blood-letting is generally necessary if the patient is plethoric, and has been accustomed to this evacuation.

Every body, says Hassenohrl, lets blood in petechial fever, repeating the operation as often as the necessity of the case seems
to require, or as the particular tenets of the physician incline him,
to do. In the strong, robust, and plethoric, it is repeated in general more than once, in some two or three times, in others once is
sufficient. In these fevers, he continues, the blood often shows
the buffy coat, but in some from the very beginning of the disease it is fluid and dissolved. Hence I learned, that the opinion
of those physicians who assert that the blood in petechial fevers,
is always putrid and dissolved, is erroneous, which opinion is,
confirmed indeed by the celebrated De Haen, who mentions a
case in which the buffy coat became firmer in petechial fever after
blood-letting. " Ex his quoque conficitur," Hassenohrl adds,
" inanem esse metum illorum, qui in febribus, sic dictis malignis,
" manum semper a venæsectione temperandam esse contendunt;
" ne scilicet debilitatem, in principio morbi jam presentem, au-
" geant ; cum enim hæc debilitas, incipientibus morbis, frequenti-
" sime ortum suum debeat sanguini spisso immeabili phlogistico;
" clare elucescit phlebotomiæ administrationem in febribus conti-
" nuis nullis circumscribi limitibus nisi conditione ægri, numero
" et vehementia symptomatum."*

The same opinion has been adopted to a greater or less extent
by Dr. Mead,† Eller, Sir John Pringle, Dr. Grant, Dr. Donald
Monro, &c.

Yet there are none of the authors that have been mentioned
who did not, in certain cases, perceive the bad effects of blood-letting in the fever we are considering. Thus Sydenham remarks,
" Quoties mihi cum ægris res est, quorum sanguis vel per se
" imbecilior existit, (uti fere in pueris) vel justa spirituum copia
" destituitur, ut in decliviore ætate, atque etiam in juvenibus di-
" uturno aliquo morbo confectis, a venæsectione manum tempe-
" ro." The candour of Huxham supplies us with ample proof of
the impropriety of his own practice. " The first blood," he ob-

* See Hassenohrl's Historia Febris Petechialis.

† We must pay little attention, Dr. Mead maintains, to the pulse, but
in general begin by letting blood in all continued fevers. " Sanguinis
" missione plerumque incipiendum est, etiamsi ex pulsu tenore vix indi-
" cari videatur."

serves, " in malignant fevers, frequently appears florid, what is
" drawn 24 hours after is commonly livid, black, and too thin, a
" third quantity livid, dissolved, and sanious ; this is frequently
" the case in malignant fevers. I have sometimes observed," he
continues, " the crasis of the blood so broken as to deposit a
" black powder like soot at the bottom, the superior part being a
" livid gore, or a kind of a dark green and exceedingly soft jelly.
" Besides the pulse in these cases sinks oftentimes surprisingly
" after a second bleeding, nay sometimes after the first, and this
" I have more than once noted to my great concern and astonish-
" ment, and that even where I thought I had sufficient indications
" from the pulse to draw blood a second time.*

In his Essay on the Ulcerous Sore-throat, the same author observes, " I have very often met with this buffy or sizy appearance
" of the blood in the beginning of malignant fevers,† and yet
" blood drawn two or three days after from the very same person
" hath been quite loose, dissolved, and sanious as it were ; too
" many instances of this lately occurred to me among the French
" captives here, who died by dozens of a pestilential fever. In this
" fever the French surgeons bled every day, or every second day,
" and I several times saw the blood of some of the officers a mere
" sanious gore on the third or fourth blood-letting.‡

, Eller observes of one of his patients who laboured under a putrid fever ; although he was bled copiously during the first days
of the complaint, the symptoms grew worse. Dr. Donald Monro says, that he was often obliged to give cordials to support the
patient's strength after blood-letting ; it is remarked by Sir John
Pringle, that many have recovered from the jail fever without
blood-letting, but very few who had lost much blood ; and Hoffman confesses, that in many cases of fever it is very difficult to
determine whether or not we ought to have recourse to this remedy. It seems well ascertained by succeeding observations, however, that it was employed by all the foregoing practitioners, in
cases where it did much harm. Dr. Monro, who is among the
latest, endeavours to support his practice less by his own experi-

---

* Huxham on Fevers.

† From these and similar observations it appears, that the buffy coat
sometimes covers the blood in cases where it certainly neither indicates a
repetition of the blood-letting, nor the propriety of having had recourse
to it.

‡ Huxham was led at length to see the impropriety of blood-letting in
most cases of typhus, and he confesses that in those fevers which arise
from contagion it is generally followed by bad consequences. He offers
the reason of this in the following manner. " The contagion being diffus-
" ed through the whole mass of blood, you will little lessen it by drawing
" off a small quantity of this fluid." On this passage Dr. Moore observes, " The reason here assigned for bleeding not being indicated, is
" unquestionably very ingenious ; but the reason which makes the strong-
" est impression on my mind for not bleeding in this fever, is simply be-
" cause it seems generally to do harm."

ence, than the authority of Hassenohrl, who again supports his, not by facts, but by opinions, such as those just quoted from his works, respecting the supposed viscidity of the blood and the means of correcting it.

Thus we find the authors who recommend blood-letting in typhus, founding their practice on hypothesis, and at the same time relating facts which invalidate every thing they say concerning the state of the blood and the modus operandi of blood-letting in fevers.

While it is acknowledged, even by the warmest advocates for blood-letting in typhus, that its bad effects are often apparent, we are led naturally to expect some account of the beneficial effects which induced them to persevere in recommending it. For these however we look in vain. It is true indeed that a few scattered instances may be collected, in which blood-letting seemed to prove serviceable in typhus. The most remarkable instance of this kind which I have met with, is a short account of an epidemic, which Dr. Donald Munro gives from Riverius. After he had attended several patients, labouring under what appeared to be a common malignant fever, attended with a swelling of the parotids, who died without these glands coming to suppuration, he formed a theory concerning morbific matter in the blood, which led him to recommend blood-letting. From the next patient he attended, he took away three ounces of blood, although the patient was so weak that the surgeon thought he would have died under the operation ; after the evacuation however the pulse rose, and in a few hours four ounces more were taken, after which the pulse continued to rise, and the patient was restored to health. Riverius asserts that all those who were treated in this manner recovered.

Nobody acquainted with the nature of fever will regard solitary instances of this kind as capable of influencing the inference which general observation warrants. Singularities are constantly observed in particular epidemics, from which no inference can be drawn respecting fever in general.

There are many reasons to induce us to believe, that the epidemic described by Riverius was attended with some abdominal inflammation ; the effects of the blood-letting were precisely such as they generally are in these inflammations. Visceral inflammations are often present, as dissection after death has shewn, when none of the symptoms seem to indicate their presence. This is particularly apt to happen in fevers. It happened frequently, for instance, in the fever of Grenada, described by Dr. Chisholm, and may account for the practice which was found most successful in that fever, and which in typhus, unaccompanied by any local affection, would prove highly pernicious. There are even cases, related by de Haen, in which inflammation of the stomach was the only or principal complaint ; and yet the patient complained neither of pain, nor the other symptoms which denote its presence.

If the above epidemic was a simple typhus, why is not blood-letting useful in other cases of this fever? Is not this circumstance alone sufficient to demonstrate that there was something peculiar in the epidemic described by Riverius?*

The inference from the facts which have been laid before the reader is very plain, namely, that blood-letting is not to be employed in simple typhus.

The most important part of the treatment in typhus still remains to be considered.

II. Of the means of increasing the excitement in typhus.

The agents which have been employed most successfully for this purpose are, opium, wine, the bark, and cold water used externally.

I have already had occasion to make some observations on the use of opium in fever as a soporific. It has also been employed in typhus as a stimulus, and some practitioners, particularly the late Dr. Brown, prescribed it in very large doses. In that kind of typhus where the delirium is considerable without partaking of coma, it is a powerful medicine, removing the delirium, diminishing the frequency, and increasing the strength of the pulse. Nor can there be a doubt that the use of large doses of opium in such cases would soon have become general, were it not that we possess another medicine, wine, capable of producing the same effects, and on other accounts, particularly the greater permanency of its good effects, preferable to opium.

On this account most practitioners have properly abandoned the practice of giving very large doses of opium in typhus, and

* Blood-letting, and other evacuations, produced the same effect as in this epidemic in the fever of Philadelphia, which we are well assured was attended with local inflammation. Purging, says Rush, raised the pulse when low, and reduced it when preternaturally tense; it revived and strengthened the patient; it often produced sweats after the most powerful sudorifics were given in vain; it sometimes checked the vomiting at the beginning, and assisted in preventing the more alarming recurrence of it about the 4th or 5th day.

Blood-letting, the same author observes, in other places, not only raised the pulse when depressed, but quickened it when preternaturally slow and subject to intermissions; it reduced its frequency and force when these were too great; checked vomiting; and lessened the difficulty of opening the bowels. Dr. Woodhouse, he informs us, often saw purging begin while the blood flowed from the arm; it removed delirium, coma, and obstinate watching; it obviated the hemorrhagic tendency; sometimes disposed to gentle perspiration; and lessened debility. The dilated pupil sometimes contracted after blood-letting. It eased pain. The pains sometimes increased after the first or second blood-letting, but yielded to the repeated use of the same remedy.

The proper treatment of the fevers of sultry climates can never be ascertained, till the nature of the local affections which accompany them is better investigated than has hitherto been done.

use it only as a soporific, while they employ as a stimulus, a medicine which from every observation on the subject is better fitted
for this purpose. But in those sudden sinkings which sometimes
happen in typhus, where the danger is great and immediate, we
have still reason to believe that large doses of opium may sometimes be useful, especially when it is impossible, as often happens,
to exhibit the necessary quantity of wine. In such cases, it is said,
a large dose of opium has sometimes snatched the patient from
the very jaws of death. But on this part of the subject our observations are at present very defective. It is only since the unguarded practice of Dr. Brown shewed what may sometimes be
done with safety, that opium has been employed with much freedom in fevers.

Some physicians run to the opposite extreme, and regard opium as hurtful in fevers, unless employed in doses so small, that
they can hardly be supposed capable of producing any important
effect. " About five and twenty years ago," Dr. Fordyce observes,
" there arose a practice in St. Thomas's Hospital of exhibiting
" opium in a much less quantity, to wit, in the quantity of a quarter
" of a grain for a dose, and repeating it at the end of every six or
" eight hours. When given in such doses it produces no imme-
" diate effect, but by degrees the patient falls into a stupor, which
" gradually increases; and although the stupor does not end in a
" complete sleep, yet it grows in a day or two into that kind of
" stupor that we find when the delirium from the fever, with ap-
" parent fulness of the vessels of the brain, begins to diminish. It is
" true indeed, that this dose of opium is obtained by adding a few
" drops of laudanum to that mixture which is called mithridate;
" but the author has often employed the opium in his private prac-
" tice with ten grains of castor with equal or rather better effect.
" Lately many practitioners have exhibited opium three or four
" times in the twenty-four hours in fevers, having borrowed their
" practice probably from that which has been pursued in St. Tho-
" mas's Hospital, the practice of the hospital being open to the
" inspection of many pupils. These practitioners have not learn-
" ed however that it is the smallness of the dose that produces
" beneficial effects; if the dose be increased so far as half a grain,
" the same restlessness, the same disturbed sleep, dreams, &c.
" as have been noticed are brought on."

Moderate doses of opium produce these effects only when given
without a due attention to the circumstances mentioned when
speaking of it as a soporific.

Upon the whole, the result of the observations on this part of
the subject appears to be, that for the purpose of procuring sleep,
moderate doses of opium may with proper care be employed in
all fevers where the excitement is not considerable, but that it is
rarely to be exhibited in these complaints with any other view.*

* It is remarkable with how much caution the older practitioners speak

For increasing the excitement in typhus, wine is the most powerful medicine we possess. It is only lately that it has been used with much freedom in fevers. Its beneficial effects in the various forms of typhus, however, are now so well ascertained, that in all cases where this fever is not cut short at an early period, it is the medicine on which we almost wholly rely.

Sydenham and his cotemporaries made little use of wine in fevers; since his time we find the practice gradually gaining ground. Most of the best later writers however, Hoffman, Boerhaave, Van Swieten, Huxham, Mead, De Haen, Hassenohrl, Eller, Pringle, Monro, &c. have erred, in recommending wine too sparingly in typhus.

Dr. Cullen is among the first who recommended it in large quantities, and to compensate for the harm which the Brunonian system has probably done, it has been a principal means of extending the use of this valuable medicine.

I have no where met with better observations on the use of wine in typhus, than in Dr. Moore's Medical Sketches; and I quote his observations, in preference to those of any systematic writer, because he is not attached to any hypothesis, and merely relates with accuracy what fell under his own observation. His remarks, however, are not here given as the result of his own observation alone, but, I may say, of the medical faculty of Great Britain for the last fifteen or twenty years; for during that period there is no British practitioner of eminence whose observations, as far as they are known to the public,* do not tend to confirm those I am about to quote. It will appear, from the remarks, which it will be necessary to make on what Dr. Moore says, that even he in certain circumstances did not employ wine with the freedom which repeated observation has now ascertained to be proper.

Of the medicines employed for the diminution of excitement it may be observed, that they are to be had recourse to only when

of the use of opium in continued fever. " Si febre jam pulsa," says Sydenham, " fractiores adhuc essent, ac magis effœtæ ægri vires, atque si " tardius convalesceret, quod hystericis frequentissime accidebat, laudano " in parva dosi exhibito, easdem restaurare et spiritus transfugos ac dissi- " patos, in desertas stationes revocare, conabar. Raro autem remedium " illud repetebam neque unquam prescripsi nisi biduo triduove a postrema " catharsi." On another occasion, however, he observes, that he often recommended opium after the operation of an emetic, " ut tumultum ab " emetico in humoribus excitatum consopiam et quietem conciliem."

In a letter to J. Bedley by Dr. Martin Wall, the reader will find an account of some cases of typhus treated with opium. For the use of opium in fevers he may also consult Dr. Lind's Treatise on Fevers and Infections; Dr. Blane's Treatise on the Diseases of Seamen, and Dr. Campbell's on the Fever of Lancashire.

* I allude chiefly to the lectures of professors in the different medical schools, and to the observations of many of the best practitioners, which have occasionally appeared in the various periodic works established in Great Britain.

they are absolutely necessary ; of those which increase excitement that they are to be employed wherever they are not absolutely hurtful. The former are often attended with the worst consequences even where necessity obliges us to have recourse to them ; the latter are often beneficial where they are not necessary. There is no remedy to which the last remark is more applicable than wine.

When the pulse is soft and frequent ; when the patient complains of weakness, and feels a desire for something to support his strength ; although these symptoms do not go so far as to indicate danger, the exhibition of wine is proper. The quantity must be proportioned to the urgency of the symptoms and the habits of the patient, but always sufficient to remove this sense of debility. Dr. Moore erred in not having recourse to the wine till the more alarming symptoms shewed themselves.

" When that prostration of strength so often mentioned has ta-
" ken place, and is followed by stupor, low delirium, twitching
" of the tendons, and other symptoms ; however proper we may
" think the bark would be, and however eager we are to give it,
" this is no longer in our power. In this state the patient gene-
" rally rejects it in all its forms, or will only take it in such small
" quantity as can be of no service. Yet the case is not entirely
" hopeless ; for even in this situation, if the lips are moistened
" with a little warm wine, sweetened with sugar, he will shew a
" relish for it ; and when given in spoonfuls will suck it into his
" mouth with signs of satisfaction, after rejecting every medicine
" with disgust, and refusing every other kind of nourishment
" whatever.

" In one particular case of this nature, which I well remem-
" ber, after a certain quantity of wine, perhaps near a pint, had
" been given in the space of an hour, I perceived the patient's
" pulse acquire strength and become slower, while the insensi-
" bility seemed to wear gradually away ; but the relations taking
" alarm at this quantity of wine, notwithstanding these flattering
" appearances, withheld it, and offered the patient some other
" kind of drink, which in their opinion was more suitable to his
" case, notwithstanding his again and again rejecting every thing
" they offered. It was not till after they plainly perceived the
" pulse begin to sink, and the delirium to return, that they could
" be prevailed on to give more wine, which on my returning to
" visit the patient, I persuaded them to do, and with the same
" success as before.

" I have known instances also where the physician, not being
" convinced that the filling of the pulse and the removal of de-
" lirium was owing to the wine, has set aside the use of it in the
" same manner, till the return of the bad symptoms obliged him
" to resume it, not without remorse for having made an experi-
" ment which had like to have proved fatal to the patient.

" It is generally necessary in such cases to begin by giv-
" ing the wine warm with sugar,. to induce the patient to
" take three or four spoonfuls, but afterwards he takes it free:
" ly cold and without sugar. The reader might be astonish-
" ed were I to mention the quantity of wine I have known some
" patients take in this fever ; and in some cases of the confluent
" small-pox, where the weakness, insensibility, and other symp-.
" toms were the same, and where the recovery of the patient was
" evidently owing to that cordial alone.*

" The proper rule is to give the wine till the pulse fills, the
" delirium abates, and a greater degree of warmth returns to the
" extremities. Upon the smallest appearance of the stupor com-
" ing back, the pulse quickening and sinking, for they all go to-
" gether, the wine must be resumed. Attentively observing this
" rule, I have often known patients, who in health were not fond
" of wine, and who would have been intoxicated with a single bot-
" tle, drink in the space of 24 hours two bottles of claret,† with-
" out any other effect but that of strengthening the pulse, abating
" the delirium, removing the tremor, and creating a moderate
" warmth on the skin. In others I have known a much greater
" quantity necessary to produce the same effect, but by giving
" that greater quantity the same effect was produced.

" As I am told that this part of my work, and many others,.
" will be exposed to censure, I refrain from mentioning the ex-.
" act quantity of wine which I have known some patients take
" with the best effects in this fever. It is sufficient to say, that it
" ought to be given in such quantity as the patient will willingly
" take till the effects above mentioned are produced, and then
" stopped." The wine ought never to be stopped till the patient
is restored to health. But as the more alarming symptoms
abate the quantity should be gradually diminished. A smaller
quantity will be required to prevent the return of these symptoms
than to remove them. There are few observations relating to the
treatment of typhus which deserve more attention than the following of Sir John Pringle. " Perhaps there is no rule more ne-
" cessary than never to let the patient when low, remain long
" without taking something cordial or nourishing ; as I have seen
" men, once in a promising condition, sunk past recovery by be-
" ing allowed to pass a whole night without any support about
" the time of the crisis." " But on the first appearance of the

* Dr. Smith sometimes allowed his patients two bottles of Madeira in
the day ; and in one instance the patient took two bottles of Port in little
more than half that time.

† More than twice this quantity of claret has been taken in 24 hours in
the more alarming forms of typhus by people unaccustomed to the use
of wine with the best effects, and without the least symptom of intoxication ; so insensible is the system in a state of atony to the most powerful
stimuli which tend to correct the atony ; whereas, by a moderate application of many of the natural agents, which acting now as atonics, increase the morbid state, life itself may be extinguished.

" pulse becoming weaker," Dr. Moore continues, " or any other
" symptoms returning, we must again have recourse to the wine,
" persevering in that quantity which is found by attentive obser-
" vation sufficient to keep up the pulse, and ward off the other bad
" symptoms. When that quantity has been continued for several
" days, it may be gradually diminished ; a little bread soaked in
" the wine, or some other simple nourishment may be offered."
Wine should always be conjoined with some farinaceous matter
when the stomach will bear it, by which the nourishment afforded
is increased, and as appears form a variety of facts relating to digestion, the wine itself better assimilated.* In extreme cases,
however, where the digestive powers are almost wholly suspended, the farinaceous matter must be omitted, as it will then only
occasion oppression, and may produce a disgust for the wine.
As soon, however, as a remission of the symptoms is procured,
sago, panada, or some other farinaceous matter, should be mixed
with it. " After the patient is able to take panada mixed with wine
" or bread soaked in it, with any degree of relish, the appetite
" sometimes becomes very keen, and he is even willing to take
" more panada, rice, or sago, mixed with wine, than is proper for
" him. This return of appetite is undoubtedly one of the
" strongest indications of returning health, but it must be indul-
" ged with caution, the patient must be allowed to eat but little at
" a time even of this kind of nourishment, and to return very
" gradually to his usual food.†

" Soon after the fever is entirely removed, and long before the

* Fluids in general are but ill digested if not conjoined with some solid matter. I have known from expericuce that the strongest decoction
of beef will not afford proper nourishment : but conjoined with any solid
matter, although the latter affords little or no nourishment, it proves sufficiently nutritious.

† There are few cautions which deserve more attention than this, particularly with respect to animal food. "Even after the disease," Dr.
Fordyce observes, " has been terminated by a crisis, animal food in a so-
" lid state should be rejected, there being no cause which has pro-
" duced relapses, as far as the author's experience has gone, so frequent-
" ly as using solid animal food too soon. Supposing even that a complete
" crisis should have taken place, and entirely terminated the disease, it
" ought to be at least five or six days before any solid animal food is ven-
" tured upon.

" The author wishes to press this more strongly, because if a perfect
" crisis should take place, the appetite often returns, and the patient is
" left in a very weak state. It has in this case been often conceived by the
" patient, and much more frequently by the by-standers, that solid animal
" food would restore his strength soon. It must however be remembered,
" that when a complete crisis takes place, and carries off the fever entire-
" ly, the depression of strength, which was a symptom of the fever, ceases,
" and the weakness which was produced by the exertions and derange-
" ment of the faculties of the system, is no longer increasing ; and that the
" patient with very moderate nourishment and the sleep and rest which
" are so apt to ensue after the fever has been completely carried off, will
" have his strength restored in a very short time, without using any thing
" that shall run any risk of reproducing the disease.

" patient has recovered his strength, he will by proper manage-
" ment be entirely weaned from the wine ; or his allowance may
" be reduced to two or three glasses in a day, if the physician
" should think that quantity more proper than noue." This part
of Dr. Moore's observations is also exceptionable. We should
not discontinue the wine when the febrile symptoms are removed, but when the patient is restored to health. Wine is not
only the most powerful means of correcting the atony; but the
best article of diet for removing the debility which succeeds it.
After the removal of the fever indeed the quantity must be greatly diminished ; it must never be sufficient to produce the least
symptom of intoxication ; a few glasses in the day will in general be found sufficient. " Indeed the third part of what formerly
" had proved a salutary cordial and a restorative, would in this
" state of convalescence occasion a dangerous state of intoxication.
" So great a difference is there in the effect of this cordial upon
" the constitution in this state of extreme weakness, when all the
" natural functions seem loaded and clogged by disease, from
" what it has in perfect health, or when the fever being just re-
" moved, the animal functions gradually resume their former
" course.

" Claret is the wine I have generally recommended, when the
" circumstances of the patient would afford it. I have seen the
" same good effects however from the use of Port, Madeira,
" and other wines. And when no kind of wine is to be had,
" brandy or rum diluted with water or milk, and sweetened with
" sugar, must be substituted in its place.

" In the state of stupor, debility, and low delirium, already de-
" scribed, spirits diluted have nearly the same effect with wine,
" and are even more relished by a certain class of patients."

We should never have recourse to distilled spirits except where
wine cannot be procured. Many practitioners fall into a serious
error who believe that provided the same quantity of alcohol is
exhibited in typhus, it is of little consequence in what form it is
given.
Porter, and the other fermented liquors of this country, which
have not been distilled, are preferable to spirits, (especially if the
patient has been accustomed to them) when the digestive powers
are not extremely weakened. In the more alarming forms of
typhus they occasion oppression and disgust. But although distilled spirits be found necessary in the height of the disease, towards its decline, when the appetite begins to return, and especially after the fever is removed, and our view is merely to restore the strength, any fermented liquor, which has not been distilled, provided it does not disagree with the stomach, is preferable to those which have.

Numberless observations have rendered it certain, that both
the more immediate and permanent effects of distilled spirits,

are very different from those of other fermented liquors. I know people who cannot take a small quantity of spirits, though much diluted, without experiencing the debilitating effects of it for several days; yet they can drink a much larger quantity of alcohol, in the form of wine or beer without inconvenience. The most violent fit of dyspepsia I ever saw, which continued for several weeks, was induced by two small glasses of spirits, taken to remove the cramp in the stomach.

. Let any one compare the state of those who indulge in the excessive use of wine, or the undistilled fermented liquors of this country, with that of the habitual dram drinker. The former are plethoric, lusty, and often vigorous; the latter, meagre and palsified. This difference is often striking between drunkards among the lower ranks in England, whose liquor is porter or strong beer, and those among the same class of people in many parts of Scotland, where they drink a spirit distilled from malt.

We have reason to believe, that the pernicious effects of distilled spirits are to be ascribed to the alcohol being separated from the milder particles which sheath it in wine and beer, and prevent it from exerting so hurtful a stimulus on the animal solid. The hurtful effects of this stimulus, is lessened by dilution, but no dilution will reduce the alcohol to the state in which it was before distillation. We bring it as nearly as possible to this state by the addition of some mucilaginous matter. Punch therefore, with a due proportion of sugar, is the form in which distilled spirits are least hurtful, and that in which they should be given to febrile patients. If the sweetness of the sugar occasion disgust, any other mucilaginous matter may be used in its stead. Popular habits are always the result of extensive experience, and much information may often be acquired by an attention to them. In those countries where distilled spirits are generally used, punch is the form in which they are taken, except by drunkards, who require the stimulus of the pure spirits. In punch all the means of obviating the hurtful effects of spirits are combined; they are diluted with a large proportion of water, sheathed by the mucilaginous quality of the sugar, and their stimulating power is diminished by the addition of an acid.

With all this preparation however the use of distilled spirits never produces the same strength and vigour which wine or beer do.

Wine seems preferable to beer only from its being less apt to clog the digestive organs. Of all wines good claret is perhaps the best in typhus; there the alcohol is neither too much diluted, as in small beer, which hardly possesses any of its invigorating property; nor too much concentrated, as in the stronger wines, whose effects approach to those of distilled spirits. Port wine diluted with nearly an equal bulk of water is a good substitute for claret. When the wine drank was port I have repeatedly seen much advantage in diseases of debility from diluting it.

The vitriolic ether has lately been employed in typhus, with the same view as wine; the reader will find it particularly recommended by Dr. Smith, Dr. Chisholm, and others. Its effects are similar to those of wine, but it is much less to be depended upon. Dr. Smith thinks it particularly useful joined with antimonials. Employed in this way it often proves a powerful diaphoretic, and is chiefly indicated when the symptoms of typhus shew themselves at an early period.

It is evident from what has been said, that no quantity of wine 'can be mentioned as forming a proper dose in typhus; the quantity must at all times be regulated by the state of the symptoms, and the change which the wine induces.

It particularly deserves attention, that we are not to be deterred from the use of wine in typhus, although the delirium run high, resembling that which occurs in the synocha; for even in these cases it is found to remove the delirium, while it lessens the frequency and increases the strength of the pulse. Dr. Walker, in his Treatise on Small-Pox, observes, that he has seen a young man in typhus, so furious, notwithstanding the pulse being weak and frequent, that he, could scarcely be kept in bed by two strong men, immediately quieted by wine. I have heard an excellent practitioner confess, that in such a case he has hesitated whether to let blood or give a large dose of opium; he adopted the latter plan, which was followed by the best effects.

Next to wine, and other fermented liquors, the bark is found the most successful medicine in typhus. In most cases of this fever, however, it is in several respects inferior to wine.

Wine we know is a powerful stimulus both to the nervous and muscular system. It is also a nourishing article of diet; it is received into, and at least in part assimilated with, the fluids of the body. The bark, on the other hand, affords no nourishment; and it is even probable, from several observations related when speaking of intermitting fever, that it is either not received into the mass of blood, or although in part received, its effects are chiefly to be attributed to its action on the stomach and intestines. On the muscular fibre the bark seems to exert but little power; the immediate action of this stimulus appears to be on the nervous matter, through which its invigorating effects are diffused to other parts of the system.

In those cases of typhus, where there is a tendency to spontaneous gangrene, the bark, if it can be taken in large quantity, is perhaps a more powerful medicine than wine, but both conjoined, are preferable to either alone. In other cases it is inferior to wine; but wherever there is a considerable degree of debility, if the stomach can bear it, it forms an useful addition to the wine, and may be given in extract or infusion, with a few drops of sulphuric acid, if the stomach will not bear the powder, in which form it is always most effectual.

Most of the authors I have had occasion to mention used the bark in fevers with more freedom than wine. De Haen gave an ounce of the extract daily in malignant fevers; and in the first volume of his Ratio Medendi, relates cases to prove its efficacy. Huxham gave it in decoction with aromatics and a small quantity of distilled spirits; and Hasenohrl is one of its strongest advocates. " Supervacaneum quidem est," he observes, " aliquid addere quod " egregiam corticis Peruviani virtutem in febribus admodum ma. " lignis demonstret."*

We found when speaking of intermittents that wherever the inflammatory diathesis is considerable, blood-letting is necessary previous to the exhibition of the bark. Some practitioners, it was observed, losing sight of the circumstances which gave rise to this practice, seem to regard venesection previous to the exhibition of the bark as necessary in all cases. This prejudice has even been transferred to the treatment of continued fever, in consequence of which blood-letting has somtimes been employed in circumstances the most improper. Dr. Cullen justly remarks, in his Materia Medica, that wherever blood-letting is proper in continued fever, the bark is universally prejudicial.

But the prejudice that has chiefly opposed the use of the bark in continued fever, and which also originates from the practice found most successful in agues, is that this medicine will not succeed unless the remissions be evident. ' " I can also affirm from " experience," Dr. Grant observes, " that the bark will not succeed " unless the fever has adopted the type of an intermittent, and " then the danger is nearly over if it is suffered to take its course." This observation is just if it be confined to those fevers in which the symptoms peculiar to synocha prevail; but in typhus the continued form of the disease is no objection to the exhibition of the bark.

When speaking of the treatment in agues it was shewn, from the observations of different practitioners, that, although wherever any degree of the inflammatory diathesis prevails the bark is only to be exhibited in the absence of fever, and wherever this diathesis is considerable it is to be delayed altogether, till the inflammatory state is removed by proper remedies; yet in all cases where the debility is considerable, the shortness and incompleteness of the remissions only indicate the necessity of using the bark more freely, and that after the fever, in such cases has assumed the continued form, the bark is still to be exhibited in smaller doses.

* See Hasenohrl's Historia Febris Petechialis. The reader will also find cases in this Treatise demonstrating the benefit arising from the use of bark in malignant fevers.

It is true indeed, that where there are no remissions we do not expect the bark to stop the fever ; but repeated experience has evinced that it tends to obviate the symptoms of debility and shorten the complaint.

From these observations it appears, that the bark is rarely to be employed at an early period of continued fever. While any degree of the synocha, which is more or less observable at the commencement of almost all fevers, is present, the bark is always hurtful. But after the typhus is fairly formed, that is, after the pulse remains weak during the exacerbations, a small quantity of bark is always an useful addition to the wine ; and when symptoms of malignity, and particularly that tendency to gangrene so frequent in the worst forms of typhus, appear, the largest quantity the stomach will receive is necessary.

(The stimulus which next demands attention, is cold water used externally. But this was treated of at length when considering the means of inducing a crisis.

Such are the principal stimuli employed in typhus ; many others have been celebrated as powerful remedies in this complaint, but they are much less used now than formerly.

It is not many years since it was a common practice to employ blisters as a stimulus in this fever, and many of the older practitioners still employ them with this view. It is now very generally admitted, however, that their stimulating effect is trifling, and never perhaps compensates for the irritation and trouble they occasion. Dr. Cullen observes, that the general stimulating effect of blisters must be inconsiderable, since they are found of so much service in cases of local inflammation.

· The serpentaria, cascarilla, and colomba have long been celebrated medicines in typhus. These seem to act in a manner similar to the bark. Like it, their stimulating effect is chiefly exerted on the nervous system. They are occasionally useful ; but in modern practice, at least in this country, they have been nearly superseded by the more powerful remedies, bark and wine. When however the bark cannot be taken in any form without oppressing the stomach, some of these often prove an useful addition to the wine.*

A new stimulus has lately been introduced into the treatment of typhus by West India practitioners, the capsicum, and from the trials which have been made with it, there is reason to believe that it will prove a valuable medicine. Dr. Wright, in his report respecting the yellow fever of the West Indies, in the 2d vol. of Annals of Medicine, observes. " We did not however

---

* When the bark or any of these medicines are given at the same time with the wine, they should not be mixed with it, but given in some other vehicle, lest the patient conceive a distaste for the medicine on which his cure chiefly depends.

" despair ; we gave capsicum pills with the most marked success,
" and even where melæna or the black vomit had taken place, the
" capsicum has snatched the patient from the most imminent
" danger." Others have made similar observations. The benefit derived from the capsicum in the cynanche maligna suggested
its exhibition in typhus, and affords as strong an argument in favour of the practice as analogy can supply.

There is a class of medicines, whose stimulus seems particularly to remove that state of debility which is attended with spontaneous contractions of the muscles of voluntary motion, occasioning subsultus tendinum, and other involuntary motions of the
trunk and limbs ; the most powerful of these medicines are
ether, opium, musk, camphire, castor, and ammonia. All of
these have been regared as powerful medicines in typhus.

Of ether and opium I have already had occasion to speak ; and
if we estimate the value of the others by the general opinion of
practitioners, we shall find them fall much short of the encomiums which some have bestowed on them. Of these, camphire,
on which Huxham placed much reliance, is the most useful in
fevers ; in small doses it often has a very considerable effect in
overcoming restlessness and anxiety, and does not interfere with
the exhibition of more powerful medicines. The mistura cam-
phorata is often a good vehicle for the bark in typhus.

Camphire combined with opium forms perhaps the most powerful medicine we possess in obstinate vomiting, which sometimes occurs in this fever, and both on account of its debilitating
effects, and because it prevents the exhibition of medicines, is always an alarming symptom.*

Dr. Lysons gave large doses of camphire with nitre at the
commencement of fevers, and when; with the assistance of a little
white wine whey, it succeeded in bringing out a sweat, it seemed frequently the means of cutting short the disease.

The ammonia and musk have been chiefly recommended when
the low delirium, characteristic of typhus, has supervened, and in
such cases they often afford relief, but their effects are transitory ;
and now that we are acquainted, with the proper mode of exhibiting the bark and wine in typhus, all this class of medicines,
with the exception of opium, are every day going more and more
into disuse.

If we contemplate the change which has been taking place in
the treatment of fevers for the last fifty years, we shall find, that
physicians have been gradually diminishing the number of their
medicines, and increasing the doses of those they retained, till
the treatment of this set of diseases, from being complicated and
feeble, has become simple and efficacious.

* Saline draughts given in the state of effervescence also frequently allay this symptom.

IT may be useful to present at one View, the Treatment of Continued Fever, when we fail to induce a Crisis at its Commencement.

I. THE indication in synocha is to change excessive into moderate excitement.

This is to be effected by avoiding the application of some of the natural agents, and by diminishing the quantity or stimulating property of others.

The natural agents to be avoided in synocha are,

1. All exercise, either of body or mind.
2. Every thing which makes an impression on the external senses.
3. All kinds of aliment and the presence of feculent or other matter in the alimentary canal.

The natural agents, the quantity of which is to be diminished in synocha are,

1. Caloric.
2. The circulating fluids.

The quantity of caloric is to be diminished by cool air, cold drink, and the external use of cold and tepid water.

The quantity of the circulating fluids is to be diminished by venesection and abstinence.

The natural agents whose stimulating power is to be diminished in synocha are,

1. Food, if any be judged proper.
2. The circulating fluids.

The means of diminishing the stimulating power of these agents are,

1. Dilution.
2. Refrigerants.

II. THE indication in typhus is to change atony into moderate excitement

This is to be effected,

1. By avoiding, as far as can be done with safety, the application of the natural agents which now act as atonics.

The natural agents to be avoided in typhus are,

1. All exercise, either of body or mind.

2. Every thing which makes an impression on the external senses.

The natural agents, the quantity of which is to be diminished in typhus, are,

1. Caloric.

2. Food.

The natural agents the quantity of which is not to be diminished in typhus, are,

The circulating fluids.

II. By applying those agents which still act as stimuli.

The chief of these are, wine, opium, the bark, and cold water used externally.

PREFACE

—♦—

WHILE I acknowledge the liberality and indulgence which the preceding volume has experienced from those who have taken the trouble to notice it publicly, the reader I hope will excuse the egotism of the following observations, since, at the same time that they tend to vindicate me from some charges, not I hope of a very serious nature, they will serve farther to illustrate the design of the present undertaking.

My manner of treating the subject, it has been said, is too diffuse, and my collection of facts too copious. To peruse five such volumes, it is maintained, would be nearly as laborious as to peruse the original writers. Can this observation be made by one who has perused these writers !! But the intention of this publication is not merely to obviate the necessity of perusing the original writers, but what is a far more difficult task, of comparing them together and arriving at the result.

" Life," it is said, is short, and we have so many things to learn, " that it is incumbent on authors to give their sense in as few " words as possible." Life, it is true, is short, and we have much to learn, but it is not those who attempt to learn most, who learn to most purpose; and on reflection it will perhaps be admitted, that he who intends to practise medicine will not have mispent his time, if after the perusal of five times five octavo volumes, he is tolerably acquainted with febrile diseases. When it is recollected that the Treatise in question is not merely an introduction, but an attempt to present at one view nearly the sum of what is known on the subject, and that a work of this nature must be adapted to those who are imperfectly or not at all acquainted with medicine, it may appear, I am afraid, that in many instances I have aimed too much at conciseness.

I have been accused of theorising. To this charge I shall only answer by asking any one who has taken the trouble to peruse the volume, if there is one page of it devoted to theory, except for the examination of prevalent opinions, the omission of which would have rendered a work of this nature extremely imperfect. With respect to the last section of the chapter on the Proximate Cause ; I have there only laid before the reader an arrangement of facts.

I have done nothing, it is said, towards ascertaining the proximate cause of fever. I did not attempt to do much. It appears, as far as I can judge, from the observations alluded to, that fever is not owing to any change induced on the fluids, their becoming too acrimonious, too viscid, &c.; nor to any change in the state of the simple solid; nor to a partial change in that of the living solid, such as relaxation or spasm of particular parts; nor to any exhaustion or accumulation of the excitability, (these as far as I know are the only rational opinions which have been maintained on the subject); but to the laws of excitability being changed not in any one, but in every part of the living solid, and equally changed in every part of it, in consequence of which the natural agents no longer produce moderate excitement followed by exhaustion, but atony or that degree of excitement which is followed by atony. This much as far as I can judge is ascertained, as will appear more clearly I think from what I am about to say, and beyond this I did not attempt to go.

The Brunonian doctrines have been so warmly contested, and so frequently mistated, that I examined them with a degree of caution and minuteness, which would not otherwise have been necessary. And aware as I was of the hypothetical manner in which the proximate cause of fever had been treated by every other writer as well as Dr. Brown, it will be admitted, I hope, that I have not departed from a due degree of caution in any of my observations on this subject.

With all the care I was capable of however, I have not succeeded in conveying the same ideas to every reader. It has been stated by one, that I espouse the general principles of the Brunonian system; by another, that I admit no part of it but that which was admitted by all physicians, before Dr. Brown's Elements of Medicine appeared. By one, many of my objections to this system are regarded as invalid; by another, their validity is admitted, and I am censured for allowing it any merit at all. I am said by one to aim at extending the Brunonian system; by another, accused of attempting to bring about a coalition between the systems of Dr. Cullen and Dr. Brown, which the critic more justly than elegantly observes, is as hopeless a task as endeavouring to milk he-goats. What shall I say in answer to such contradictory objections? I shall only observe of the two last, that I am perfectly unconscious of having made either the one attempt or the other. All I have attempted is to give an accurate view of the Brunonian system, to separate the true from the false parts of it, and to arrange certain facts relating to the laws of excitability without reference to any system whatever. I shall here endeavour in a few words to place the result of what was said of the proximate cause of fever in a clearer point of view.

When a state of excessive excitement* or atony† exists inde-

---

* See the definition of excessive excitement, p. 215.
† See the definition of atony, p. 212.

pendently of the continued application of some artificial agent ; one of two changes must have taken place, either the quantity or. quality of the natural agents or the state of the living solid is different from that which prevails in health. If it can be shewn that the state of the living solid remains the same, it follows that the deviation from health is owing to some change in the natural agents ; if it can be proved that the state of these agents remains the same, it then follows, that the deviation from health is owing to some change in the state of the living solid. We may go a step farther ; if it can be proved that some of the natural agents remain unchanged and yet produce effects different from those they produce in health, it not only follows that the state of the living solid is changed, but also that, if this change in the state of the living solid will account for the changes observed in the effects of other natural agents, we are not in any degree to attribute such effects to a supposed change in these agents, there being no occasion for any such hypothesis to explain the phenomena.* In fever, many of the natural agents, caloric, food, light, noise, for example, evidently remain untouched, the difference in their effects therefore is owing to a change in the state of the living solid. But this change is capable of accounting for the change we observe in the effects of those agents whose condition we cannot with precision ascertain, the circulating and other fluids. It follows therefore, that whatever change may take place in these during the progress of fever, and however this change may modify the symptoms of fever,† too great lentor, acrimony, or other morbid condition of the fluids, is not the proximate cause of fever.

With respect to the hypothesis of fever depending on a change in the state of the simple solid. As the natural agents act not on the simple but on the living solid, it is necessary to suppose a change in the state of the latter ; and as this change accounts for the phenomena of fever, there is no occasion for any other supposition.‡

And farther, as all the natural agents excite a morbid action, and as this effect is not confined to any one, but observed equally in every part of the system, what room is there for supposing that any one part is more particularly affected than every other?‖

Lastly with regard to fever being a state of accumulated or exhausted excitability in the sense in which Dr. Brown uses these terms, it is only necessary to refer to the facts which prove that no such morbid states exist.§ It is true that the phenomena of synocha are such. as we should expect from an accumulation of excitability ; but will a surfeit or an excessive quantity of distil-

* See p. 209.   † See p. 211.
‡ See p. 211.   ‖ See p. 220.
§ See p. 198.

led spirits, frequent causes of synocha, occasion an accumulation
of excitability? It appears then, that in fever the living solid is
so changed, that a change is effected in the laws of its excitability,
and that this admitted, there is no occasion for any of the foregoing hypotheses to explain the phenomena essential to fever.*
Upon the whole then the following, as far as it goes, would appear to be a just view of the nature of fever.

　Every agent acting on the system in general is capable of producing three effects, moderate excitement,† excessive excitement, or atony, according to the degree in which it is applied.
The first operation of agents constitutes health; the two last
general disease,‡ which has been called fever. If, by the application of artificial, or the excessive application of natural agents,
either of the two last states be maintained for a sufficient length
of time, the living solid is so changed, that is, such a habit is formed, that the natural agents applied in the usual degree produce
the same morbid effects till the diseased habit has been counteracted; which, as in the case of other habits, is the more easily
effected, the shorter its duration has been. Hence it is that almost any thing making a strong impression will sometimes remove fever at an early period; and hence the difficulty of removing a fever is generally proportioned to the time it has lasted.
The means which cure a fever at an early period, that is, produce a crisis, seem either to expel the offending cause before the
morbid habit is effected, as vomiting during a fit of drunkenness;
or break the morbid habit before it has gained force, as cold-
bathing during the first days of fever. In a more advanced stage,
as the morbid habit is corrected with more difficulty, it is corrected more slowly. When in synocha we succeed in changing
excessive into moderate excitement,‖ h. e. into that excitement
which is followed by exhaustion, we have removed the morbid
habit, and consequently cured the fever. The cure of synocha
therefore depends on the abstraction of stimuli. But as atony
is the consequence of excessive excitement, if excessive excitement has lasted for a considerable length of time, atony will always
be evident previous to the restoration of health. Hence it is, that
the symptoms of typhus succeed those of synocha. When we
succeed in changing atony into moderate excitement,§ we have
corrected the morbid habit, and consequently cured the fever.
The cure of typhus therefore depends on the addition of stimuli.

　I have been indirectly accused of having ascribed too much
importance to the study of nosology. It is fashionable at present
to regard nosology as a very useless branch of medicine. Will
the knowledge of a nosological system, it is said, enable you to

* See p. 210; &c.
† See the definition of moderate excitement p. 213.
‡ See the definition of general disease p. 218, 219.
‖ See p. 219　　　　　　　§ See p. 219.

cure a disease? It certainly will not, but it greatly assists in acquiring the knowledge that will. Let those who slight the labours of the nosologist, recollect that it is his province to point out the symptoms which distinguish one disease from another, and to arrange diseases in such a way as may best shew their affinity, and consequently assist the memory in recollecting their modes of treatment. The anatomist detects the changes induced by internal disease; but of what use would this knowledge prove, did not the nosologist point out the means of ascertaining the presence of such morbid states previous to death. In vain might the chemist and botanist supply us with medicines, did not the nosologist enable us to distinguish the cases in which they are useful,*

It has been asserted, that the practice of medicine would be improved by attending to symptoms individually, without attempting to ascertain their various combinations, and applying to these combinations particular names. Those who make this assertion maintian, and if the assertion is true, justly maintain, that nosology is an useless study. Is the assertion true? Does any symptom at all times require the same mode of treatment? Nay, is not the same symptom in one case salutary, in another pernicious? We must therefore be influenced in treating each symptom by an attention to those which accompany it, that is, an attention to the combinations of symptoms is necessary, and consequently nosology of the first importance. By far the greater number of mistakes I have witnessed in practice, have originated from the neglect of nosology. It often happens that an opinion, at first maintained on no other account than its singularity, becomes current among those who are unable, or will not be at the trouble, to think for themselves. Many exclaim against nosology, but cannot tell why. The truth is, an accurate knowledge of it is acquired with difficulty, and the indolent are glad of an apology for neglecting it altogether.

Having experienced so many instances of indulgence, I am wrong perhaps to notice some in which the preceding volume has been unfairly censured. I have been accused of inaccuracy in point of arrangement, but the only instance adduced is one for which I apologised, and for the admission of which I offered my reasons. The inaccuracy is commented upon, but the apology is unnoticed. The definition of atonics, it is said, is not *luculent*. "Atonics are those agents which produce atony." As thus quoted by the critic, it is indeed far from luculent. He neglects to mention that the definition of atony precedes that of atonics, on the precision of which it depends whether the definition of atonics is luculent or not. A few similar instances I omit to mention.

* See the 20th and 21st pages of the preface to the first volume.

Contrary to my first intention, the present volume includes all the species of eruptive fevers, and consequently finishes the first part of the work, comprehending idiopathic fevers. The two volumes now published therefore form a Treatise on Idiopathic Fevers, and may be regarded as independent of those which are to follow.

The Symptomatic Fevers will form the three remaining volumes. In the first of which, that is, the third volume of the work, the inflammations of the skin, head, and neck, will be considered ; in the fourth, those of the thoracic and abdominal viscera, and of the joints. The last volume will comprehend hemorrhagies and profluvia, with a more detailed view of the nosology of febrile diseases.

It is my intention when the present work is finished to commence another, (which will consist of two volumes, and for which the materials are already collected) on the Nervous Complaints most frequently complicated with Febrile Diseases.

A TREATISE, &c.

CHÁP. V.

Of the Varieties of Continued Fever.

CONTINUED fever, or, as it has been termed, Synochus, is divided into five varieties; the Synochus Simplex, that which is not accompanied by any eruption, the Synochus Petechialis, the Synochus Miliaris, the Synochus Aphthosus, the Synochus Erysipelatosus, and the Synochus Vesicularis.

The symptoms, causes, and treatment of the synochus simplex have been considered. I am now to p n out the circumstances in which the other varieties of synochus differ from this.

SECT. I.

Of the Petechial Fever.

THE Synochus Petechialis may be defined,

Synochus, incerto morbi die, plerumque post varia debilitatis signa, apparent maculæ parvæ, rubræ, circulares, minime eminentes, per cutem, præcipue colli et pectoris, sparsæ.

There is little to be added to what was said in the first volume of this variety of synochus. Petechiæ* seldom appear in the first, very frequently in the second, stage of synochus (the typhus). They are most apt to appear when there is a tendency to the hemorrhagies characteristic of this species of fever.

This eruption appears in other complaints besides fever, particularly in scurvy, and sometimes supervenes without any previous disease. But wherever it appears, we still find it accompanied with a tendency to the worst forms of hemorrhagy.

* See Petechiæ described in the first volume.

All that is known of its causes is, that whatever debilitates, disposes to it.   It nevertheless now and then shews itself where the
excitement is considerable ;* and on the other hand, we often meet
with extreme debility in fevers, as well as other complaints, unattended by petechiæ.

As petechiæ generally denote debility, their $_a{}_{pp}{}^{ea}{}_r{}^{an}{}_c{}^e$ in typhus indicates a strict attention to the invigorating plan ; and antiphlogistic measures should be employed with caution when they
shew themselves in synocha, which, however, rarely happens.

When petechiæ appear as an idiopathic affection, stimulants,
and particularly those which are termed astringents, are most useful, the chief of which are the bark, port wine, sulphuric acid, and
alum.   It will be necessary to consider the other varieties of synochus at greater length.

SECT. II.

Of the Miliary Fever.

THE Miliary Fever is defined by Dr. Cullen,

" Synochus cum anxietate, frequenti suspirio, sudore olido, et
" punctionibus cutis.   Incerto morbi die, erumpunt papulæ ru-
" bræ, exiguæ, discretæ, per totam cutem, præter faciem, crebræ,
" quarum apices, post unum vel alterum diem, pustulas minimas,
" albas, brevi manentes, ostendunt."

It appears from what was said of the miliary fever in the introduction, that it is to be regarded only as a variety of synochus,
characterized by a particular eruption and a certain train of symptoms which attends that eruption, whether it appears in fever or
other diseases.   In laying down the symptoms then of what has
been termed Miliary Fever, it will be the most distinct plan, in the
first place, to describe the eruption ; secondly, to enumerate the
symptoms which generally precede or attend it ; and lastly, to
point out the febrile states in which it is most apt to shew itself.

1. Of the Symptoms of the Miliary Fever.

Of the Miliary Eruption.

The first appearance of this eruption is sometimes a roughness
of the skin, resembling that produced by cold ; soon after which,
or without having been preceded by this appearance, a number of
small red pustules shew themselves, about the size of millet seeds,
from which they are termed miliary.   They often lose their redness, and appear of the ordinary colour of the skin.   Their pro-

* See Eller de Cognosc. et Cur. Morb. and Dr. Grant's Treatise on
the Fevers most common in London.

mlnence is so inconsiderable that it can scarcely be seen ; to the touch it is always sufficiently evident. For the most part they are distinct, but now and then appear in clusters. After they have remained for ten or twelve hours, sometimes longer, a small vesicle appears on the top of each, which at first is of a whey colour, but soon after becomes white.*

Such is the appearance of the white miliary eruption, and the red only differs from it in the pustules retaining their red colour, and the matter formed in them being yellow.

In two or three days the vesicles break; if they have not been rubbed off, and in either case are succeeded by small crusts, which fall off in scales.

The miliary eruption generally first appears about the neck and breast, gradually spreading to the trunk and extremities, but rarely appearing on the face. The white and red eruptions generally appear separately ; sometimes however they are intermixed. In both, the matter formed in the vesicles, like the sweat which we shall find constantly attends this eruption, has an offensive smell, and, it is said, a very acrid taste.

The miliary, like other symptomatic eruptions, often appears repeatedly in the course of the disease, and it is not uncommon for one crop immediately to succeed another for many days ; new pustules appearing while the former advance to maturation and decline.

. We are assisted in forming the prognosis in Synochus Miliaris, by the appearances of the eruption. The red generally indicates a milder disease than the white ; and it is frequently observed, that the greater the inflammation that attends the eruption, the better is the prognosis. " Exanthemata rubra," Dr. Mead[†] observes of this eruption, " minus periculum afferunt quam albi-" da, iliaque quo vividiora perstant, eo sunt tutiora." . Quarin however remarks, that both kinds of miliary eruption appearing at the same time indicates a worse disease than either singly. It has been observed, that a very numerous eruption indicates more danger than a scanty one.[‡] The eruption being steady is more favourable than its frequently disappearing and coming out again ;[||] and it is more favourable when the places covered with the eruption appear swelled and stretched, than when they remain flaccid.

The prominence of this eruption sufficiently distinguishes it

---

* The matter of the pustules at first appearing of a whey colour and afterwards white has given rise to a very improper division of the white miliary eruption into pellucid and white. See the 388th paragraph of Burserius's Institut. Med. Pract. where the reader may also see some other divisions of the miliary eruption which are equally useless.

† Monita et Præcepta Medica.

‡ Quarin. || Burserius.

from petechiæ. The circumstances which distinguish it from other eruptions will be pointed out as we proceed in describing those
eruptions.*

Of the Symptoms which precede or attend the Miliary Eruption.

It is not uncommon for the symptoms of febrile diseases, a
short time before the miliary eruption shews itself, to suffer an
evident exacerbation, which appears chiefly in an increase of temperature and restlessness. The eruption is generally preceded by
oppression, and a sense of tightness about the præcordia, the
breathing becomes laborious and interrupted with sighing or a
cough,† while the spirits are oppressed with sadness and ti-
midity.

With the increase of temperature, there is generally a sense
of pricking and itching in the skin, which is also sometimes felt
in the bowels,‡ now and then accompanied with a degree of numb-
ness in the extremities, particularly in the fingers';|| and for
sometime before the eruption comes out, the patient is frequently
bathed in a profuse sweat of a sour rank odour, during which,
Allionius observes, there is a contracted pulse.

There are other symptoms, which, though less constantly, are
sometimes observed to precede this eruption. The dejection is
often attended with pains of the head or internal ear, and tinnitus
aurium, now and then with delirium. The eruption is sometimes
preceded by pains in the back, limbs, and loins,§ and, in some
cases, by a pungent heat referred to the back.¶ ' Before the miliary eruption appears, the belly now and then swells and becomes
tense, the whole face is swelled and red,** and the eyes inflamed
or watery.†† The internal fauces also are frequently inflamed, and
there is sometimes a considerable flow of saliva. In many cases
the miliary eruption is preceded by that of aphthæ; between
which and this eruption there is often, we shall find, an evident
connection. Like most other eruptions, the miliary is sometimes, though very rarely, preceded by an epileptic fit.‡‡

Upon the whole, dejection of spirits and anxiety, with unusually fetid sweats, are the most common forerunners of the miliary eruption.

Most of the foregoing symptoms are usually relieved on its appearance. The sweating however, if means are not used to

---

* The white miliary eruption has been termed purpura alba; the red,
purpura rubra.

† Quarin.   ‡ Vogel.

|| Allionius. Vogel.   § Quarin. Vogel.

¶ Hoffman observes, that a pungent heat in the back is often a sign
that the miliary eruption is about to appear.

** Burserius.   †† Quarin.   ‡‡ Burserius.

check it, generally continues, and then fresh crops of the eruption will probably continue to come out for many days.

The more severe the preceding symptoms, and particularly the greater the debility and depression of spirits, the more unfavourable is the prognosis. If the sweat is moderate, Vogel observes, and the respiration not oppressed, the prognosis is good. A degree of itchiness, instead of the sense of pricking, on the coming out of the eruption, has been regarded as unfavourable.[*]

Such are the symptoms, more or fewer of which precede and attend the miliary eruption in whatever kind of fever it makes its appearance, and even when it is unaccompanied by fever of any kind. The miliary eruption, says Burserius, may appear without being attended by fever, but it is still preceded by the same restlessness, sickness, and anxiety. When the miliary eruption, Hoffman observes, appears as a chronic complaint, unattended by fever, it is almost always accompanied with a copious excretion of thin serum by sweat or urine, sometimes by spitting, and sometimes by watery stools.

The red miliary eruption, the rash as it is vulgularly termed, appears unaccompanied by fever more frequently than the white. "The miliary glands of the skin," Huxham remarks, "appear "very turgid, and mimic a rash upon profuse sweating, even in "the most healthy." The white however, as well as the red, now and then appears without fever.[†]

Of the Febrile States in which the Miliary Eruption most frequently appears.

It is when debility prevails that the miliary eruption is most apt to shew itself. The robust and sanguine, Quarin observes, are rarely seized with the miliary fever, but in them it is most dangerous. That species of synochus therefore, in which typhus forms the principal part of the complaint, is most frequently accompanied with this eruption ; and in the works of those who treat of the miliary fever as a distinct disease, and consequently endeavour to point out its characteristic symptoms, those are enumerated which have been mentioned as attending this species of synochus.

The cold stage, it has been observed, is generally very evident, often attended with considerable langour and depression of spirits, which sometimes, Hoffman remarks, proceeds to syncope. The pulse during the chills is for the most part very small and weak ; after the heat is generally diffused, it becomes stronger and fuller ; but never, it is observed, acquires a great degree of strength, and generally in a few days becomes small, soft, and

[*] Burserius.
[†] See Mr. White on the Diseases of Lying-in Women, and other writers on Miliary Fever.

depressed. The various symptoms denoting much debility, such as tremors, cramps, subsultus tendinum, delirium, &c. enumerated among the symptoms of typhus, have been regarded as characteristic of this fever. When we consider the nature of the fever in which this eruption generally appears, the irritation of the eruption, and the profuse sweats which attend it, it will not appear surprising that these symptoms very frequently accompany the Synochus Miliaris.

Such is the complaint which has been termed the Miliary Fever. In what does it differ from other cases of typhus, except in the eruption and certain symptoms connected with it, which, as will be evident in considering its causes, are accidental appearances, that may often be prevented by a proper mode of treatment?

Some allege that the miliary eruption generally shews itself on a certain day of the fever, demonstrating an essential connection between the fever and eruption. Allionius says that it appears on the third or fourth day; Huxham says it appears on the seventh, ninth, or eleventh day; and other days are mentioned by other writers; from which it is sufficiently evident, and practitioners indeed now admit, that it may appear on any day of the fever; it is not common however for it to appear before the third or fourth day, probably because the debility is seldom considerable before this period.

The foregoing observations apply chiefly to the white miliary eruption, the form in which it generally appears in typhus. The red is a slighter affection, and often appears in synocha. When the red miliary eruption appears, Lobb* observes, the pulse is commonly strong, the tongue dry, and the febrile heat great. Even in this case however, the eruption is generally attended with oppression and sinking of the spirits.

The symptoms connected with the miliary eruption, it has just been observed, for the most part suffer a remission on its appearance, and in some instances it also relieves the febrile symptoms;† in general however the miliary eruption, and the sweats and other symptoms that attend it, only increase the debility, and we shall find that they are always if possible to be prevented. An increase of the symptoms of debility, on the coming out of the eruption, affords an unfavourable prognosis; but the prognosis is still worse, if such symptoms shew themselves or suffer a considerable exacerbation on its sudden disappearance. When in this case, exces-

* See his practice of Physic.

† Quarin observes, that it is chiefly in catarrhal and rheumatic fever that the miliary eruption brings relief. We shall afterwards find that sweats, however induced, more frequently bring relief in these, than in most other febrile diseases. But Planchon (in his Dissertation sur la Fievre Miliare) justly remarks, that when this eruption does relieve the febrile symptoms, the favourable change is not to be depended on, the symptoms often returning with equal and sometimes greater violence.

sive anxiety and dejection, obstinate vomiting, delirium or convulsions supervene, the danger is very great; and if we do not
succeed in removing such symptoms, death is to be regarded as
almost inevitable.

Dropsical swellings of the legs and sometimes of the belly have
been observed frequently to supervene on miliary fevers, and are
regarded by some as part of the complaint; they seem however
merely the consequence of debility. For the most part as the
patient gains strength, the swellings disappear without the assistance of medicine, especially if they are merely anasarcous. Any
degree of ascites is always to be dreaded. In some cases they
are suddenly removed by a spontaneous flow of sweat. We shall
soon have occasion to consider a species of eruptive fever, almost
uniformly succeeded by anasarcous swellings, which are rarely
attended with any danger.

From the great debility which prevails in the synochus miliaris,
it is apt to be followed by the various consequences of protracted
fevers, enumerated among the consequences of continued fever.
See the observations of Vogel and Burserius on the consequences
of the miliary fever.

2. Of the Causes of the Miliary Fever.

A fever, says Allionius,* which may be considered a new disease from the miliary eruption which attends it, in which, if the
eruption subsides, the patient falls into convulsions and soon expires, appeared at Leipsic about the middle of the last century.
And the generality of writers agree with Allionius, that the miliary fever which appeared at this place in the years 1652, 1653,
and 1654, is the first fever of this kind of which we have any account. The eruption first shewed itself in that fever which frequently attacks women after delivery, termed puerperal; but soon
spread, and appeared in various fevers, attacking persons of every
sex and age. " Ita ut," says Allionius, " pueros cum juvenibus,
" adultos cum senibus, viros cum fœminis, aggrediretur."

Many, however doubt of the miliary fever having appeared at this
period for the first time. " It seems to me very improbable," Dr.
Cullen observes " that this should have been really a new disease
" when it was first considered as such; there appear to me very
" clear traces of it in authors who wrote long before that period,
" and if there were not, we know that the descriptions of the an-
" cients were inaccurate and imperfect, particularly with respect
" to cutaneous affections, whilst we know also very well that those
" affections which usually are symptomatic were commonly neg-
" lected or confounded together under a general appellation."
Burserius thinks, that the miliary eruption has been confounded
with petechiæ by some of the older writers; and Mr. White, in his

* See his Tractatio de Miliarium-Origine, &c.

Treatise on Pregnant and Lying-in Women, observes, that it is highly probable, if not certain, that the miliary fever has occurred to practitioners ever since the days of Hippocrates. The reader will find in Planchon's Treatise sur la Fievre Miliare, quotations from Hippocrates and Ætius, to prove that the miliary fever was known to these authors. This dispute is of little moment.

In speaking of the causes of synochus miliaris, we must take the same view of the complaint as in enumerating its symptoms, endeavouring to trace the causes, not of the fever, but of the eruption which attends it.

There is no symptom which more constantly attends the miliary eruption than sweating, and the causes of both are often the same ; thus it frequently happens in the same epidemic, that in those treated with the cool regimen no sweat appears, and the eruption is prevented ; while in others, treated with the hot regimen, sweats are forced out, and the eruption soon makes its appearance. Sweating indeed is so frequently accompanied with this eruption in febrile diseases, that some assert we may induce it in any fever, if we force out sweats by keeping the patient warm, and obliging him to swallow heating medicines.* Dr. Cullen considers the miliary eruption merely as a disease of the skin, produced by heat and forced sweats, and little connected with the general affection of the system ; this opinion he thinks is further confirmed by the eruption never appearing on the face, although it affects every other part of the body, by its appearing chiefly on those parts which are most covered, and by its being possible to bring out the miliary eruption on particular parts by external applications.

It is certain however that in some fevers, as in the puerperal, it is more apt to appear than in others. It will be necessary therefore to inquire into the circumstances which predispose to its appearance.

" As this symptomatic affection," Dr. Cullen observes, " does " not accompany every instance of sweating, it may be proper to " enquire what are the circumstances which especially determine " this eruption to appear." " There is only one observation," he remarks, " I can offer to the purpose of this inquiry, and it is " that, of the persons sweating under febrile diseases, those are " especially liable to the miliary eruption who have been previ- " ously weakened by large evacuations, particularly of blood." Quarin and others make the same observation ; thus it is that lying-in women are more frequently attacked by it than others.

Those also who have laboured under frequent and copious men-

---

* Even in the writings of foreign authors, who generally contend for the miliaria being an exanthema, and particularly in those of Vogel and Quarin, there is sufficient proof of the miliary eruption being generally the consequence of forcing out sweats by warmth and stimulating medicines,

struation or a long continued fluor albus; are frequent subjects of
this complaint. It has often been remarked, that the miliary
eruption is apt to appear in fevers arising from wounds, where
the loss of blood has been considerable. But every debilitating
cause, as well as loss of blood, predisposes to it. In lying-in women, Vogel observes, it often makes its appearance before delivery. Not only every excessive discharge, but the interruption
of any habitual discharge, such as that of the menses, even habitual
costiveness, is ranked among its causes. A bad diet from a deficiency either in quantity or quality, or intemperance, predisposes
to the miliary eruption ; to the last cause, and also to excessive
venery, it is attributed both by Hoffman and Planchon ; even the
debility produced by a damp atmosphere seems sufficient to give
the predisposition. The miliary eruption, Quarin observes, is
often endemic in marshy countries.

Persons of a lax habit of body, Hoffman remarks, and of a sanguine temperament, are more subject to it than others ; children
more than adults ; old people than such as are in the vigour of
life ; women more than men ; and in child-bed more than at other
times. And those, he might have added, who have formerly laboured under the disease, are more subject to it than others.

Though these causes of the miliary fever, Hoffman continues,
have always existed, the disease itself has made its appearance
only of late years, since the introduction of tea and coffee, and it
is chiefly among the drinkers of these that miliary fevers are frequent. I may observe, in confirmation of this remark, that I have
repeatedly known fetid sweats, anxiety, and an intolerable sense
of pricking in the skin, induced in dyspeptic people by drinking
tea. Nor is this effect, as Hoffman supposes, to be ascribed to
the warm water ; for the same or even a much larger quantity of
warm milk and water was not found to produce the same effects.

A variety of observations point out a striking connection between the appearance of the miliary eruption and the state of the
stomach. Van Swieten, Quarin, and Zimmerman have all observed, that it is occasioned by an accumulation of irritating matter in the stomach ; and Quarin even remarks, that on evacuating
such matter from the primæ viæ, he has observed the eruption
immediately disappear ; an observation which has not been sufficiently attended to. We shall find other eruptions, particularly
the erysipelatous, equally connected with the state of the primæ
viæ. The necessity, Planchon observes, of clearing the primæ viæ
in the miliary fever is pointed out by the nausea, vomiting, bitter
taste in the mouth, furred tongue, fetid breath, and eructations,
(all symptoms denoting derangement of the primæ viæ) which
occur in the beginning of this fever. In another place, he observes that an intermitting pulse often attends the miliary eruption, indicating an accumulation of bile in the stomach and intestines.

r

All these, and other debilitating powers, should be regarded, perhaps chiefly as predisposing causes, while the hot regimen is to be looked upon as the principal exciting cause of this eruption. At least we shall not err much by forming this opinion, since it is found, that whatever the state of the patient may be, the miliary eruption is very generally avoided by cool drink, and exposure to cool air.

It is not to be denied however, that by the former set of causes, or others less known, the body is sometimes so predisposed to this eruption, that no attention to the cool regimen is capable of preventing its appearance. In spite of every thing that can be done, sweating sometimes supervenes, and is followed by the miliary eruption. In 1758, Quarin observes, this eruption was epidemic. Almost all that were confined to bed were seized with it, although the primæ viæ were cleared, the patients kept cool, and all heating medicines avoided. Van Swieten has also observed that the miliary eruption is sometimes epidemic, and both Stork[*] and Planchon[†] mention instances where this eruption occurred after every precaution had been used to prevent its appearance. Such cases however are rare.

Moist variable weather is most favourable to its appearance. It appears most frequently in spring, and more frequently in autumn than in winter and summer; winter is least favourable to its appearance.

The reader will find a variety of causes of miliary fever enumerated by authors, particularly by Burserius in the 2d vol. of his Institut. Med. Pract. But these are rather the causes of the fevers in which this eruption most frequently appears, than of the eruption itself; such authors regarding the miliary fever as an idiopathic disease.

Some dispute has arisen concerning the contagious nature of the miliary fever, some asserting that it is always contagious, and others denying that it ever is so. The dispute could only have arisen from regarding it as an idiopathic disease. When it is known that the miliary eruption is an accidental appearance in all kinds of fever, the cause of this difference in opinion, and the means of reconciling it, are sufficiently apparent. It is one of the inconveniences which has arisen from a wrong view of the nature of the disease.

3. Of the Treatment of the Miliary Fever.

As what has been termed the miliary fever is nothing more than the occurrence of the miliary eruption with the peculiar symptoms that always attend it in continued fever, and as the

[*] Anni Medici.
[†] Sur la Fiev. Mil.

treatment of continued fever has already been considered, we have only at present to point out how far this treatment is influenced by the appearance of the miliary eruption.

When a sweat appears in any continued fever, especially where the debility is considerable, if the symptoms are not relieved by it, we have reason to fear that its continuance, among other bad effects, will induce the miliary eruption, with the anxiety, oppression, &c. that generally attend it.

Concerning the propriety of checking such sweats there can be no doubt. A dread of this practice, especially where there is particular reason to expect the miliary eruption, is expressed in the writings of a variety of authors. It seems however to have, arisen less from cases in which they observed the bad effects of the practice, than from certain opinions respecting the eruption which, according to these writers, is the means employed by nature to throw out the morbific matter, from which they suppose the fever to arise.

The effects of the practice indeed fully warrant the assertion just made. Using proper means to check sweats which do not relieve the symptoms, has never been attended with any bad consequence.

The most effectual means of checking sweat is the application of cold, and in many cases it is the best. But the employment of it requires some caution.

If the fever be typhus, in which however the increase of temperature is considerable, and steady, the application of cold may be free. The same may be said of synocha, if we have no reason to dread a tendency to local inflammation. In the synocha however, sweats rarely occur without relieving the symptoms. The application of cold requires much caution in the exquisitely formed typhus, where the temperature is little, if at all, above the natural degree. In such cases, attempting to diminish sweating by the application of cold, would often produce an alarming diminution of temperature. Here we must trust chiefly for moderating this sweating, a consequence of debility, to the means of invigorating the system, the best of which in this case are wine, bark, sulphuric acid, and alum.

When the propriety of applying cold to check the sweating is determined on, it should be applied gradually. The air of the bed-room should be cooled, part of the bed-clothes removed, the patient desired to lie with his arms bare, and allowed cold drink ; by these means we at the same time avoid the miliary eruption, and check sweats which serve no purpose but that of diminishing the strength ; for no salutary sweat ought to be checked, nor in such is the miliary eruption to be feared. " Whatever the miliary eruption may be, the sweats which attend it," Mr. White observes, " are by no means critical."

When these means prove insufficient for checking the sweat, we must at the same time employ a gentle cathartic. An equal prejudice has prevailed against this practice, as against the last; and for similar reasons it is equally groundless. It appears from the foregoing observations respecting the connection between the state of the primæ viæ and the miliary eruption, that wherever we have reason to suspect the presence of irritating matter in these cavities, much is to be expected from evacuating it, and consequently that a cathartic is particularly indicated. We should inquire therefore whether the patient feels a sense of weight about the stomach, whether the breath be offensive, whether he is troubled with head-ach, eructations, or nausea, swelling of the belly, or tormina.

When the stomach is oppressed, Quarin recommends diluents, and if these fail, an emetic. Much dilution however is evidently improper where we wish to avoid sweats;* emetics are doubly hurtful, by promoting the perspiration and increasing the debility, and should be avoided unless considerable advantage is to be expected from evacuating the stomach, as in cases where the eruption is evidently caused by the irritation of its contents. Mild cathartics in general answer much better the different indications in this case.

When it happens that notwithstanding our endeavours the sweat continues, and the miliary eruption appears, or, what more frequently happens, when the eruption has been induced by improper treatment, what mode of practice is to be adopted?

" But it may happen," Dr. Cullen observes, " when these pre-
" cautions have been neglected, or from other circumstances, that
" a miliary eruption does actually appear, and the question will
" then be put, how the case is to be treated. It is a question of
" consequence, because I believe that the matter here generated
" is often of a virulent kind. It is frequently the offspring of pu-
" trescency, and when treated by increasing the external heat of
" the body, it seems to acquire a virulence which produces those
" symptoms mentioned in the 719th paragraph, and proves cer-
" tainly fatal.

" It has been an unhappy opinion with most physicians, that
" eruptive diseases were ready to be hurt by cold, and that it was
" therefore necessary to cover up the body very closely, so as
" thereby to increase the external heat. We now know that it is
" a mistaken opinion, that increasing the external heat of the bo-
" dy is generally mischievous, and that several eruptions not only
" admit but require the admission of cool air. We are now per-
" suaded, that the practice which formerly prevailed in the case
" of miliary eruptions of covering up the body close, and both by

---

* Hoffman cautions against the use of warm diluting liquors, unless the eruption has been repelled.

" external means and internal remedies encouraging the sweating
" which accompanies this eruption, was highly pernicious, and
" commonly fatal. I am therefore of opinion, even when a mili-
" ary eruption has appeared, that in all cases where the sweating
" is not manifestly critical, we should employ all the several means
" of stopping it that are mentioned above, and I have sometimes
" had occasion to observe, that even the administration of cool air
" was safe and useful."

From the observations of other writers we might be inclined
to infer, that however uniformly safe the application of cold previous to the appearance of the eruption may be, it is a more doubtful practice while the eruption is present. Cases are recorded
in which it did harm.*

But in these, the application of cold was unguarded, and the
state of the patient such that sudden exposure to cold might have
induced the same train of symptoms, had there been no eruption.
Even those who saw the eruption repelled by cold, warn us against
the more dangerous extreme of heat; for while an unguarded application of cold now and then proves hurtful, keeping the patient
warm never fails to be so. On the first breaking out of the miliary fever amongst us, Hoffman observes, when it was treated with
warm alexipharmics and a hot regimen, almost every one who
was seized with it died, whereas by the temperate mode of treatment now pursued, numbers escape. While the older practitioners oppressed the patient with bed-clothes, they were not
aware that the eruption may be repelled by whatever debilitates,
and that much heat may have this effect, as well as imprudent
exposure to cold. There is reason to believe indeed that the latter cause often produced the effect in consequence of the previous application of the former.† Delirium, subsultus tendinum,
dyspnœa, anxiety, convulsions, and often death, says Burserius, is
the consequence of repelling the miliary eruption, and this may
be done, he adds, by too much heat or too free an exposure to
cold, by keeping the patient too long in the erect posture, by violent affections of the mind, particularly by anger, terror, or grief.‡
Quarin and others make similar observations, and what sufficiently
demonstrates that debility is a principal, perhaps the only cause
of retrocession, is that the various symptoms of debility which

* The reader will find cases in which this eruption was repelled, and
an alarming train of symptoms induced, by exposure to cold, mentioned
by Hoffman and others.

† The retrocession of the eruption rarely happens when the cool regimen has been employed from the beginning of the complaint.

‡ If a sudden and copious evacuation follows the retrocession of the
eruption, he observes, such as much sweating or copious diarrhœa, the bad
effects are prevented. There is no eruption according to Burserius which
is so readily repelled as the miliary.

attend it, and which have been erroneously regarded as its consequences, in many cases precede it.*

Upon the whole then, it may be observed that the application of cold, while the sweat continues threatening the appearance of the eruption, should be as free as the symptoms of the fever admit of, and that we have reason to believe that the same observation applies to those cases, where the eruption is actually present.†

It appears from the foregoing observations, that it is in the typhus gravior where the debility is great, and the temperature little or not at all above the healthy degree, that the retrocession of the eruption is most to be feared, and the application of cold in such circumstances often induces the foregoing train of symptoms, whether the miliary eruption be present or not.

Some of the medicines which have been termed refrigerant, tend to check sweat, and are therefore useful in the miliary fever. Acids, and the neutral salts composed of a fixed alkali and mineral acid, are best suited to this indication; those into the composition of which ammonia or vegetable acids enter, being too apt to promote perspiration. Nitre and other neutral salts however are not well suited to typhus. Acids in general, (and particularly the vitriolic) are employed with more advantage where the miliary eruption is to be feared.

Allionius, Hoffman, and others, forbid the use of acids in the miliary fever, for which the latter has been justly censured by Planchon and others. It is the worst of prejudices, says Quarin, which has instilled itself into the minds of some practitioners, that because the sweat in miliary fevers is acid, absorbents should be employed, and acids of every kind avoided.

It seems to be the same hypothesis that led to the exhibition of alkalis in the miliary fever.‡ The ammonia is that which has been most employed, and is often serviceable; but its good effects are rather to be attributed to its cordial than alkaline property.

With regard to saffron, castor, elder-flowers, milfoil, and many other such medicines, frequently recommended in miliary fever, they seem to be of little or no use, and as they tend to excite disgust and oppress the stomach, ought to be avoided.

When the miliary eruption brings no relief to the febrile symptoms, it may be regarded as the accession of a new disease, which combines its influence with the disease already present to reduce the patient's strength. Its appearance therefore renders neces-

* See the observations of Planchon and others. Subsultus tendinum, syncope, convulsions, delirium, &c. Planchon observes, often shew themselves a short time before the eruption recedes.

† See what is said of the doctrine of repelled eruption in speaking of the treatment of the synochus aphthosus.

‡ See this part of the subject considered at length by Burserius.

sary a strict adherence to the tonic plan; for the irritation of the miliary eruption, and the debilitating sweats which attend it, will even at an early period of the fever induce the symptoms of typhus; besides, it has just been observed, that tonic medicines are sometimes the principal means of checking such sweats, and in this way they are always useful after the typhus has commenced; the sweating being often protracted by the debility it occasions. Opium however, from its tendency to promote perspiration, should be avoided. Tralles, in his work on opium, alleges that the miliary eruption may often be induced by the use of this medicine.

As the appearance of miliary eruption in continued fever renders the tonic plan more necessary, it follows as a consequence that it renders the opposite plan more pernicious. The bad effects of blood-letting and much purging in the miliary fever have often been observed; and they are ranked by the generality of authors among the principal causes of retrocession.

Without attending to the antiquated theories of repelled eruption, of this we are assured, that whatever debilitates, in most cases of miliary fever, is pernicious; whatever supports the vigour of the system, beneficial. It is not to be overlooked however that there are cases, where notwithstanding the sweatings and miliary eruption, the excitement is such as in all kinds of fever warrants blood-letting. In these cases the theory of retrocession deserves as little attention as in the former. In the one case we avoid blood-letting, because the excitement is already sufficiently low; in the other we employ it, because the excitement is such that its continuance would occasion a greater degree of debility than the blood-letting which relieves it; nor, reflecting on what has been said, need we fear that blood-letting in such circumstances will repel the eruption. It is determined by experience, says Burserius, that if while the miliary eruption is present, an inflammation of the viscera be feared, or if the fever be very vehement, a large blood-letting may be employed without repelling the eruption. Quarin and others make similar observations. Blood-letting, says Quarin, is particularly necessary in the miliary fever, when it has arisen from the abuse of spirituous liquors, or the suppression of the lochia, that is, he might have added, where the excitement runs high. In such cases, however, the evacuation should be less in proportion to the excitement than in cases of simple synochus.

Reviewing all that has been said we shall find, that the change which the appearance of the miliary eruption and the symptoms that attend it render proper in the treatment of synochus, consists in employing tonic remedies more liberally, and evacuations more sparingly, than in cases unattended by an eruption; the miliary eruption tending constantly to overcome excitement and produce debility. The nature of the complaint thus leads to the practice which experience has proved to be most successful.*

* In considering the treatment of the synochus miliaris I have taken no

The remedies which have been employed, when a retrocession of the eruption, attended by various symptoms of debility, happens, are the same as those recommended in similar circumstances in other eruptive fevers, and which we shall presently have occasion to consider more at length. In the disease before us, musk and camphire are particularly recommended where convulsions supervene; opium, blisters, and frictions of the skin, in all cases. But our principal view should be to bring out and support a sweat, and if the retrocession be followed by any considerable evacuation, we must be careful not to check it. Different means, it is evident, will be proper in different cases, according to the cause of the retrocession.* See what has been said of the causes of retrocession.

SECT. III.

Of the Aphthous Fever.

THE Aphthous Fever is defined by Dr. Cullen,

" Synochus. Lingua tumidiuscula, linguæ et faucium color
" purpurascens; ascharæ in faucibus, et ad linguæ margines,
" primum comparentes, os internum totum demum occupantes,
" albidæ, aliquando discretæ, sæpe coalescentes, abrasæ cito re-
" nascentes, et incerto tempore manentes."

This definition, we shall find, does not include all the affections which have been known by the name of aphthæ; but it describes with sufficient accuracy that to which, by the general consent of physicians, the term is now confined.

It appears from what was said in the introduction, that the aphthous fever is to be regarded in the same point of view as the miliary, being nothing more than the common synochus accompanied with an eruption of aphthæ, and the peculiar, symptoms that attend it, whether accompanying fever or other diseases, or appearing as an idiopathic affection.

In detailing the symptoms of the synochus aphthosus, I shall pursue the same method followed in detailing those of the synochus miliaris; in the first place giving an account of the eruption, then enumerating the symptoms which precede or attend it, and lastly pointing out the febrile states in which it is most apt to shew itself.

notice of blisters, which have been warmly recommended in this fever, as there is nothing to be added on this part of the subject to what was said in speaking of the treatment in the synochus simplex. It appears from what was then said, that their cordial property, for which they seem chiefly to, have been recommended in the miliary fever, is very inconsiderable.

* Quarin thinks that the retrocession is the more dangerous the more copious the eruption.

1. Of the Symptoms of the Aphthous Fever.

Of the Aphthous Eruption.

The aphthæ infantum* is the same eruption which occasionally appears in synochus ; and whether it attacks the infant or the adult, and whether it appears with or without fever, it is attended with the same train of symptoms. As a symptom of synochus it has not demanded so much attention as where it appears as an idiopathic affection, which it seldom does in adults. In the writings of those who treat of the aphthæ infantum therefore we find the best account of this eruption. I shall describe the idiopathic affection as it appears in children, and then shew that all the symptoms of aphthæ infantum occasionally attend this eruption when it shews itself in synochus.

The local affection of the fauces is often the first symptom of the aphthæ infantum ; certain symptoms however now and then precede it even in the youngest children From appearing in health they sometimes, very suddenly, shew signs of uneasiness ; they either refuse the breast, or if they receive the nipple, do not suck ; they appear restless and anxious, cry much, sleep less than usual, and what sleep they have, is disturbed. They become pale and emaciated, and are often troubled with hiccup, and diarrhœa in which the stools are acrid and fetid. Curdled milk is sometimes past by stool, and bile evacuated by vomiting.†

Such are the symptoms which Arnemann says he frequently observed to precede the appearance of aphthæ.‡

They are sometimes preceded by other symptoms. If the child is not very young, the pulse is often considerably affected, becoming more frequent than in health, the temperature is increased, and a sleepiness sometimes approaching to coma supervenes. Upon the whole however, in children, the affection of the mouth and fauces is generally the first symptom, the mouth becomes redder than natural, the tongue swelled and rough, and the nurse perceives an increase of temperature in the child's mouth. Sometimes the mouth becomes pale instead of red previous to the eruption of aphthæ, which generally presages a worse form of the complaint.

Soon after these appearances, the aphthæ begin to shew themselves in the internal fauces, and about the edges of the tongue. " Pustulæ sunt albicantes," says Ketelaer,‖ who saw as many ca-

* The thrush.

† Arnemann's Commentatio de Aphthis.

‡ It will appear, as we proceed in considering the symptoms of this complaint, that those here enumerated by Arnemann as frequently preceding the affection of the fauces, arise from the aphthous eruption first seizing upon the œsophagus.

‖ Ketelaer's Treatise de Aphthis Nostratibus.

ses of this disease as perhaps any other practitioner, " summis
" ac internis oris, et interdum vicinis respirationis partibus insi-
" dentes." The true aphthæ are described in nearly the same
manner by most authors who practised in those countries where
the disease is common. Armstrong compares their first appearance to that of broken curds.

Even on their first coming out, aphthæ sometimes so run together that they look like a white compact crust, covering a great
part of the internal fauces, and often arising as it were from the
œsophagus. At first, Boerhaave* observes, solitary pustules often appear here and there on the tongue, angles of the mouth,
fauces, and neighbouring parts ; these are generally of a favourable kind. Sometimes they appear first in the deepest part of the
fauces, as if ascending from the œsophagus, in the form of a white
dense shining crust† gradually spreading over the fauces. These
are of a bad kind and generally fatal. Boerhaave adds another
appearance which they sometimes assume, " Aliquando duris
" crassis densis tenacibus crustis, totum cavum oris ubique, us-
" que ad labia obsident, omnia tegentes simul : et ab his raro re-
" surgent ægri."

In short, aphthæ are small whitish eschars, appearing in the
fauces and about the tongue or lips, sometimes few and distinct,
at other times numerous and confluent. Their number and degree of confluence are particularly to be attended to, as the prognosis rests much upon them.

In determining the number of aphthæ we may sometimes be
deceived, since they are often numerous on the deeper seated
parts, while they are but thinly scattered on the tongue and other
parts of the mouth. It also happens, though rarely, Van Swieten
observes, that although there be few aphthæ on every part which
can be seen, yet on the more internal parts (for we shall find that
the seat of aphthæ extends much farther than the fauces) they
are very numerous, and may often therefore prove fatal when the
physician least expects it, if he forms his judgment from the appearance of the fauces alone.

But even in this case, a person acquainted with the nature of
the disease can hardly be mistaken, for wherever the aphthæ are
numerous in internal parts, sickness, hiccup, oppression, and
generally pain referred to the stomach, with much debility, point
out the danger, which when these symptoms occur is always urgent, whatever be the state of the fauces. The presence of
this variety of the disease, it is evident, is not so easily ascertained in children as in adults. Whatever be the attending symptoms, however, when the crust mentioned by Boerhaave, appears
to ascend from the œsophagus, it is probable that the more inter-

* Aph. 984.

† It is in this case that the symptoms mentioned by Arnemann most frequently precede the appearance of Aphthæ.

tal parts are considerably affected, and the prognosis therefore
is had. Nor is the case more favourable when the whole mouth
appears covered with a crust and becomes dry, the process which
ought to throw off this crust being absent or extremely languid.
If this state of the fauces continues for a considerable length of
time, the power of swallowing is lost, and the danger becomes
very urgent. Van Swieten met with cases of this kind in which
the tongue, lips, and cheeks were rendered almost rigid by the
crust; so that a liquid could not even be retained in the mouth;
at length, he observes, the same complaint spreading to the fauces, the patients were suffocated.

The colour of the aphthæ has occasioned some dispute, which
seems to have arisen from the same aphthæ changing their colour
and becoming darker the longer they adhere; for there seem to
be, no well authenticated cases in which the aphthæ on their first
appearance were of a dark brown or black colour, as some writers
have alleged. Boerhaave indeed observes, that the colour of
aphthæ is various, being either of a pellucid or shining white, like
pearls, or of an opaque white or yellow colour, livid, or even black.*
But Boerhaave speaks here not of the difference of aphthæ on
their coming out, but of the appearance of the same aphthæ at
different periods; for his commentator Van Swieten, Arnemann,
Ketelaer, Armstrong, and others, who had extensive opportunities
of seeing this disease, declare that they never saw aphthæ dark
red, brown, or black on their first appearance. " Non enim veri-
" simile est," Ketelaer observes, " ut in rebus sibi adeo vicinis, et
" cognatis, fors tantum polleat, cum albæ plus millies nobis obla-
" tæ sint, ut rubrarum, nigrarumve, ne umbræ quidem unquam
" apparuerint." We therefore see the propriety of Dr. Cullen's
making whiteness one of the distinguishing marks of this eruption; and giving it a place in the nosological character.

But although aphthæ on their first appearance are never of a
dark brown or black, they sometimes, though not very frequently,
appear of a light brown or ash colour. Arnemann terms the colour of these " flavæ vel fuscæ cineritiæ."

. The white pellucid aphthæ, like pearls, are always the safest,†
and when they are few in number the disease is scarcely attended
with any danger; but when aphthæ appear from the first of a
brownish colour, the prognosis is very bad. Van Swieten says,
that he has uniformly found such cases fatal. The prognosis is
between these extremes; when the aphthæ appear at first of a
pearl colour but in considerable number, and soon begin to assume
a brownish hue; when they become black the danger is very urgent; they are then to be considered as nothing less than small

* Aph. 985.

† When they appear of an opaque white, like lard, they are less favourable.

gangrenous sloughs, which often reduce the whole internal fauces
to a state of mortification.

It has just been observed that it is only after the aphthæ have
remained for a considerable time that they become brown or
black; hence the time they adhere becomes a point of consequence in forming the prognosis; but when they begin to fall,
we shall often be deceived if we look for the immediate termination of the disease, since it frequently happens, that a fresh crop
succeeds that which has fallen or been rubbed off.

If this crop appears more numerous and crowded together than
the first crop, the prognosis is worse than when the aphthæ appear fewer and more distinct. But upon the whole one crop falling off and another appearing affords a more favourable prognosis,
than one crop continuing for the same space of time, and becoming brown or black, which is always indeed the effect of its continuance.

Aphthæ sometimes fall off in the space of ten or twelve hours,
at other times they remain attached for many days; nor do they
fall from the whole fauces at the same time, nor always first from
any one part, but in this respect they are as variable as in their
duration.

Although when the disease continues for a considerable time,
repeated crops of apthæ afford a more favourable prognosis than
the same crop remaining throughout the whole course of the disease; yet the prognosis is still better, when the aphthæ fall early,
as in the former case, and are not succeeded by a fresh crop or only by a very scanty one; it is therefore a matter of much consequence in forming the prognosis to be able to foresee whether or
not a fresh crop of aphthæ is about to come out, and this in some
measure may be learnt from the appearance of the places which
the former occupied.

If they be clean, red, and moist, the aphthæ either do not reappear, or only reappear in a small number; but if the parts the
first crop occupied appear foul and parched, then we may very
certainly except a renewal of the eruption, and in such cases the
separation and reproduction of the aphthæ often take place a
great number of times before the final solution of the disease.
Both Ketelaer and Van Swieten observed this process repeated to
the sixth, seventh, or eighth time; and the latter remarks that
he has sometimes known an interval of several days between
the separation and reproduction of the aphthæ; but upon the
whole, however frequently they return, those aphthæ which fall
off the soonest are the safest.

There are two seemingly opposite extremes, which are now
and then equally dangerous. The one when the new crop supervenes before the old crop is thrown off; this not only gives rise
to a great number of aphthæ adhering at the same time, but also

shews that they have little tendency to separate, which is always an unfavourable sign. [*] The other, and no less dangerous, case is when the first crop falls off, and from the appearance of the fauces we are led to expect another, which however does not come out, or, at least, is delayed for some days. If, along with this symptom, much anxiety, oppression, and other marks of debility, or a degree of coma, supervene, the danger is very considerable, this case generally proving fatal if a fresh crop of aphthæ do not make their appearance, which in most instances is attended with relief.

In the most favourable cases then, the aphthæ appear of a white pearly colour, fall off early, leaving the places they occupied clean, red, and moist ; and upon the separation taking place, all the symptoms begin to abate, and in a short time wholly disappear. On the other hand, the more the aphthæ assume a brownish tint, the longer they continue to adhere, the more foul and parched the places which they occupied appear, the sooner the first crop is succeeded by another, or the more alarming the symptoms of debility or the coma when a second crop does not make its appearance, the greater is the danger.

We have hitherto considered the course of aphthæ in the fauces, where it may be seen, but this disease sometimes extends to the more internal parts, and seems to run the same course in them as in the fauces. " Latius quandoque propagantur aphthæ," Lieutaud [*] observes, " quæ œsophagum, ventriculum et " intestina haud sine presenti vitæ discrimine nonnunquam invadunt." The same observations have been made by all who have been conversant in this disease.

The symptoms which indicate that the disease has extended to the stomach and alimentary canal, are various. Many of these however cannot be detected in the aphthæ infantum, since infants cannot describe what they feel. In treating their complaints we must trust to our own observation and that of the attendants.

The symptoms to be discovered in this way, and which teach us that the complaint is extending along the alimentary canal, are, an appearance of much anxiety, oppression, and debility, vomiting, hiccup[†], what Armstrong calls watery gripes,[‡] and convulsions. What places the matter beyond a doubt is finding aphthæ about the time they are observed to separate in the fauces, thrown up from the stomach, or passed by stool.

Ketelaer saw them thrown out in both ways in astonishing

---

[*] Synopsis Med. Pract.

[†] Hiccup attends aphthæ in the œsophagus or stomach. See Van Swieten's Commentary on the 659 Aph. of Boerhaave.

[‡] This is one of the most fatal symptoms, as we shall see more particularly in considering the treatment in this complaint, which must be so regulated as carefully to prevent the appearance of this symptom.

quantity. " Aphthas quando jam maturuerunt et excernuntur,
" tanta copia aliquos dies per os et per alvum nonnunquam rejici,
" ut aliquot pelves vel matulæ congestas eas vix capiant." Vogel
makes a similar observation. This is almost incredible, and denotes the very worst form of the disease. Were there nothing
to destroy the patient but the debility which so profuse an evacuation must occasion, he could not long support it.

Aphthæ have also been found in the trachea extending, as Lieutaud* observes, even to the bronchiæ. They are known to have
extended to the trachea, and bronchiæ by the presence of dyspnœa,
and by their being thrown up by coughing. This is perhaps the
most dangerous form of the disease, the aphthæ often accumula-
ting in the wind-pipe or its branches so as to occasion suffocation.

Besides the symptoms which have been enumerated, there are
others, which, though less essential, often accompany this disease.
When the aphthæ of the mouth fall off, a salivation often ensues,
in part at least caused by the high degree of sensibility which remains, the whole internal fauces sometimes appearing as if the
cuticle had been abraded.

About the same time also, a diarrhœa frequently supervenes,
which may either be produced by the affection of the stomach
and the intestines themselves, if the disease has extended to
them, or by the acrid matter secreted in the mouth being swallowed. As these symptoms supervene towards the termination
of the disease, when the patient is much debilitated, they often
prove alarming, sometimes carrying him off when the attendants,
and even the physician, judge the danger nearly passed.

When these discharges are moderate, they have been looked
upon as salutary. This opinion, however, is as much perhaps an
inference from hypothesis as from facts ; it being a favourite
maxim with the older physicians, that the dregs of the fever, as
they were termed, should be carried off by catharsis or venesection. The patient indeed often recovers about the time the salivation and diarrhœa appear. But at this period the aphthæ fall,
and the complaint generally remits, whether such symptoms supervene or not.

It will appear however in considering the treatment, that a moderate diarrhœa at the time the aphthæ fall is often useful, especially when the disease has spread to the stomach and bowels, by
preventing a relapse, which the irritation of the fallen aphthæ in
the bowels frequently occasions.

The taste in general is nearly lost, and deglutition is often prevented while the aphthous incrustation remains. After it is separated, on the contrary, the taste is so acute, and the whole internal fauces so sensible, that the mildest food gives pain, and the

* Synopsi Med. Pract.

patient is now, although from a different cause, often as incapable of swallowing as before.

The aphthæ indeed frequently leave the parts so sensible, that they bleed on the slightest occasion ; hence it is that bloody saliva and bloody stools frequently attend this disease. Boerhaave justly observes, that if we reflect that the seat of aphthæ is in the stomach and intestines, as well as in the fauces, we shall not be surprised at the variety of symptoms which attend, or follow them. This indeed readily explains the greater part of these symptoms, bloody or dysenteric purging, symptoms denoting inflammation, excoriation, or mortification, in the alimentary canal. "Aphthæ igitur " vulgatiores, et ori coercitæ," says Lieutaud,* ," minime sunt " pertimescendæ, et facile evincuntur, sed ubi œsophago infigun-" tur, ad ventriculum et intestina se spargere solent, hinc subori-" untur febris, tormina, diarrhœa, dysenteria, aliique graviores " morbi : si vero laryngem subeant, et ad tracheam bronchia et " pulmones diffundantur ; tussem ferocem, spirandi difficultatem, " alique truculentiora symptomata concitant."

Notwithstanding what Lieutaud says in the first part of this quotation, aphthæ, even when they extend no further than the fauces, are often a very alarming disease. For besides proving dangerous in the ways already mentioned by impeding deglutition and tending to interrupt respiration, even where the disease has not spread to the trachea,† aphthæ often induce mortification on the palate and neighbouring parts ; for it frequently happens that when the aphthæ adhere longer than usual, the parts beneath become gangrenous, and the mortification sometimes extends to the palate bones.‡

The aphthæ infantum are sometimes complicated with other diseases, most frequently with worms.

Such are the symptoms of idiopathic aphthæ, the aphthæ infantum. Idiopathic cases of aphthæ rarely occur in adults. Kelaer indeed declares that such cases are very common ; but it was observed in the Introduction that Boerhaave had seen but two cases of this kind, that neither Van Swieten nor Cullen had seen one, and Arnemann very few. When aphthæ appear as an idiopathic affection in adults, the symptoms do not differ from those of the aphthæ infantum, and the treatment in both cases is the same.

Of the Symptoms preceding and accompanying Aphthæ.

Although the complaints in which the miliary eruption occurs, are no less various than those occasionally attended by aphthæ, yet it appears from what was said of the former eruption, that in

* Synopsis Med. Pract.

† Aphthæ, Vogel observes, often occasion suffocation merely by the swelling of the fauces which attends them.

‡ Aph. Boerhaavii, Aph. 989.

whatever complaint it appears, a certain train of symptoms generally attends it. The same is true of aphthæ, although the accompanying symptoms in this instance are less uniformly present.

When aphthæ begin in internal parts (which is sometimes the case in the symptomatic as well as idiopathic aphthæ) their appearance in the fauces is consequently preceded by the various symptoms denoting their presence in other parts of the alimentary canal. In this case the aphthæ appear to ascend from the œsophagus in the same manner as in the worst cases of aphthæ infantum.

Anxiety, oppression, and debility however often precede the appearance of aphthæ, when they are about to make their first attack on the fauces, and like most other eruptions, they are now and then preceded by a degree of coma, less frequently by delirium.

But such symptoms frequently occur in fevers where no aphthæ are about to appear, and aphthæ sometimes appear without being preceded by these, or indeed any other symptoms, which can be supposed particularly connected with their appearance; so that although there are certain symptoms which frequently precede this eruption, especially when it begins in internal parts, yet there are none from which we can with much certainty predict its appearance.

If however the foregoing symptoms occur in fever, while at the same time the fauces appear unusually red or pale, there is reason to expect an eruption of aphthæ.

It is almost unnecessary to observe, that when aphthæ spread from the fauces along the alimentary canal, they are followed by the same symptoms which precede their appearance, when they make their first attack on internal parts. "But of much more " uncertain and dangerous event," Huxham observes, speaking of malignant fevers, " are the brown dark coloured aphthæ. Nor " are those which are exceedingly white and thick, like lard, of a " very promising aspect; they are soon succeeded by great diffi- " culty of swallowing, pain and ulceration of the fauces, œsopha- " gus, &c. and with an incessant singultus; the whole primæ viæ " become at last affected; and a bloody dysentery comes on fol- " lowed by a sphacelation of the intestines, as is evident from the " black sanious bloody stools, horribly fetid and extremely infec- " tious."

Upon the whole, the symptoms of the symptomatic aphthæ are not different from those of the aphthæ infantum, except that the former generally occurring in adults, we have a more distinct account of many of the attending symptoms; and that these symptoms are occasionally modified by the idiopathic disease in which the aphthæ appear.

Of the Febrile States in which Aphthæ most frequently appear.

In some fevers there is a remarkable tendency to dysenteric affections. The symptoms of dysentery are afterwards to be considered; it is sufficient at present to observe, that in fevers attended by much griping and mucous and bloody stools, the appearance of aphthæ is more frequent than in most others.

The first mention of aphthæ which occurs in the works of Sydenham, is in his account of the dysenteric fever of the years 1669, 1670, 1671, and 1672. The aphthæ generally supervened in those cases in which the fever proved obstinate, and chiefly, he observes, where the hot regimen had been pursued, and diarrhœas checked by the unseasonable use of astringents. " Præ-" sertim si, præter regimen calidius, evacuationes etiam per al-" vum medicamentis astringentibus prius fuerint coercitæ." Arnemann makes the same observations.

Sydenham further observes of this fever, in which aphthæ were more frequent than he had found them in any other, that it was seldom or never attended with sweats, while in fevers, unaccompanied by aphthæ, the sweating was often profuse. The latter remark has been confirmed by many succeeding observations. Ketelaer even goes so far as to maintain, that it is the deficiency of perspiration that renders aphthæ more frequent in cold than in warm climates; and in support of this opinion he asserts, that he has found aphthæ rendered milder by a copious flow of sweat or urine, and that every thing tending to check these discharges, increases the virulence of the aphthæ.

Notwithstanding the truth of these observations, aphthæ are apt to appear in the miliary fever, where there is generally much sweating. There is such similarity between some of the symptoms attending aphthæ, and those attending the miliary eruption, that some have believed these eruptions to arise from the same cause,* and that when the appearance of the one is prevented, that of the other, the general state of the symptoms remaining the same, is a necessary consequence; and to this circumstance Van Swieten thinks we may ascribe the frequent appearance of aphthæ in cold countries, where the flow of sweat, and consequently the appearance of the miliary eruption, is checked; and on the other hand, the frequency of the latter eruption, with the rarity of the other, in warmer climates.

The frequent concurrence of the miliary eruption and aphthæ, certainly points out some connection between the two affections. Sydenham seldom met with aphthæ in fevers, except in the one just mentioned, remarkable for its dysenteric tendency; and in that which was mentioned when speaking of the synochus miliaris, in which he frequently observed both eruptions. " In the

* " Materiem aphthosam et miliarem eamdem esse judicabam." Stoli's Ratio Medendi.

" course of many miliary fevers," says M'Bride,* " it is frequent
" to see aphthæ in the mouth and ulcerations in the fauces preying
" upon the tonsils and uvula."

This fact however does not certainly warrant the opinion, that
both affections arise from a cause lurking in the body, that must
produce the one eruption or the other. We are well assured
that the miliary eruption may be prevented without inducing
aphthæ. It will appear more clearly from what will be said of
the causes of aphthæ, that irritation of the primæ viæ and skin,
seems, from a well-known sympathy which subsists between the
different parts of the alimentary canal, and between every part of
it and the skin, often to give rise to this affection of the fauces,
and it is in this way that we may account for aphthæ being so
common in dysenteric fevers, and in those where the skin is unusually parched, or covered with so irritating an eruption as the
miliary.

Aphthæ are also most apt to shew themselves where the debility is considerable ; and particularly when those symptoms, which
have been termed putrescent, make their appearance. In adults,
says Arnemann, aphthæ very frequently follow putrid, continued,
and intermitting fevers ; " præcipue febres autumnales, quæ cum
" diarrhœa et dysenteria incipiunt, imprimis si ægroti, calido re-
" gimine fuissent usi, vel materiæ peccantis evacuatio adstringen-
" tium usu intempestivo foret impedita." Francis, he adds, met
with aphthæ in putrid continued fevers ; Bosch in putrid intermitting fevers ; Grant in the irregular quartan and tertian ; Hillary in the malignant dysentery ; Huxham in the low nervous fever ; Sims in a similar fever ; Kloeckhoff in an epidemic continued fever ; Untzer in putrid and hectic fevers.

Such are the fevers in which aphthæ frequently appear. The
characteristic marks of these fevers are morbid affections of the
skin and bowels, and much debility.

There are many other complaints, occasionally attended with
this eruption, and as in fevers, so in these, it is still most apt to
appear where debility prevails. Among the principal of these
are worms and dysentery, further denoting the tendency of aphthæ to accompany affections of the alimentary canal ; and scurvy,
phthisis pulmonalis, and the last stage of all kinds of dropsy further denoting their tendency to appear in debilitated states of the
system.†

Such are the aphthæ properly so called, the symptoms which attend them, and the fevers in which they are most apt to appear.
The term aphthæ however has been used to express complaints
very different from the true aphthæ. Most of these are local af-

* Introduction to the Theory and Practice of Medicine.

† Boerhaave remarks, that aphthæ are apt to accompany all visceral
inflammations.

fections of little consequence ; it will be sufficient to mention a few of the most remarkable.

The indefinite use of the term aphthæ is chiefly met with, in the works of the ancients, " Nam quæ a priscis medicinæ con- " ditoribus aphthæ describuntur, adeo a nostris diversæ sunt, ut " toto cœlo distent."* It has already been observed that aphthæ are less a disease of warm, than of cold climates ; so that many doubt whether the true aphthæ were at all known to the ancients, and think that we have borrowed a term from them for the name of a disease, which was unknown in the times and countries in which they practised.† In the works of Hippocrates, Arctæus, and Galen, we not only find, mentioned under this term, affections of the mouth different from aphthæ (small sores for instance on the inside of the cheeks and about the lips)‡ but also similar erup- tions in other parts of the body, particularly in the genitals. A pustulary eruption of these parts, independent of any venereal affection, is not uncommon, and seems frequently the consequence of cold, of which I have known several instances.

Besides these, there are other eruptions termed aphthæ by the ancients. The reader will find an account of many of them in the works of Fernelius,‖ and in those of Sennertus in his chapter entitled, de Oris Inflammationibus et Ulceribus.

2. Of the Causes of the Aphthous Fever.

'It has just been observed, that this disease is more frequent in cold, than in warm and temperate climates. In the southern parts of Europe indeed it is hardly known ; while in Holland and other northern countries there are few diseases more frequent. Van Swieten observes, that while he practised in his native coun- try (Holland), there were few symptoms which more frequently occurred to him in acute diseases, whereas at Vienna he had not met with a single instance of aphthæ in the space of five years.

Aphthæ are most frequent in low marshy situations, and in spring and autumn, particularly in the latter when it is unusually moist, and follows a warm and moist summer. In short, cold

* Ketelaer de Aphthis Nostratibus.

† Sennertus asserts, on the authority of Aretæus, that aphthæ were common in Syria and Egypt ; but the complaint mentioned by Aretæus is not the same with that now termed aphthæ.

‡ Van Swieten describes a thrush of a peculiar kind, which he thinks the same with one of the species of aphthæ mentioned by Aretæus. It was epidemic in Holland in the 18th year of the present century, appear- ing in small ulcers about the lips, cheeks, and gums, and when neglected on account of the little uneasiness it gave at first, quickly eroding the parts it occupied, and forming putrid sores. This complaint, like the true thrush, was most apt to attack children, and when it appeared in adults was generally milder.

‖ Fernelii Universa Medicina.

and moisture are among the principal causes of this complaint. In Zealand, which lies lower than the surface of the sea, which is prevented from overflowing it by raised banks, aphthæ are so frequent, that Ketelaer calls them the endemic distemper of the island.

Although aphthæ appear in people of all ages, infants and old people, Boerhaave observes, are most subject to them. In many parts of Holland, it is unusual for a child to escape aphthæ during the first month ; but they are generally of so favourable a kind, that in most cases medical assistance is not necessary. In old people, in whom they generally appear during fevers, they are for the most part of a bad kind, and often prove fatal.

Such are the circumstances which may be regarded as the predisposing causes of aphthæ, for although cold and moisture have a principal share in producing the disease, the application of some other cause in general seems necessary, since the majority of children in most countries, however cold and damp, escape it.

One of the principal exciting causes appears to be derangement of the primæ viæ. It was observed that aphthæ are frequently preceded by symptoms indicating such derangement. It has been an observation, says Arnemann, from the days of Hippocrates even to our own times, that impurities of the primæ viæ are conjoined with exanthemata and other cutaneous diseases ; and daily experience evinces, that derangement of these passages tends to vitiate the skin in various ways. " Signa præterea aphtharum," he adds, " eruptioni præcedentia et socia symptomata sat super- " que declarant, mali nostri fomitem in primis viis unice " quærendum esse, communi omnium cutis exanthematum sca- " turigine. Indicant aphtharum ex abdomine originem nauseæ, " vomitus, diarrhœæ male olentes, fecium color viridis, mucus et " colluvies ovorum albumini quandoque non absimilis. Quin adeo " prædixit cl. Oosterdyck futuram aphtharum eruptionem, ex " anxietate, pondere stomachi, sensuum confusione, somnolentia, " singultu, tussicula sicca, et frequenti screatu." But these things, he observes, are so well known, that I might appear tedious were I any longer to dwell on them.

We shall also find, that some arguments in support of the opinion, that aphthæ are occasioned by impurities of the alimentary canal, may be drawn from the mode of treatment.

It does not appear, that such affections of the primæ viæ do always, by their local irritation, first produce the aphthæ in the stomach and bowels, which afterwards spread to the fauces ; but from the sympathy of parts, they occasion their first eruption in the fauces.

From what has just been said it follows, that the various causes of derangement in the alimentary canal are to be regarded as occasional causes of aphthæ. One of the chief of these is worms, and it appears to be in this way that these two complaints are so frequently conjoined. Bad milk often has the same effect; Lieutaud observes, that a drunken nurse often occasions aphthæ in the infant, and the same may be said of whatever else disturbs the nurse's health, such as anxiety, violent passions, &c.

Some suppose that bad milk may operate in another way in producing aphthæ, by irritating the fauces, and it would be difficult to ascertain that aphthæ proceed from the action of the milk on the stomach and intestines alone, although there are many reasons to believe that this is the case.

- There can be little doubt however, that more powerful irritations of the fauces are sometimes the exciting cause of aphthæ. Sennertus indeed esteems local irritation in the mouth a frequent cause of the complaint. " Gignuntur aphthæ interdum primario " in ore, dum ibi pravi humores collecti sunt, quos natura foras " expellat." And Dr. Home in his Principia Medicinæ enumerates among the causes of aphthæ " Frictio oris ab externis cau- " sis," and violent exertions in sucking. Nay the former author even thinks that where they arise from the morbid contents of the stomach, they are occasioned by these, or an acrid vapour arising from them, being thrown upwards and immediately applied to the fauces. When we reflect however, that derangement of the alimentary canal frequently occasions, eruptions on the skin, as well as in the fauces, this opinion appears very improbable.

In the same way, we may account for an increased secretion of bile proving the cause of this complaint. Fernelius considers this one of its most frequent causes. It has not however been generally so regarded; an immoderate secretion of bile being rare in those countries where aphthæ prevail.

Such are the chief circumstances which have been determined respecting the causes of the aphthæ infantum; yet in many cases they do not seem to proceed from any of those which have been mentioned; and in a still greater number of instances, these causes are present, without producing the disease.

Still less is known respecting the causes which give rise to aphthæ in adults. The presence of the different diseases in which they occur may doubtless be looked upon as the predisposing causes, and in considering in what kinds of fevers they most frequently make their appearance, we found certain circumstances, besides affections of the primæ viæ, namely, unusual deficiency of perspiration, and the presence of the miliary eruption, favourable to their appearance.

How these circumstances tend to produce them, or whether or not they and the aphthæ arise from the same unknown cause, it is impossible for us positively to determine. It has already been hinted, that the sympathy which subsists between the different

parts of the alimentary canal and the skin, may explain why affections of the latter are frequently accompanied by aphthæ. We
know that derangement of the stomach and bowels produces aphthæ, and nothing injures the functions of these organs more than
causes affecting the perspiration.

3. Of the Treatment of the Aphthous Fever.

The treatment of aphthæ may be divided into two parts. In
the first, we shall consider the cure of idiopathic aphthæ, the aphthæ infantum ; and in the second, the mode of treatment when
aphthæ appear in fever. As for those cases in which aphthæ supervene in dropsy and other complaints, unaccompanied by fever,
their treatment is in no respect different from that of idiopathic
aphthæ, except as far as the treatment of the primary disease
renders it so.

We are in the first place then, to consider the treatment of
idiopathic aphthæ.

The first thing to be done is to remove the remote causes, if
they still continue to be applied. It appears from the foregoing
observations, that we have often reason to suspect the disease to
arise from bad milk. The state of this should therefore be examined, and if it be found that no attention to diet renders it mild
and sweet, it is necessary to change the nurse.

Wherever we suspect the disease to have arisen from the ingesta, we must begin the treatment by clearing the primæ viæ.
Both emetics and cathartics are recommended by those who have
been most conversant with the disease.

The exhibition of the latter requires much caution, very gentle
cathartics in this complaint having sometimes induced a fatal hypercatharsis. Children who die of aphthæ indeed, even where
no cathartic has been exhibited, are very frequently carried off by
a profuse diarrhœa.

This ought not however to deter us from employing gentle
laxatives at the commencement of the complaint, especially when
it seems to arise from the cause just mentioned. It is in fact one
of the best means of preventing profuse purging, since the irritating matter, when suffered to accumulate in the alimentary canal,
increases the morbid affection of the intestines. Sydenham, it
was observed, remarks, that he has often seen aphthæ induced by
stopping a diarrhœa, and thus confining irritating matter, which,
together with that produced by the disease itself, often gives rise
to the fatal purging just alluded to. But whether it has this effect or not, the retention of irritating matter in the primæ viæ
must increase a complaint, which it is capable of causing. These
were the worst and most dangerous cases, Ketelaer from very
extensive experience observes, in which evacuations were not
employed in the beginning.

Thus far then the practice seems well ascertained: a gentle cathartic is proper in all cases when we see the patient at the commencement of the disease, particularly where there is reason to suspect irritating matter in the alimentary canal. Nor should the disease appearing in the mildest form, induce us to neglect this precaution, which can never do harm.* If there is much acid in the primæ viæ, absorbents are proper, and magnesia is preferable to chalk, as it forms with the acid generated in the bowels a cathartic salt. Dr. Aery, in the second volume of the Medical Museum, says that he has almost entirely laid aside other remedies in the thrush, confining himself to magnesia in small doses; and with this practice for many years he had lost only one in thirty. Dr. Underwood also trusts chiefly to absorbents in mild cases.†

Should the purging, however induced, shew a tendency to become excessive, which is always attended with danger in this complaint, we need not hesitate to exhibit a gentle anodyne, after the matter we wish to expel is evacuated. Lieutaud remarks, that anodynes are not only innocent but useful in this complaint, when cautiously administered, even where they are not used with a view to check immoderate catharsis.

It sometimes though rarely happens, that symptoms denoting a tendency to visceral inflammations shew themselves. In such cases it is better to permit the purging to continue till the symptoms are relieved, and at all events not to check it by opiates. But children are much less subject than adults to such inflammations, and the chief danger in the aphthæ infantum arises from debility.

When there is no tendency to excessive purging, opiates perhaps may be omitted, unless they be necessary to procure sleep,

* The syrup of rhubarb has been recommended as one of the best cathartics in this case. The preparations of rhubarb, while they evacuate the intestines, tend at the same time to strengthen the digesting organs. They are all apt however, especially when given alone, to occasion much griping. Rhubarb and magnesia are much recommended as a cathartic for children by Dr. Underwood, in his Treatise on their Complaints. Manna and the cassia fistularis, recommended by Dr. Cadogan in his work on the Management of Children, as less irritating than rhubarb, in the present case are perhaps preferable to it. Myrobalans are possessed of virtues in some degree similar to those of rhubarb, and are recommended by Van Swieten in this disease. Myrobalans are the dried fruit of a tree growing in the East Indies, with which botanists are not well acquainted. Their taste is astringent; they strike a black colour with chalybeate solutions, and are even employed by the Indians for tanning leather. Their purgative virtue is trifling. To the case before us, where much purging is dreaded and the patient very young, they seem well adapted, and the authority of Van Swieten, who was well acquainted with the aphthæ infantum, in their favour is not to be overlooked. They have been rejected however from the catalogue of simples by the colleges of London and Edinburgh.

† See Underwood on the Diseases of Children.

when they are always to be employed, except in the inflammatory cases just mentioned, proper means being used to prevent costiveness.

But the practice which is proper at the commencement of the complaint, is by no means suited to the advanced stage of it. If the disease has been properly treated from the beginning, there cannot at this period be any occasion for cathartics. But even in those instances, in which proper evacuations have been omitted till the disease is far advanced and the stomach and bowels are loaded with irritating matter, even in such cases, which seem more than any other to demand the employment of cathartics, we are not warranted to recommend them. They have often at this period induced a fatal hypercatharsis. The fæces may be evacuated by clysters, but it is dangerous to go further.

Arnemann proposes to give cathartics in small doses till the desired effect is produced, in order to guard against hypercatharsis; but we have reason to believe that neither this nor any other precaution can render their exhibition safe at the height of the disease. Ketelaer, whose opinion must have great weight, makes some excellent observations on the use of cathartics. "Eædem " rationes etiam contra purgationem eam militant, quæ cacochy- " miæ propria et accommodata, ab universo corpore et ulteriori- " bus viis, noxios quosque humores trahit. Ea hic funestissima " est, et intra paucas horas hypercatharsi finem vitæ plerumque " facit." But there is another kind of purging, he adds, if so it can be called, which may be employed with propriety, as it only evacuates the fæces, namely that induced by clysters. These medicines, he continues, are excellently suited to this disease in which costiveness is frequent; they not only empty the intestines, thus removing a noxious irritation; but they often relieve oppression, and what is of equal consequence frequently restore the other excretions, particularly those of the skin and kidneys, and tend to loosen the aphthæ.

Notwithstanding these observations of Ketelaer however, the indiscriminate use of clysters in this complaint is often dangerous; they have the same tendency with cathartics, though in a less degree, and should never perhaps be employed at this period, where the body is moderately open, unless the complaint be mild and the inflammatory tendency evident; and Ketelaer in other places makes nearly the same remark. In short, we recommend clysters at this period of the aphthæ infantum, to obviate restlessness, oppression, &c. occasioned by costiveness; and we ought not perhaps to recommend them till these symptoms begin to shew themselves.

It is to be recollected, that we do not at this period attempt to evacuate the stomach and small intestines, since the risk of inducing hypercatharsis more than counterbalances the chance of advantage from it. If the intestines have not been cleared at the beginning of the complaint, this must be looked upon as an irremediable error, and we must patiently wait its consequences. Hypercatharsis is chiefly to be dreaded when the disease has spread to the stomach and bowels.

Reflecting on what has been said, we readily perceive the effects to be wished for, and those to be dreaded, from clysters. By an attention to these, we determine what the composition of the clyster ought to be.

The first thing we have in view is to evacuate the fæces, with as little irritation as possible ; the clyster must therefore be mild, it should consist chiefly of water gruel or some other mucilaginous decoction. Some have recommended the addition of a cathartic, but this should only be had recourse to when a milder clyster is found insufficient. We have also in view to relax the excretories. Few things tend more to promote diaphoresis than a quantity of diluting fluid received into the stomach or intestines, and we have seen that according as the perspiration is free, the disease is often mild or otherwise. On this account the quantity injected should be considerable. When the aphthæ spread to the great intestines, which it was observed they often do, and even appear externally about the anus, clysters serve a further use, in lubricating and softening the parts to which they are immediately applied, and thus disposing the aphthæ to fall. In short they produce effects similar to those of gargles in the fauces, and should therefore in these cases be gently detergent as well as mucilaginous.

When such clysters are found to produce but little evacuation of the fæces, which is often the case, they may be repeated frequently.

That I may give at one view what is to be said of the employment of cathartics in the aphthæ infantum, which forms a very principal part of the treatment, it is to be observed, that there is a period of the disease, which succeeds that I am speaking of, in which their exhibition again becomes proper.

We must, says Arnemann, be careful not to exhibit purgatives while the aphthous crust still adheres to the intestines and their surface is raw and excoriated ; but they are necessary in the beginning of the complaint, and in its decline, when the aphthæ begin to fall, and are passed by stool. They are then serviceable by expelling the fallen aphthæ which, when allowed to remain, soon begin to corrupt and produce a new train of morbid symptoms.

But even after the aphthæ begin to fall, the danger of hypercatharsis, as might be supposed from the observations of Arnemann, is by no means passed, and sometimes scarcely at all lessened. There are several circumstances to be attended to in recommending cathartics at this period. We must not, as soon

as a few aphthæ are thrown out by stool or vomiting, order a cathartic ; we must wait at least twenty-four hours after this appearance, in order to learn whether the separation of the aphthæ
be really the solution of the disease, or merely partial and succeeded by a fresh crop, which is known by the symptoms suffering no abatement. In this case nothing more than an emollient
clyster is to be recommended.

. When on the other hand the symptoms abate, and particularly
if the aphthæ of the fauces fall, leaving the parts they occupied clean and moist, which is a sign, it was observed, of their
not being about to return, a cathartic is not only safe but necessary. If irritating matter in the primæ viæ is capable of producing
the disease, where it had not previously existed, it may certainly
be the means of renewing it.

In short, cathartics are to be employed in the decline of the
disease as early as can be done with safety.

However flattering the state of the patient may be, hypercatharsis may be induced by a rough cathartic. The intestines
are often left by this disease in a very irritable state, and the
proper choice of a cathartic is therefore a point of much consequence. On this subject there is little to be added to what has already been said. Rhubarb we still find particularly recommended
by those who have practised extensively in this disease. Calomel has been much recommended, but this, and still more scam-
mony, which is also employed, are certainly exceptionable.* o

Such are the circumstances to be attended to in the employment of cathartics in aphthæ, without an attention to which, the
practitioner must often be guilty of fatal errors.

Emetics may also be beneficial or otherwise.

At the commencement of the complaint they serve the same
purpose as cathartics, by evacuating the morbid contents of the
alimentary canal. At this period however they are on many accounts preferable to cathartics; their operation tends to weaken
less, and is particularly easy in young children, who seem often
to vomit with scarcely any uneasiness. Besides, the cause of
the disease seems often lodged in the stomach rather than in the
intestines. It is an organ of greater sensibility. Its affections
produce greater and more sudden effects on distant parts. If aphthæ be ever produced by acrid matter applied to the fauces, it is
chiefly from the stomach that such matter comes. A pain in the
stomach and vomiting more frequently precede the appearance
of aphthæ, than a griping or diarrhœa ; in short the stomach is
that part of the primæ viæ which seems most connected with the

* Has calomel any specific power in this disease as we shall find it has
in many other inflammatory affections ? If not, less irritating cathartics
are certainly preferable.

state of the disease, ' It is not 'surprising, therefore, that at its commencement emetics are often attended with the best effects.'

Arnemann extols them above every other remedy... " Emeti- " ca infantibus præscripta, omnibus medicamentis reliquis palmam " præripere videntur, quando morbi fomes in ventriculo adhuc la- " tet, et anxietas, singultus, ructus male olentes vel vomituri- " tiones ipsæ adsunt." Nor are they, he adds, to be preferred to cathartics, only because they seem better calculated for removing the cause of the disease, but also because they are found to weaken much less. They seem also serviceable, he might have added, by promoting perspiration, and it is probably in this way that they often relieve the disease, where the stomach is not loaded.

If however the first emetic does not bring relief, it is not prob- able that its repetition will be attended with much benefit.[a]

Emetics in the more advanced stages are either unnecessary as in mild cases, or they may do much harm where the aphthous in- crustations have spread to the œsophagus and stomach, by produ- cing hemorrhagy, excoriation, or inflammation.

Dr. Armstrong and Ketelaer recommend antimonial prepara- tions both as emetics and cathartics in this complaint. At an early period antimony is perhaps the best emetic we can employ, but in more advanced stages of the disease, should it be necessary to recommend an emetic, which is seldom the case, we must employ one which we can venture to prescribe at once in such a dose as secures its success. In this case therefore, ipecacuanha is preferable to antimony which must be given in small doses and may consequently pass the pylorus and excite purging.

Disputes have arisen respecting the propriety of blood-letting in the aphthæ infantum. Some asserting that all periods of the complaint are equally proper for the employment of this remedy, should inflammatory symptoms appear; others deeming it so dangerous to let blood after the appearance of aphthæ, that there is scarcely any symptom which will induce them to recom- mend it.

Reflecting on the nature of the complaint, the question seems a priori easily decided, and the judgment we are thus led to form is sanctioned by experience. Whatever other effect venesection produces, it always diminishes the strength. The question then is, are there any of the symptoms of the aphthæ infantum which we would endeavour to remove at this risk? In perhaps ninety of a hundred cases there are not. In by far the majority, the cau- ses of debility are more to be dreaded than any other. And in these circumstances who would think of adding one more to the number, and that the most powerful of all?

If the excitement is such as threatens danger, or visceral in- flammation has supervened, we must have recourse to blood-letting; but the latter seldom, and the former almost never, occurs in the aphthæ infantum.

When such symptoms do occur, blood-letting may be employed at any period of the disease, but with the more caution the more it is advanced. Such is the practice warranted by experience, and with respect to assertions which pre-conceived opinions have extorted, even from the best writers, they deserve little attention. " Omnem igitur, præsentibus aphthis," says Ketelaer, " incisionem venæ huc usque damnamus, atque proscribi: " mus." But in another place the same author admits, that plentiful blood-letting is necessary when an internal inflammation supervenes at any period of the disease, and gives a case in which it saved the patient's life.

The diet in this complaint requires some attention ; on this however there is little to be added to what was said of diet in synochus. When fever is present, the diet must be regulated by an attention to the febrile symptoms. If the excitement be considerable, it must be light and diluent ; if too low, as happens in the majority of cases, the diet must be more nourishing ; but in all cases it should be mild and mucilaginous.

In most cases it is proper to give cordials* composed of a little wine and aromatics, and sweetened with sugar. If the patient be at the breast and can suck, good milk of course must form the principal part of the diet. Where deglutition is wholly prevented, mild nourishing clysters have been recommended, and are, often serviceable.

It only now remains to make some observations on the local remedies employed in the aphthæ infantum ; and these, in the mildest cases where the aphthæ spread no farther than the fauces, and where there is no general affection of the system, are all that is necessary.

As it is impossible to make infants wash the mouth with any thing and then spit it out, the applications made to the internal fauces must either be such as may be swallowed, or they must be applied in very small quantity, by means of the finger or a bit of rag. The former are not only useful by their effects in the fauces, but serve a similar purpose in the stomach and intestines when the aphthous eruption has spread to them. They are generally composed of mild mucilaginous and gently stimulating decoctions. The decoction of turnips or turnip-radishes, or their expressed juice mixed with water, and sweetened with sugar, or honey which is better, may be given in the quantity of a dram or two every half hour. The common people in Holland use small beer or ale sweetened with sugar. Van Swieten recommends

* For the use of the bark in this complaint, see what is said of it when speaking of local remedies. It will then be necessary to mention it, and it will save repetition to throw together the few observations to be made on it.

veal broth,' boiled with rice and bruised turnips, which has the advantage of being an excellent article of diet in this complaint.

It has already been hinted that when the rectum is affected, mild injections are proper, and produce effects similar to those of gargles in the fauces ; they should consist of such decoctions as those just mentioned.

The ingredients left, after the preparation of some of these decoctions, are often applied to the external fauces by way of cataplasm, and sometimes relieve the internal parts.

More stimulating remedies than those just mentioned, seem in many cases to produce better effects. Dr. Armstrong found a solution of white vitriol, in the proportion of about half a scruple to eight ounces, very successful, occasionally adding a little more of the vitriol. And about a dram of this mixture, he observes, now and then swallowed is of service by cleansing the stomach and bowels. He generally applied it however by means of a piece of rag three or four times in the twenty-four hours.

We shall have occasion to consider more particularly the different applications to the internal fauces, indicated when a tendency to gangrene shews itself, in speaking of the cynanche maligna.

Much difference of opinion has arisen concerning the use of refrigerant and astringent gargles in aphthous affections. Practitioners having observed, that in certain cases an alarming train of symptoms sometimes attend the sudden retrocession of aphthæ, have avoided such gargles. Ketelaer reprobates them in the strongest terms.

This is not only reasoning a priori, but reasoning also on very bad grounds. It is a mode of reasoning however that has been very generally adopted by Physicians, and it may not be improper to take this opportunity of making a few remarks upon it.

In almost all the exanthemata it now and then, though rarely, happens, (for such cases are much less frequent than the fears of some writers have inclined them to suppose) that the eruption suddenly disappears, a train of symptoms supervening, which, if effectual means for restoring the eruption are not speedily employed, often terminates in death. This accident I shall frequently have occasion to notice in considering the exanthemata, and shall point out its causes, and the means to be employed when it happens. It has been inferred, that the train of symptoms which attends the retrocession of eruptions, is its consequence ; and that the same effect will follow if we repel, or even retard the eruption, whatever be the means employed for this purpose.

This mode of reasoning is similar to, and equally fallacious with, that employed respecting the solution of fevers by crises. From observing that a spontaneous flow of sweat, for instance, of ten attends the change from fever to health, it was inferred, that the same beneficial effects are to be expected from a sweat however excited. This inference, it was remarked, when speaking of the crisis of fevers, is invalidated by reflecting, that the sweating, instead of causing the solution of the disease, may only be a symptom of recovery; and that it is so seems probable since forced sweats rarely induce a crisis.

· There is precisely the same fallacy in the reasoning employed in the case before us. Although dangerous symptoms are sometimes observed to supervene on the eruption spontaneously disappearing, it is by no means an inference from this, that the train of unfavourable symptoms is occasioned by the retrocession of the eruption; both may be the effects of a common cause, the disappearance of the eruption being the one of the unfavourable symptoms, and having no share in producing the others. And that this is generally the case appears highly probable, when we know, that the accompanying symptoms often appear a short time before the retrocession, and that it is in debilitated states of the system, and after debilitating causes have been applied, that the retrocession generally happens; circumstances sufficient to account for the symptoms that attend it, and which often produce the same train of symptoms in cases where there is no eruption.

And that such symptoms will not follow the retrocession or retardation of the eruption, except the body be somehow or other peculiarly predisposed to them, appears from numberless facts, which seem at first accidentally to have obtruded themselves on the attention of physicians. Thus we know that retrocession in the small-pox or miliary fever has been accompanied by the same symptoms which attend the retrocession of aphthæ. In a thousand cases however the most vigorous means for repelling the eruption in the small-pox and miliaria are every day employed, and they are actually impeded and kept back, and yet no bad consequences, but on the contrary, the best effects, ensue.

It is true indeed, that when the eruption is recalled, the unfavourable symptoms generally disappear; but what are the means of recalling the eruption? Those which obviate the debility that occasioned its retrocession; and we have reason to believe, that the relief obtained is not the consequence, but the cause of the reappearance of the eruption.

. In considering the propriety then of astringent gargles in aphthæ, let us appeal from the doctrine of retrocession to simple facts.

Have astringent gargles been employed in this complaint, and what have been their effects? They were employed in cases of aphthæ as early as the days of Sydenham; for this author used the bark in fevers, while aphthæ were present, and found that the fever yielded and the separation of the aphthæ was promoted by it. Such was the dread of astringent applications while aphthæ were present, that, even in typhus, long after the ben-

efit derived from the bark in this fever was ascertained, the appearance of aphthæ was deemed a sufficient reason for avoiding it, till
Sydenham and some other practitioners ventured to 'employ it.
I was encouraged to give the bark in debilitated aphthous patients,
says Van Swieten, in whom the incrustation often became very
thick. It was given in decoction, because the powder is not easily
swallowed when the fauces are covered with aphthæ. I did not
give the bark in those cases without some fears that by its astringency it might do harm; of two evils however the best that could
be done was to choose the least. I therefore continued to give
the bark, interposing between the doses emollient decoctions, to
correct any hurtful tendency it might have. I had not, he adds,
continued this practice long, before I was astonished to find that
the aphthæ terminated favourably in those patients who took the
bark, sooner than in those who did not, although the latter were
not only stronger but had also less fever.

So thoroughly now are practitioners convinced of the safety
of the bark in aphthous complaints, that they not only use it occasionally as a gargle, but give it internally in-large doses, even
where there is no fever, if the disease threatens to be alarming ;
and its decoction is very generally recommended in the mildest
cases.*

The same objections have been urged against the use of acids,
tending, it was supposed from their refrigerant power, to repel
the eruption, and particularly against the sulphuric acid on account of its astringency. Some practitioners however have been
bold enough to employ them, and have established the propriety
of doing so.† The muriatic acid properly diluted, has been found
particularly useful.

Such is the treatment of the aphthæ infantum, and from what
has been said may be readily collected the treatment in every other form of the disease.

With regard to the treatment of symptomatic aphthæ, it seems
to be much more simple than many have imagined. It is not difficult to perceive how hurtful many of the prejudices just mentioned must prove, if permitted to influence our practice in every
complaint in which this eruption occurs. What would be the
consequence, were we, for instance, in synocha to abstain from
blood-letting, or in agues and typhus from the bark, as soon as
aphthæ make their appearance. If these prejudices demand no
attention while the aphthæ are the only complaint, they certainly
demand as little when they are merely a symptomatic affection,

* See the observations of Boerhaave, Van Swieten, Ketelaer, and
those of Vogel in his Prælectiones de Cog. et Curand. Morbis.

† For a variety of applications to the internal fauces, see Vogel and
others on Aphthous Fever. For easing the pain of the excoriated fauces,
Burserius recommends a mixture of the yolk of eggs, cream, and syrup
of poppies ; when the salivation is considerable, a decoction of agrimony
with honey ; when it is obstinate and profuse, gentle astringents.

and when neither their appearance nor falling materially affects the primary disease.

When indeed aphthæ prove critical in fevers, which rarely happens, it would be improper to employ any means which might tend to impede the eruption. The use of astringent gargles even in this case has not, as far as I know, been found injurious. From analogy however we should be inclined to avoid them. It is improper, we know, to check other critical discharges, those for instance by sweat or stool.

It only remains to make a few observations on certain symptoms, the treatment of which does not fall under the general plan of cure.

Those which chiefly demand attention, are profuse diarrhœa or hypercatharsis, and the symptoms which attend retrocession. It often happens indeed that in neither of these we can be of any service. In the latter we must trust chiefly to tonic medicines. The eruption seems to recede in consequence of debility, and when this is obviated, it often reappears. Bark and astringent wines are the remedies chiefly to be depended on. Thus the remedies which have been supposed capable of occasioning retrocession, are not only the best means of preventing it, but also of obviating the danger which attends it. Gently stimulating applications to the internal fauces are also sometimes of service in recalling the eruption.

With regard to hypercatharsis, we must endeavour to check it by opiates and astringents. Of the latter, gum kino and the extract of logwood seem the best for this purpose. Where there are symptoms of acidity, the mistura cretacea should be joined with these medicines ; but caution is requisite in checking purging, and the diarrhœa which occurs in the decline of the disease and throws out the fallen aphthæ, if not profuse, is salutary.

SECT. IV.

Of the Vesicular Fever.

CONCERNING the characteristic symptoms of this fever there has been some dispute. It is defined by Dr. Cullen,

" Typhus contagiosa, primo, secundo, aut tertio, morbi die, in " variis partibus vesiculæ avellanæ magnitudine, per plures dies " manentes, tandem ichorem tenuem effundentes."

Dr. Cullen never saw the disease but once, and some of those who have had more frequent opportunities of observing it have proposed considerable alterations in his definition. Dr. Dickson* observes, that he doubts much whether this disease should be

* See his paper on Pemphigus (the name by which this fever is generally known), in the Transactions of the Royal Irish Academy in 1787.

considered, contagious. He saw six cases of the complaint, in none of which it was received by contagion, nor communicated, to those who attended the sick.

He also objects to that part of the definition in which it is said that the eruption appears on the first, second, or third day, as he observed it appear on other days of the complaint. *Per plures dies manentes, he also thinks exceptionable, as he never found them remain for many days.

The fluid of the vesicles, instead of being a thin ichor, as mentioned by Dr. Cullen, was a bland, inodorous, and insipid fluid; and lastly he observes, instead of being poured out, it was generally absorbed. He therefore proposes the following instead of Dr. Cullen's definition.

" A fever accompanied with the successive eruption from dif-
" ferent parts of the body, internal as well as external, of vesi-
" cles about the size of an almond, which become turgid with a
" faintly yellowish serum, and in three or four days subside.

This definition is certainly preferable to that given by Dr. Cullen, not because the disease never appears in the form described by the latter, but because it sometimes does not, and it is necessry to have a definition including every form of it.

Notwithstanding the observations of Dr. Dickson, Dr. Cullen's definition applies perhaps to the generality of cases. On the Continent, where the disease is more frequent than in these kingdoms, it seems generally to assume the appearance described by Dr. Cullen. The blisters in particular are generally filled with an acrid serum, which is discharged not absorbed.‡

Mr. Blagden, in a Letter to Dr. Simmons, relates two cases of pemphigus which fell under his care, and seemingly with a view to Dr. Dickson's observations makes the following : " And now " I may be permitted to draw the following conclusions, that the " pemphigus is contagious,‖ that new vesicles in every case do " not arise after the end of the fourth day, that the fluid they con- " tain does not in every case, even of pemphigus simplex, ap- " pear to be of a bland nature, and that in some instances no ap- " parent absorption takes place." In short, the cases which Mr. Blagden saw, very accurately correspond to Dr. Cullen's definition.

There is another letter indeed on the same subject also addressed to Dr. Simmons by Mr. Christie, whose observations agree better with those of Dr. Dickson. He thinks the disease ought

* Sauvages remarks, that the vesicular eruption sometimes appears on the fourth day.

† We shall find that this eruption is not confined to the skin.

‡ See the observations of Burserius and other foreign writers on this disease.

‖ One of his patients seemed to take the disease from the other.

to be divided into two species, pemphigus simplex, and pemphigus complicatus. But our knowledge of this variety of fever is not sufficiently extensive for rendering such a division of much consequence. As we proceed in considering the symptoms of the complaint, its varieties will of course be mentioned.

1. Of the symptoms of the Vesicular Fever.

Of the Vesicular Eruption.

This eruption appears in the form of small pellucid blisters, similar to those produced by burning. They are of different sizes, sometimes as large as walnuts, more frequently about the size of almonds, and often considerably less, surrounded by more or less inflammation. They appear on the face,* neck, trunk, arms, and sometimes over the whole body,† as in a case given by Dr. Stewart in the Medical Commentaries, in which the vesicles were of the size of a walnut, and the distance of any two of them from half an inch to three or four inches. They sometimes run into each other.

It has just been hinted that external parts are not the only seat of this eruption. The mouth and fauces, where it now and then makes its first appearance, are particularly apt to be attacked with it. This happened in a case related by Dr. Dickson; in which on the third day of the fever, the patient complained of a smarting itching, and, as she termed it, tingling in her tongue and through the whole inside of her mouth. Her tongue was of a florid red colour, dry and clean. On the day following there appeared upon it a large pellucid vesicle filled with a faintly yellowish serum, a smaller one of the same kind appearing on the inside of the cheek.

In some instances the complaint spreads along the whole alimentary canal. "No person," Dr. Dickson remarks, " has noticed an extraordinary peculiarity in this disease, that the vesicles have taken possession of the internal parts of the body, and proceeded in succession from the mouth downward through the whole tract of the alimentary canal; some rising while others decayed."‡

The following are the symptoms which indicate that this erup-

* Burserius observes, that they are particularly apt to appear on the face and neck.

† When they have appeared on the scalp, the hair generally falls from the places they occupied.

‡ He first observed this in the case of a woman treated by Dr. Gregory in the Edinburgh Infirmary. In this instance, the menses had been interrupted for a year and a half, during which period the patient had been twice before subjected to the same complaint, and each time it followed a vomiting of blood. The other case in which Dr. Dickson met with this eruption spreading along the alimentary canal, he relates very minutely. In this case the first appearance of the eruption was in the mouth.

tion is spreading along the alimentary canal. Great difficulty of swallowing, the vesicles in the mouth, when there are any there, at the same time beginning to shrivel and crack, the eruption being apt, in spreading to neighbouring parts, to leave those it first attacked. From these symptoms, especially if accompanied with hiccup, we infer that vesicles are coming out in the œsophagus.

When they have spread to the stomach, the patient complains of pain referred to that organ, and nausea ; whatever is taken is rejected by vomiting, and often mixed with blood.

. Similar symptoms attend their presence in the intestines, a general sense of soreness is felt in the abdomen, and the stools are often bloody.

After the blisters have remained for an uncertain time, from one to several days, they either break, discharging in some cases a yellowish bland, in others a sharp ichorous fluid ;* or they begin to shrink, and in a short time disappear. And this perhaps is the most favourable termination, since when they break they sometimes leave troublesome ulcers.†

The foregoing process does not proceed on every part of the body at the same time, for the vesicles which first appear soonest subside.

· From perusing the cases of pemphigus, which have been accurately described, we should be inclined to think that the eruption in this complaint is most apt to attack internal parts when the matter of the vesicles on the surface is absorbed ; from one or two instances however no general conclusion can be drawn. It is said, that in a pemphigus which raged in Switzerland, in which the eruption often attacked the fauces, these parts were always most affected when the skin was least so ; but there is reason to believe that the vesicular fever has sometimes been confounded with the scarlatina, and from this circumstance perhaps the foregoing observation took its rise.

ᵇPemphigus resembles the small-pox, in frequently leaving pits in the skin ; and in the parts which the vesicles occupied, remaining for a considerable time afterwards of a dark colour.‡

* It sometimes happens in the same case, that the fluid in some of the vesicles is ichorous, in others bland. See the Observations of Dr. Stewart, above alluded to.

† Mr. Blagden observes of one of his patients, in whom the vesicles broke, " It was very evident that the child had suffered extremely from the soreness of those on the waist, which were not completely healed in less than two months." It is uncommon however for them to be troublesome for so long a time.

‡ Dr. Winterbottom, in the third volume of the Medical Facts and Observations, observes of one of his patients, " When I first saw him," which was some time after he had had the disease, " his face and legs were co- " vered with spots nearly of the size of a six-pence, resembling the marks " left by the small-pox: Many of these were attended with considerable

The time during which new vesicles continue to come out is as uncertain as their duration. According to Dr. Cullen's definition, no fresh vesicles appear after the third day, but this we have seen by no means applies universally.*

Swellings and abscesses of the parotid, inguinal, and axillary glands, have frequently accompanied this eruption; and as in other cases of continued fever accompanied by these swellings, the safety of the patient seems often to depend on the matter formed in them being discharged.

The vesicular eruption seldom brings relief to the febrile symptoms, but the prognosis in this variety of fever is in some respects influenced by its seat and appearance. When the vesicles are not numerous and only appear on external parts, they demand little attention; when they are numerous, when they attack the alimentary canal and are attended with a small hard pulse, the danger is considerable and is, cet. paribus, proportioned to the degree of these symptoms.

When the ulcers left by the vesicles, although external, appear livid, shewing a tendency to gangrene, which seldom happens unless in well marked typhus, the danger is very great. Even in idiopathic cases of this eruption, where there is no fever of any kind, gangrene sometimes supervenes, and then there is danger;† though in general, Burserius observes, where there is no fever, the vesicular eruption is unattended by danger.

Of the Symptoms preceding and attending the Vesicular Eruption.

In some cases this eruption is preceded, like those which have been considered, by anxiety and depression, but more generally it appears without being preceded by any peculiar symptoms.‡

A degree of coma, it was observed, frequently precedes the appearance of the miliary and aphthous eruption, and this we shall find is a frequent forerunner of most of the eruptions we shall have occasion to consider. It has not been observed however particularly frequent in the vesicular fever, nor is this eruption general-

" depression of the skin, in so much as to produce suspicion, among per-
" sons not much acquainted with the disease, of his really having had the
" small-pox. The discolouration of the skin," he adds, " was not entirely
" removed for a twelvemonth after the disease had left him, but was still
" very evident in cold weather." Mr. Blagden makes similar remarks.
" The vestiges of five of the largest of these vesicles and of two on the
" forehead will ever remain."

* In chronic cases they have continued to come out for a great length of time. See a case related by Mr. Christie.

† Burserius relates a case of this kind which terminated fatally.

‡ It appears, from what was said of one of Dr. Dickson's patients, that when the eruption is about to appear in the mouth, it is sometimes preceded by a peculiar sensation and change of colour in the parts which it is about to occupy.

ly accompanied with any peculiar symptoms, besides those already enumerated, which the eruption itself occasions.

Of the Febrile States in which the Vesicular Eruption most frequently appears.

We still find the symptomatic eruptions most apt to shew themselves in those fevers in which the typhus prevails. This will appear from the following account, extracted from authors who regard the vesicular fever as an idiopathic complaint.

In the commencement of pemphigus, as in other fevers, the patient droops and is averse to every kind of exertion. The symptoms of the cold stage are generally well marked, attended with head-ach, sickness, and oppression, the pulse is frequent, seldom strong and full, and delirium is a frequent symptom.

It appears from what was said of the definition of the synochus vesicularis, that there is no particular period of the fever at which the eruption shews itself. It now and then appears in other complaints as well as in the synochus. See an account of the Cynanche Maligna in the Acta Helvetica, by Dr. Langhans. There is reason to believe, that in several epidemics which raged in different parts of the Continent, the vesicular eruption attended this complaint, but the accounts of them are far from being distinct.

It has just been hinted, that the vesicular eruption has appeared as an idiopathic affection unaccompanied by fever. Cases of this kind are related by Dr. Winterbottom, and Mr. Gaitstkell in the 4th vol. of the Mem. of the Med. Soc. of London. Burserius speaks of this eruption without fever as a frequent occurrence.

2. Of the Causes of the Vesicular Fever.

The vesicular fever was unknown to the Greek, Roman, and Arabian writers.

Some indeed assert, that mention of the pemphigus is to be found in the writings of Hippocrates and Galen; but this seems to be a mistake. There is reason to rank it among those varieties of disease which have only made their appearance in modern times. Sauvages considers it as described by Bontius in his Medicina Indorum; but Dr. Dickson asserts, that, except one case related by Carolus Piso, he can find no distinct account of it in any author before the days of Morton, who took notice of this disease towards the end of the last century,* but without describing it particularly.

Sauvages met with it himself in the hospital of Montpelier, near the beginning of the present century, and gives the following

* Burserius even doubts whether the complaint mentioned by Morton be the pemphigus; of this however there can be little doubt. See what is said in the 37th and 38th pages of the Introduction.

account of it, " Pemphigus, febris est acuta exanthematica bollis
" seu ampullis pellucidis avellanæ magnitudine, per corpus enas-
" centibus insignita " Since his time this disease has been described by various authors; most of what they say of it however
consists in the narration of particular cases, if we except some;
for the most part indistinct accounts of it, as it raged on different
parts of the Continent.

As little has been determined concerning the causes of the vesicular eruption, as those of perhaps any other complaint. There
is one case in which it occurred three times in the same patient,
during a long interruption of the menses, and another in which it
occurred twice, each time attacking the patient on a visit to a cold
climate ;* yet there are thousands exposed to these causes
without having this eruption. It appears from these cases, as well
as one related by Dr. Hall, in Dr. Duncan's Annals of Medicine,
that the disease is apt to attack the same person more than once,
and that it probably, like some other symptomatic eruptions, particularly the erysipelatous and miliary, leaves behind it a predisposition to future attacks.

As with respect to other eruptive synochi, some disputes have
arisen concerning the contagious nature of vesicular fever. Most
foreign writers regard it as contagious, and some of the cases mentioned by British practitioners seem to support this opinion. Mr.
Blagden thought that one of his patients received it from the
other.

Many, on the contrary, under this disease, have been admitted
into public hospitals without communicating it to their fellow patients; and in most of the cases of pemphigus that have occurred
in Britain, it has appeared in a single person and spread no farther.
In none of those mentioned by Dr Dickson, Dr. Stewart, Dr.
Winterbottom, and Mr. Christie, did this complaint appear contagious, nor was it so in the case which Dr. Cullen saw. Dr. Hall
inoculated with the matter of the vesicles without producing the
disease.†

It has been proposed to divide pemphigus into two kinds, the
one contagious, the other not so. The reader will find an attempt
of this kind in the 106th paragraph of Burserius's Institutiones
Med. Pract. The contagious pemphigus, he observes, is always accompanied with much fever, and symptoms of malignity;
whereas in that which is not contagious, the fever is either moderate or absent. For several reasons however, which will readily
suggest themselves from what has been said, this division seems
to be inadmissible. It is more than probable, that it has in part

---

* See the observations of Dr. Winterbottom and Mr. Christie.

† See Observations on the Pemphigus Major of Sauvages, by Dr. R.
Hall, in Dr. Duncan's Annals of Medicine for the year 1799.

arisen from confounding the cynanche maligna with the synochus vesicularis.

The truth seems to be, that the vesicular, like other symptomatic eruptions, appears both in fevers which are and are not contagious; and it seems probable, that like these also it will sometimes be propagated with the fever and sometimes not, but it does not appear, as in the case of the miliary eruption, what the circumstances are which determine the vesicular to appear in fever.

3. Of the Treatment of the Vesicular Fever.

The same prejudices which for many centuries did, and in many places s ill, influence the treatment of other fevers, have been extended to that of pemphigus. " In Switzerland " says M'Bride,* " the physicians began the cure with one or two large bleedings, " then blistered the head, laid cataplasms on the neck, and en- " deavoured to raise sweats by sudorific medicines."

As the pemphigus was considered a complaint essentially different from common fever, particular modes of practice have been tried, and specifics looked for. " In Bohemia," Dr. M'Bride continues, " the only medicine which did service was the acetum be- " zoardicum, and this is said to have cured all who took it, while " those who trusted to other things died." It seems more surprising, that Dr. M'Bride should credit this assertion, than that Thierry the practitioner who makes it, should either himself have been deceived, or wished to deceive others.

Calomel in small doses, followed by a saline purge, has been employed by British practitioners. Small doses of tartar emetic have also been recommended, and these medicines, as in other cases of fever, are often serviceable. There is at least more to be hoped from them, than from the acetum bezoardicum, and much less to be apprehended than from profuse and repeated blood-letting, in a complaint where debility is what we chiefly dread.

The result of all that has been written on the treatment of pemphigus, as far as I am capable of judging, seems to be, that it is the same as in simple synochus, with the addition of local remedies for the eruption, which in general seems very little to modify the fever.

With regard to the local remedies, the larger vesicles are generally opened,† and kept clean; when any have appeared in the mouth and formed ulcers there, demulcent and detergent gargles are to be employed. When the ulcers either there or on other parts of the body become obstinate, they are to be treated by the surgeon, and therefore do not fall to be considered here.

* See his Introduction to the Theory and Practice of Medicine.
† The propriety of opening them is doubtful.

If there is reason to think, that the eruption has spread to the alimentary canal. copious draughts of some mucilaginous decoction are proper. and when the irritation is considerable and prevents sleep, if the symptoms of the fever admit of it, opiates should be exhibited, except inflammation of the stomach or bowels has supervened; cases which will be considered when speaking of the phlegmasiæ.

SECT. VI,

Of the Erysipelatous Fever.

THE Erysipelas* is defined by Dr. Cullen,

" Synocha duorum vel trium dierum, plerumque cum somno-
" lentia, sæpe cum delirio. In aliqua cutis parte, sæpius in facie,
" phlogosis† erythema."

It was observed in the Introduction, that, although I have arranged the erysipelas as a variety of synochus, because, like the foregoing complaints, it has been arranged among the exanthemata, yet if the view there taken of it be just, and that it is so will I think appear more fully in considering its symptoms, causes, and mode of treatment, it should be regarded as a combination of two complaints, of synochus, and Dr. Cullen's second species of plogosis, the erythema, and consequently should have no place in a system of nosology. We shall here find the eruption forming a much more important part of the complaint than in the preceding varieties of synochus, modifying the general plan of treatment as well as the symptoms of the fever.

* Erysipelas is the name given this complaint by the Greeks; by the Romans it was termed ignis sacer, or merely, ignis, by which appellation it is known in many parts of the Continent; but none of these terms have been used in a very definite sense. Sennertus calls it rosa; authors however have not adopted this name. By the vulgar of this country it is called the rose or St. Anthony's fire; foreign writers generally confine the latter appellation to Dr. Cullen's second species of it, which is also termed zona or zoster; and the erysipelas of the face has been termed sideratio.

† Phlogosis Dr. Cullen defines, " Pyrexia, partis externæ rubor, calor, " et tensio dolens."

The erythema is his 2d species of phlogosis, which is defined, " Phlogosis " colore rubicundo, pressione evanescente; ambitu inæquali serpente; tu- " more vix evidente, in cuticulæ squamulas, in phlyctænas vel vesiculas, abe- " unte; dolore urente." Dr. Cullen makes pyrexia part of the definition of phlogosis, and yet introduces synocha into the definition of erysipelas, in which phlogosis is mentioned. If pyrexia and synocha are not synonimous terms in these definitions, the definition of erysipelas contains a contradiction; if they are synonimous terms, synocha in this definition is evidently superfluous. This inaccuracy proceeds from a defect in Dr. Cullen's mode of arrangement, considered at length in the Introduction. See the 24th and following pages of the Introduction.

1. Symptoms of the Erysipelatous Fever.

Of the Erysipelatous Eruption.

This eruption appears in the form of a red blotch or stain, which spreads with more or less rapidity. The redness sometimes disappears on pressure ; sometimes it does not, arguing the inflammation having spread deeper.

It is generally attended with a sense of burning and a pungent pain, but for the most part without tension or pulsation ; and the inflamed skin is not raised above that which surrounds it. The parts beneath however, as well as those in the neighbourhood, are generally affected with some degree of swelling, which often remains after the redness has disappeared or removed to some adjacent part ; for this eruption is apt to leave, or become less considerable on, the parts it first occupied, when it spreads to others. But in this respect there is much variety.

After the redness has been present for an uncertain time, blisters of various sizes sometimes rise on the skin, generally containing a thin, sometimes limpid, sometimes yellowish fluid. In some cases the fluid is viscid,* and instead of running out, as generally happens, when the blister is broken, adheres to and dries upon the skin.

In unfavourable cases these blisters sometimes degenerate into obstinate ulcers, which now and then become gangrenous. This however is a rare accident, for although it is not uncommon for the surface of the skin. in the blistered places to appear livid or even blackish ; yet the tendency to gangrene seldom spreads deep, and generally disappears with the other symptoms of the complaint.

The red colour changes to yellow as the eruption goes off, and the parts on which no blisters arose often suffer a desquamation. If the colour of the eruption change from a red to a purple or blackish hue, the prognosis is bad ; but this is comparatively rare.†

When the eruption has spread deeper than usual, suppurations sometimes take place, and it has sometimes happened, that erysipelas has renewed ulcers which had been long healed ‡

The period of the eruption at which the vesicles shew themselves is quite uncertain ; the same may be said of the duration of the eruption. In mild cases it often gradually disappears, or

* See Tissot's Avis au Peuple.

† Platerus, Hoffman, and others, mention cases in which erysipelas terminated fatally by grangrene in old people. In the typhus gravior it is apt to terminate in this way, as will presently be more particularly observed.

‡ See a case of this kind in the 6th number of Desault's Chirurgical Journal.

is carried off by spontaneous sweating, in a day or two. In some cases it continues without beginning to decline for twelve or fourteen days, or longer.

The erysipelas has had different appellations according to the appearance of the eruption, erysipelas benignum, malignum, grangrenosum, tuberculosum, scabrum, vesiculosum, pustulare, &c.*

Such is the general appearance of the erysipelatous eruption, but there is some variety in its appearance, according to the part of the body it occupies.

In the mildest cases it appears on the extremities; often on the feet, and then if the febrile symptoms are moderate, if the eruption does not spread rapidly, and is only attended with a degree of itchiness or burning, or slight pain resembling the stinging of nettles, there is reason to believe that it will not prove troublesome, and will be of short duration.

In more severe cases the eruption gives more uneasiness and spreads with more rapidity. If it has appeared on the foot, it extends along the leg, the skin over the tibia becoming highly inflamed, stretched, and glossy.

In such cases the patient sometimes complains of tension and a sense of pulsation. This kind of pain however, as will be observed more particularly in considering the different kinds of inflammation, is not characteristic of the erysipelatous.

When the inflammation of the extremities is considerable, sharp pains, increased by the slightest touch, often shoot along the muscles, and the limb is generally much swelled. Erysipelas of the feet and legs sometimes leaves an obstinate œdema.

If the eruption attacks the trunk, the complaint is generally more severe. When it attacks the breasts of women, it is often attended with much pain, the breasts swell, become hard, and sometimes suppurate. The pain is also severe when it attacks the arm pits. In these and other glandular parts it often leaves the glands in a state of induration.†

Upon the whole, the erysipelatous eruption much less frequently attacks the trunk than the extremities. There are two varieties of it however, which appear on the trunk and deserve to be particularly mentioned.

The first may be termed the erysipelas infantum. This appears in children soon after birth, begins about the umbilicus, and

---

* See Burserius's Institut. Med. Pract.

† Erysipelas in glandular parts, Schroeder observes, especially if cold astringent and spirituous applications have been made to it, sometimes leaves behind it schirrus of the part. See Schroeder de Febre Erysipelatosa, in his Opuscula Medica.

often spreads over the whole abdomen.* It is not very uncommon indeed for children to be born with the face or belly, particularly the parts about the umbilicus, uniformly red and swelled.
It is more common however for the erysipelas to appear a few
days afte. birth, and it frequently makes its first attack about the
genitals.

The inflamed skin is hard, and apparently very painful to the
touch.

This species of erysipelas is more apt than others to terminate
in gangrene. The belly often becomes uniformly tense, and
sphacelated spots make their appearance. Dr. Bromfield relates
one case in which the gangrene in the extremities spread so
deep that several joints of the fingers were separated. Any appearance of gangrene in this form of the disease affords a bad
prognosis, and recovery is very rare when it spreads so deep as
in the case just alluded to.

Suppuration also, though more rarely, occurs in the erysipelas
infantum.

It appears from dissections mentioned by Dr. Underwood,
that in this form of the disease the inflammation frequently spreads
to the abdominal viscera.

The other species of erysipelas, attacking the trunk, which deserves particular notice, is Dr. Cullen's second species, the erysipelas phlyctænodes,† which he defines " Erysipelas erythemate
" ex papulis pluribus, trunci corporis partes præcipue occupanti-
" bus, et protinus phlyctænas, sive vesiculas parvas, abeuntibus."

·· This complaint, it was observed in the Introduction, is not very
properly ranked as as a variety of erysipelas, the appearance of
the eruption differing considerably from that above described.
Instead of appearing an uniformly inflamed surface, it consists of
a number of little pustules,‡ which in a short time have vesicles
formed on them. It generally surrounds the trunk, and appears
like a red belt thrown around the body a little above the umbilicus, from which it has got the name of zona. It is not always
however confined to this part. Dr. C. Smith says, he has seen it
spread round the neck and shoulders.

This is generally regarded as more dangerous than other forms
of erysipelas affecting the trunk and extremities. And Schroe-

* See an account of this species of erysipelas in two papers, one by
Dr. Bromfield, and another by Dr. Gartshore, in the 2d vol. of the Medical Communications, and also in Hoffman's Practice of Medicine, and
in Dr. Underwood's Treatise on the Diseases of Children.

† It is this species of erysipelas which has been termed zona or zoster.
In English it is called the shingles. See the 2d vol. of Burserius's Instit.
Med. Pract. Scroeder de Feb. Erysip. in his Opusc. Med. and Vogel,
Prælect. Acad. de Cog et Cur. Morh.

‡ When narrowly inspected however, the erysipelas on other parts of
the body sometimes has more or less of the same appearance.

der indeed regards it as the most fatal of all the varieties of this disease. Dr. Smith however remarks, " This species of erysi-
" pelas has been accounted extremely dangerous, which charac-
" ter it surely does not deserve, unless where the patient is in the
" decline of life, or the liver or some of the viscera are in a dis-
" eased state, or the patient is in other respects in a bad habit of
" body. I have frequently seen the disease in children and in
" young people," he adds, " without a single alarming symptom."

When the erysipelatous eruption attacks the face and head, it its most dangerous. It has then the same appearance as when it attacks other parts of the body.

A red spot appears on some part of the face, generally of no great extent, but which spreads till it sometimes covers, not on-ly the whole face, but the scalp also, now and then descending a considerable way down the neck, and occasioning what Tissot calls, " Esquinancie tres facheuse."

As in other cases, it often leaves the part it first attacked, when it spreads to neighbouring parts.

The face and frequently the whole head swell, sometimes to such a degree that the eyes are closed, so that Sydenham* ob-serves, the patient looks like a person under the small-pox, only there are no pustules. The tumors of the eye-lids sometimes terminate in suppuration.

The duration of the eruption on the face, as on other parts of the body, is various. It generally lasts eight or ten days, some-times longer. Desault in his Surgical Journal mentions a case in which it lasted 23 days. The uncertainty of the duration of symptomatic eruptions is another circumstance 'in which they differ from the exanthematic.

"The greater danger of erysipelas when it attacks the face, arises chiefly from the inflammation being apt to spread to the brain." There is reason indeed to believe, from symptoms that will pre-sently be enumerated, that the inflammation sometimes attacks the brain at the same time, or even before, it appears on the face.

More rarely the erysipelas of the face spreads to the fauces and along the alimentary canal, which is also a very alarming acci-dent. This form of erysipelas is also apt to spread to other in-ternal parts. Sometimes, Schroedert observes, it spreads to the nares, trachea, and thence to the lungs, producing all the symp-toms peculiar to inflammation of these parts.

It has just been observed, that when the erysipelatous eruption attacks the neighbouring parts, it often leaves that it first occu-pied; sometimes it removes suddenly to distant parts, what phy-

* See Sydenham de Feb. Erysipel.
† Opuscula Med.

sicians have termed Metastasis takes place; the inflammation leaving the skin, seizes on some of the viscera.

The viscus most commonly affected is the brain, but for the most part, Dr. Cullen observes, the brain is not affected by metastasis, but merely by a spreading of the inflammation; as in all the cases he saw, the external affection continued and increased with the internal.

Other viscera are sometimes but more rarely affected, on the sudden retrocession of the erysipelatous eruption, whether of the face or other parts. In metastasis of this disease, Schroeder observes, the inflammation also seizes the intestines, liver, uterus, and bladder. I shall hereafter have occasion to make some observations on attempts which have been made to distinguish erysipelatous inflammation of internal parts from what is called phlegmonous. In the latter, the inflammation extends deeper, and differs otherwise from the erysipelatous, particularly in being more apt to terminate by suppuration.

The erysipelas sometimes is not confined to any particular part of the skin, but spreads equally over the face, trunk, and extremities. Cases of this kind are rare; the reader will find such mentioned by Vogel and others. Sometimes, says Schroeder, the erysipelas spreads over every part of the body, from the head to the ends of the fingers. This most frequently happens in the erysipelas infantum.

In certain countries the erysipelas seems most disposed to attack particular parts of the body, thus Sauvages observes, that in Germany, the erysipelas generally seizes on the groin, thighs, and arm pits; in England and in France it more frequently attacks the face.

Such is the appearance of the erysipelatous eruption and the manner of collecting the prognosis, as far as it depends on the eruption.

It appears from what has been said that the prognosis is particularly influenced by the seat of the eruption; in the extremities it is safer than in the trunk, in the trunk than in the face, and, cet. par. the more extensive the inflammation the greater is the danger.

Suppuration in general is to be regarded as an unfavourable termination, as it frequently, especially in the face, leaves troublesome ulcers. For when erysipelas produces suppuration, it is seldom of the favourable kind.* Quarin however, on the authority of Strack, mentions an epidemic erysipelas, in which those recovered in whom suppuration took place, those died in whom it

* See an account of the Epidemic Erysipelas, by Tissot and others.

did not. We have reason to believe that suppuration will occur, when we find the inflammation spreading deeper than usual, which is known by the redness not disappearing on pressure, the pains being deeply seated, and the swelling considerable and hard.

It was observed above, that a degree of gangrene often appears on the blistered parts, and if the habit of body be good, and particularly if the eruption still retains the florid appearance, this tendency to mortification is generally superficial; but if the patient is much debilitated, especially if he is advanced in life,* and the eruption assumes a purple or livid hue, the mortification often spreads deep, and the danger is very great.†

Of the Symptoms which precede or attend the Erysipelatous Eruption.

The symptoms which frequently precede the erysipelatous eruption are similar to those which precede the foregoing eruptions; and this, like the others, sometimes appears without being preceded by any peculiar symptoms.

Before the appearance of the erysipelatous eruption, the oppression and anxiety are often considerable, and frequently attended with other symptoms denoting derangement of the primæ viæ, a bitter taste in the mouth, foul tongue, head ach, confusion of thought, vertigo, nausea, and even vomiting and purging, generally of bile. Most of the foregoing eruptions we have found connected with the state of the primæ viæ; this connection is not more remarkable in any than in the erysipelatous. Anxiety, pain of the stomach, eructations, dyspnœa, nausea, and bilious vomiting, are enumerated by Burserius among the symptoms preceding this eruption. "Accedit non raro," Schroeder observes of the same period of the disease, " ciborum fastidium, sapor amarus, nausea, conatus vomendi, aliquando etiam vomitus ;" and in another place, " Sæpissime autem signa colluviei vitiosæ, præ sertin, biliosæ ad primas vias apparent." Dr. Smith says, he has often seen erysipelatous blotches in fever, where the redundancy of bile was apparent. Tissot and others make similar observations.

Such are the principal forerunners of the erysipelatous eruption when about to appear on the trunk and extremities. But when it is about to attack the face, some of these symptoms, (particularly the affections of the head, which in such cases often rise to delirium) are almost always accompanied with a greater or less degree of coma,‡ and the eruption generally appears upon the

* See the observations of Platerus on what he terms Macula Lata.
† See Vogel de Cog. et Cur. Morb.
‡ More or less coma, as in other eruptive fevers, often precedes the eruption in erysipelas, whatever be the part of the body which the inflammation is about to occupy; but if the eruption is about to appear on the

face one, or two, at most three days after these symptoms shew
themselves.

It is from the state of the brain in erysipelas of the face, that
we chiefly collect the prognosis. When neither delirium nor coma have preceded the eruption, which indeed is rarely the case,
nor supervened after its appearance, there is generally little or
no danger, if the symptoms of the primary disease, whether it be
fever or any other, are not alarming. But when a considerable
degree of coma or delirium has preceded the eruption, and still
more when the coma, which often happens, rather increases than
abates after its appearance, there is reason to believe that the inflammation has spread to the brain, and the danger is then very
great.

When the coma is considerable from the beginning of the disease, it indicates that the inflammation first seized on the internal
parts, and then, in a nosological point of view, the complaint must
be regarded in the same light as when the external inflammation
is the first symptom of the complaint, that is, it must be regarded
simply as a case of phlegmasia; and we shall find that the treatment which experience has established as most successful, is the
same as in other phlegmasiæ.

From what was said of the tendency of erysipelas to attack internal parts, it will readily be perceived, that the symptoms which
occasionally attend this eruption must be very various. We shall
have occasion to consider at length the various symptoms which
accompany inflammation of the different viscera, when considering the phlegmasiæ.

*Of the Febrile States in which the Erysipelatous Eruption
is most apt to appear.*

The erysipelatous eruption differs from the eruptions we have
been considering, and agrees with inflammations, in appearing
more frequently in synocha than in typhus. On this account it
generally appears early in fevers; so that although we find authors differing about the time of its appearance, it seems to be
generally admitted, that it seldom shews itself later than the
fourth or fifth day; but within this period the time of its appearance is as uncertain as that of any other eruption which has been
mentioned.

It sometimes appears after the fever has lasted only a few
hours, in many cases on the second, third or fourth day; and
when the fever has begun to assume the form of typhus before
the eruption shews itself, if the patient's strength is not much
reduced, it resumes that of synocha, the strength and the fullness

trunk, or extremities, the coma is much less uniformly present, and generally less considerable, than when the inflammation is about to appear on
the face

of the pulse increasing, often attended with a considerable degree of hardness. Other inflammations supervening on the typhus mitior, often have the same effect, a consequence that never attends any of the preceding eruptions, which all tend to increase the symptoms of debility.

As the erysipelatous eruption is most apt to attend the synocha, and as the more alarming fevers generally incline to typhus at an early period, it is in the milder forms of fever that this eruption most generally appears. But in erysipelas of the face, the brain is often affected before the inflammation shews itself externally.* This inflammatory affection of the brain, while it induces coma, often preceded by severe head-ach, sometimes by a greater or less degree of delirium, at the same time increases all the febrile symptoms ; so that although the fever which precedes erysipelas of other parts of the body is seldom alarming, that which precedes erysipelas of the face frequently is so.

In such cases we have every reason to believe that the inflammation, although it does not show itself externally for some days after the commencement of the disease, is in fact the primary complaint, the fever being only symptomatic of it ; and the treatment which has been found most successful, which is by no means that of an idiopathic fever, sufficiently warrants this opinion.

The erysipelas of the face sometimes appears without any previous affection of the brain, and then it is often observed to appear also without previous fever. Sydenham mentions an erysipelas in which the affection of the face was the first symptom of the disease. " Facies siquidem ex improviso in tumorem attollitur, " qui subito exorsus cum dolore ruboreque summis, denso minimarum pustularum ordine distinguitur, quæ, aucta magis inflammatione, vesiculas subinde facessunt."

This eruption, like other inflammations, instead of relieving, increases the febrile symptoms, the pulse becomes harder, the nostrils, fauces, and skin more parched, and the breathing more laborious, so that the general, keeps pace with the local, affection. " Procedente morbo," says Sydenham of the erysipelas, " ut " plurimum febris, dolorem, tumorem, atque alia peperit sympto- " mata (quæ indies ingravescentia nonnunquam in gangrena ter- " minatur); ita hæc invicem haud mediocrem ad febris augmen- " tum conferunt operam, donec remediis idoneis utraque restin- " guantur." " The pain," Dr. M' Bride observes, " from the in- " flammation, keeps up the fever, until both are taken off by pro- " per remedies."†

---

* As has just been observed, in enumerating the symptoms which precede this species of erysipelas, and will more fully appear when we consider the diagnostic symptoms of phrenitis.

† In some rare cases however, the erysipelatous eruption has proved critical. The reader will find cases mentioned by Van Swieten and others in which the fever ceased on the appearance of this eruption.

Nor is the affection of the brain in general relieved by the appearance of the inflammation externally, the coma often increasing as the inflammation extends; so that as this inflammation, when it makes its first attack on the face, sometimes spreads to the brain without leaving the face; when it makes its first attack on the brain, it is apt in like manner to spread to the face without leaving the part it first occupied, which always affords an unfavourable prognosis.

When the fever does not increase much after the appearance of the eruption, and the coma begins to abate, the prognosis is good. Soon after this the eruption generally begins to assume a yellowish hue, and all the symptoms, both local and general, gradually abate.

Such is the general course of erysipelas of the face, and the circumstances which influence the prognosis. But Van Swieten justly observes, that it is no mark of ignorance in the physician, although he may have considered the patient in a state of safety, when he was within a few hours of death; he has often seen cases. he continues, which from being accompanied with no alarming symptom, often suddenly indicated so much danger that death was hourly expected, the inflammation having attacked the membranes of the brain. It sometimes happens, Tissot observes, that without any apparent fault of the patient or practitioner, the inflammation suddenly changes its seat, attacking the brain or lungs, and then the patient is often carried off in a very short time, although, previous to the metastasis, there seemed little or no danger.

It has been observed above, that the erysipelatous eruption often makes the fever resume the character of synocha after the typhus had commenced; this however is only where the symptoms of typhus are not strongly marked. When this eruption appears in the typhus gravior, which is not a very frequent occurrence. instead of changing the nature of the fever, the eruption partakes of its nature, shewing a strong tendency to gangrene, increasing the debility, and consequently adding to the unfavourable prognosis. The complaint is then, what has been termed by foreign authors, febris erysipelatosa maligna or pestilens : A form of the disease little known in this country. On different parts of the Continent it has sometimes been epidemic, as at Thoulouse in the year 1716, where it appeard in so dreadful a form, that it was compared to the plague, and proved little less fatal. This epidemic is analogous to those mentioned by De Haen,[*] Bartholine,[†] Professor Silvius de la Boe,[‡] and others, in which an inflammation of the stomach and duodenum accompanied the fever.

The erysipelatous eruption is apt to appear in other complaints besides fever. Among the chief of these, Schroder enumerates

[*] Ratio Medendi.   [†] Hist. Anatom. Rar. hist. 56.
[‡] Prax. Med. Append. tract. x.

dropsy, jaundice, wounds, particularly those of the cranium* injuring the membranes of the brain, fractures, or considerable
abscesses in any part of the body. Erysipelas from wounds,
Quarin observes, affords a bad prognosis. Erysipelas also frequently attends schirrus, and cancerous or other considerable ulcers. It also frequently accompanies diseases, occasioning derangement of the primæ viæ, particularly worms, and is often
one of the effects of poisonous injesta.

The terms erysipelas and erythema have been used by authors
in a very vague sense, the former having been assumed both as
the name of the complaint, and of the eruption which characterises it. Sauvages and Cullen however have confined the term
erysipelas to the former ; and the eruption, with its consequences, they have termed erythema   But this eruption frequently
occasions fever, so that Dr. Cullen has found much difficulty,
both in his nosology and practice, in distinguishing the erysipelas
and erythema, and this difficulty will be readily perceived when
the reader is informed that the eruption termed erythema is often
preceded by slight indisposition, hardly, and sometimes not at all,
affecting the pulse, so that it is difficult to say whether it has been
preceded by fever or not, and consequently whether, according
to Dr. Cullen's definitions of these complaints, it is to be regarded
as a phlegmasia or exanthema.

If we confine the term erythema to those cases where no symptoms of general derangement have preceded the eruption, we
shall include under the term erysipelas a disease which hardly at all differs from erythema. Yet we must distinguish between the erythema, a disease evidently referable to the phlegmasiæ, and in which the mode of treatment is the same as in other phlegmasiæ, the fever being merely symptomatic ; and the
erysipelas, in which the fever is as evidently idiopathic, and must,
as experience has taught, be treated as such, except as far as it
has been modified by the appearance of the local affection.

The only way, as far as I can judge, to remove the difficulty,
is either altogether to lay aside the term erysipelas, regarding
what is at present called erysipelas as a combination of erythema
and simple fever ; or, what would be preferable, to confine the
term erythema to express the local affection, the simple inflammation which sometimes occurs without fever, and apply that of
erysipelas to the phlegmasia, namely, to those cases in which the
inflammation occasions fever,† giving no name to the combination
of synochus and erysipelas, which never assumes the appearance
of an exanthema ; we might as well give a name to the combination of worms and erysipelas. According to this view of the com-

* Gunshot wounds are particularly apt to produce erysipelas, and all
wounds, Dr. Smith observes, which are attended with much laceration.

† The reader will find, in perusing the works of those who treat of erysipelas, that the nature of the complaint constantly leads them uninten-
tionally to use these terms nearly in this sense.

plaints, the term erysipelas would be confined to the cases in which the local affection is either preceded by no symptoms of general derangement, or by such as frequently precede the local affection in the other plegmasiæ.

The inaccurate use of the foregoing terms forces Dr. Cullen into a mode of arrangement in his System of Practice, by which the consideration of that form of erysipelas in which the eruption appears on the trunk or extremities is altogether omitted, for Dr. Cullen, finding the symptoms which precede the eruption on these parts often so trifling as hardly to be perceived, and sometimes altogether wanting, so that the complaint had little if any appearance of an exanthema ; but observing at the same time, that the preceding symptoms were very generally considerable when the eruption was about to appear on the face and head ; in treating of erysipelas he considers this case alone. He expresses the difficulty in the 697th paragraph as follows : " I suppose the " erysipelas to depend on a matter generated within the body, and " which, analogous to the other cases of exanthemata, is in con- " sequence of fever thrown out on the surface of the body. I " own it may be difficult to apply this to every particular case of " erysipelas, but I take the case in which it is generally supposed " to apply, that of the erysipelas of the face, which I shall there- " fore consider here." Dr. Cullen therefore leaves other cases of the disease, if they are considered at all, to be arranged among the phlegmasiæ. According to his view of the disease then, if the eruption in erysipelas appears on the face, the complaint is an exanthema ; if on the trunk or extremities, a phlegmasia. Can this view of the disease be accurate ? Besides, how shall we arrange the case above described in a quotation from Sydenham's Treatise on Erysipelas, in which the eruption on the face was the first symptom of the complaint ?

The foregoing view of this disease obviates every difficulty, and is supported, as far as I know, by every fact on the subject. The erysipelas is a phlegmasia, which like gastritis, enteritis, or any other phlegmasia, sometimes occurs in idiopathic fevers.[*]

Different divisions of erysipelas into varieties have been proposed by authors, none of them however are of much use in practice. I have already had occasion to allude to the division into febris erysipelatosa benigna, and febris erysipelatosa maligna. A variety of divisions of this complaint has been adopted by Celsus, Fernelius, Hoffman, and others, founded on the appearance of the eruption, according as the inflammation is more or less superficial, as vesicles do or do not supervene, and do or do not leave ulcers behind them ; and the ulcers being superficial or deep, — mo[...] of the view of the com-

* The justness of this view of the complaint will be sufficiently apparent, I hope, on comparing what is about to be said of the causes and treatment of erysipelas, with what will be said in the next volume of the nature of the phlegmasiæ, and the maxims which conduct our practice in this order of symptomatic fevers.

well conditioned or otherwise, have also afforded other useless divisions.*

2. Causes of the Erysipelatous Fever.

In the causes, as in the symptoms of erysipelas, we still find it partaking of the nature of the phlegmasiæ; with these it agrees, and differs from symptomatic eruptions, in having been known from the earliest times.

With regard to the predisposing causes, those most disposed to this complaint are the young and people in the vigour of life, especially those of a sanguine and choleric temperament, and of a plethoric habit. Like the other phlegmasiæ, it is most apt to attack those who formerly laboured under it.

The exciting causes of erysipelas also are the same with those of the phlegmasiæ. One of the most frequent, particularly in those who have formerly laboured under it, is cold, especially if alternated with heat, as in variable weather. It is sometimes the consequence of excessive heat, too full a diet, particularly the abuse of fermented liquors, the suppression of any habitual discharge, as the drying up of an issue, suddenly checking hemorrhois, or abstaining from habitual blood-letting, or any other cause of plethora.

It is frequently re-produced by local irritation, whether chymical or mechanical. "As I have known erysipelas," Dr. Cullen observes, " with all its symptoms, arise from an acrimony applied " to the part, as it is commonly attended with a full and frequency " with a hard pulse, as the blood drawn in this disease shews the " same crust upon its surface as appears in the phlegmasiæ, and " lastly, as the swelling of the eye-lids in this disease frequently " ends in suppuration; so from these considerations it seems " doubtful, if this disease be properly in nosology separated from " the phlegmasiæ; at any rate I take the disease I have described " to be what physicians have named the erysipelas phlegmonodes, " and that it partakes a great deal of the nature of phlegmasiæ."

In some of its other causes the erysipelas appears to bear a stronger analogy to other symptomatic eruptions. It has been observed of all these, that they seem frequently to arise from derangement of the primæ viæ. This is not more remarkably the case with any eruption than the erysipelatous. Such derangement indeed seems one of its most frequent causes. Purging, says Tissot, is in general necessary to evacuate the corrupting bile from the primæ viæ, which is the most frequent cause of erysipelas. Such is the connexion of this complaint with the primæ viæ, says Schroeder, that we often wholly remove the disease by

* See the 3d chap. of the 4th book of the Pathology of Fernelius, and Schroeder's Opusc. Med. See also a division of erysipelas, equally objectionable, in Burserius's Institut. Med. Pract.

removing the irritating matter, which is generally bilious, from the stomach and intestines.*

The redundancy of bile in the stomach and intestines so frequently accompanying erysipelas, gave rise to the hypothesis of erysipelas being occasioned by a bilious st te of the fluids, a doctrinet long mainta.ned, and adopted by so late an author as Quarin. But other noxious matter in the primæ viæ al-o produces erysipelas, and other eruptions we have seen, not suspected to depend on a bilious state of the fluids, arise from the same cause.

It is perhaps by affecting the state of the primæ viæ, that the passions of the mind, particularly rage, terror, and vexation, frequently excite erysipelas, and that pregnant women are observed to be particularly liable to it.

But even in these causes we find erysipelas resembling other phlegmasiæ, which, it will appear in considering these complaints, more frequently arise from derangement of the primæ viæ than is generally supposed.

Erysipelas seems also now and then to arise from other affections of the abdominal viscera, particularly affections of the liver.‡ In this respect also we shall find that the erysipelas resembles some of the phlegmasiæ.‖

Erysipelas in general is not contagious, yet like other symptomatic eruptions, as well as certain phlegmasiæ, it sometimes attends the prevailing epidemic, and then the fever is generally the typhus gravior. It has already been observed that such epidemics seldom occur in Britain. Dr. Bromfield, in his Surgical Cases

* Schroeder has been at the pains to collect a number of authorities to prove that this complaint frequently arises from the presence of irritating matter in the alimentary canal; the fact indeed is generally admitted to be unquestionable. In confirmation of this opinion we are referred to the works of Hippocrates, Galen, Ballonius, Hoffman, Lieutaud, Tissot, Bagliviys, Bianchus, Friend, Richa, Mead, Brocklesby, Zimmerman, Molinarius, and others of less note, to which Quarin, Vogel, Burserius, Desault, and other late writers may be added. Desault in his Surgical Journal relates several striking cases of erysipelas arising from, or supported by, derangement of the primæ viæ.

† See this doctrine considered at length in Bureau's Treatise on Erysipelas.

‡ The erysipelas infantum in particular has been observed to arise from this cause.

‖ It will appear from a variety of observations, that inflammations of the viscera, of the thorax in particular, are apt to arise from various affections of the abdominal viscera. See an Account of the Pleuritis Verminosa, in the 43d, 44th, and 45th sections of the 21st Epistle of Morgagni. See also an Account of Dissections by Wendt in his Treatise de Pleuritide in Sandifort's Thesaurus; an Account of the Pleuritis Filiosa in Bianchus's Historia Hepatica, and in the fifth volume of the Edinburgh Medical Essays; and several papers, in the second volume of Haller's Disputationes ad Morb. Hist. et Cur. pertinent. on the Pneumonia Putrida which seems often influenced, if not caused, by affections of the primæ viæ.

and Observations, mentions an erysipelas of the head, which was epidemic for two years, in which it was necessary to employ cordials and Peruvian bark, anti-phlogistic measures generally proving fatal. Instances of epidemic erysipelas are also to be found in the works of Sydenham, Burserius, Tissot, and others.

It is remarkable that erysipelas sometimes returns periodically, attacking the patient once or twice in the year, or even once every month, and then by its repeated attacks it often gradually exhausts the strength, especially if the patient be old and of a bad habit. Hoffman mentions several cases of this kind. In one of these, the return of erysipelas was prevented by an issue and low diet; two of the most powerful means, we shall find, of preventing the appearance of the phlegmasiæ. Vogel and Schroeder mention cases of the same kind, and the former observes, that those who are subject to erysipelas are generally free from other complaints. Schroeder mentions several instances, in which the erysipelas constantly supervened at the time the menses should have appeared.

3. Of the treatment of the Erysipelatous Fever.

From what has been said of the symptoms and causes of erysipelas it appears, that in those cases where the affection of the skin has been present from the beginning of the complaint, or where the complaint has been attended from the first with coma or delirium, it is to be regarded as a phlegmasia, and universal experience has ascertained, that the treatment in these cases is the same as in other phlegmasiæ. The treatment in such cases therefore will be considered when we come to speak of the phlegmasiæ.

To the same place it is proper to refer the local treatment in erysipelas.

We are at present to consider, how far the appearance of the erysipelatous eruption in the progress of synochus, influences the treatment of this fever.

The appearance of the erysipelatous eruption in the first stage of synochus, that is, while the inflammatory symptoms prevail, the period at which it most frequently supervenes, occasions but little change in the mode of treatment, except that as the inflammatory affection of the skin increases the symptoms of synocha, the means of moderating the excitement must be employed with greater assiduity. They are also safer than in other species of synochus.

It has been observed, that if the typhus has commenced before the appearance of this eruption, the symptoms of synocha are often recalled by it. They are not only recalled, but maintained, for the typhus which supervenes towards the end of an erysipelatous fever is less considerable, in proportion to the preceding symptoms, than in other varieties of synochus; the erysipelatous fever in this respect also approaching to the nature of a phlegmasia, hence the effects of evacuations are less to be dreaded than in cases of synochus where no erysipelatous eruption supervenes. Sydenham did not scruple to employ blood-letting in erysipelas almost as freely as in any of the phlegmasiæ;[*] how we are to proportion the evacuations to the state of the local affection will appear more fully in treating of the phlegmasiæ.

All that need be said at present is, that the more severe the local affection, that is, the greater the swelling, heat, pain, and the further the inflammation extends, especially if its seat be the head or trunk, and the greater the coma or delirium, the more powerful must the antiphlogistic measures be ; provided the pulse continues full and strong, still more if it be hard, which is generally the case when the local affection is considerable. " Upon " this conclusion," Dr. Cullen observes, " the erysipelas of the " face is to be cured very much in the same manner as phlegmo-" nic inflammations, by blood-letting, cooling purgatives, and by " employing every part of the antiphlogistic regimen, and our " experience has confirmed the fitness o this method of treatment. " The evacuations of blood-letting and purging are to be em-" ployed more or less according to the urgency of the symptoms, " particularly those of the pyrexia, and those which mark an af-" fection of the brain. As the pyrexia continues and often in-" creases with the inflammation of the face, so the evacuations " mentioned may be employed at any time in the course of the " disease."

When erysipelas appears as a simple phlegmasia however, more copious evacuations are proper than in the case before us, where a phlegmasia supervenes on continued fever, particularly if the fever has arisen from contagion or shewn a tendency to' typhus.

There is another caution which deserves attention in the employment of evacuations in the synochus erysipelatosus. This, like other affections of the skin, which appear in continued fever, has been known suddenly to recede, an alarming train of symptoms, of which debility is the characteristic feature, supervening. This is comparatively a rare occurrence ; as in other eruptive fevers, it is most apt to happen where debilitating causes have been applied. It is also to be remembered, that when retrocession takes place, the patient is seldom out of danger till the eruption is recal-

* " Hæc ut fiant, ubi primus accedo, satis largam sanguinis quantita-" tem e brachio extrahi præcipio, qui quidem pleuriticorum sanguinem " fere semper æmulatur;" and after mentioning the other means he employed after blood-letting, he observes, " Hac methodo tum febris, tum " alia symptomata citissime fugantur. Sin aliter, rursus venam seco, quod " et tertium nonnunquam fieri debet interposito semper die uno, si prava " nempe adsit sanguinis diathesis et febris intensior." Sydenham de Feb. Ersipel.

led, which is done with the greater difficulty the more he is debilitated.

The advantages of blood-letting over other evacuations for moderating the excitement have been pointed out.; but the erysipelatous eruption frequently indicating derangement of the primæ viæ. and being often increased if not caused by such derangement, a small evacuation by the bowels in the erysipelatous fever often produces more powerful effects than a larger evacuation by venesection. We shall find, in considering the phlegmasia. that in all inflammatory affections of the head, purging is particularly useful ; in the erysipelas of the face therefore it is doubly indicated. and in all forms of the complaint, when the symptoms are moderate, generally renders the employment of blood-letting unnecessary.

Schroeder justly observes, that catharsis should always precede blood-letting in the erysipelas. One caution however is to be kept in view. if the local affection proceeds from. or is in any degree caused by, affections of the primæ viæ, the beneficial effects of purging will very quickly be observed, so that if it does not produce a favourable change. we should not persevere in the use of this remedy. Frequent purging, says Quarin, especially where the habit is debilitated and the pulse frequent and small, renders the erysipelas more alarming ; but even where the pulse is strong and hard, if the first exhibition of cathartics is not attended with beneficial effects, it is better, for the reasons given in speaking of the modus operandi of blood-letting, to reduce the excitement by this remedy than by repeated purging. And with regard to the opinion, that venesection is apt to occasion a retrocession of the eruption and make it sieze upon internal parts, the observations made on the same objection to it in other eruptive synochi, are applicable here. We need not fear, says Schroeder, that blood-letting will occasion a retrocession of erysipelas or make it fall on internal parts.*

If the erysipelatous eruption appears at an early period of the fever, vomiting should precede catharsis, except in erysipelas of the head, in all cases of which an emetic is at least a doubtful remedy.

While we endeavour to evacuate the morbid contents of the alimentary canal, we should at the same time correct what part

* When the eruption recedes, blisters and cordials, with diaphoretics, have been found the best means of restoring it See the observations of a variety of authors, particularly those of Hoffman and Schroeder. " If the " swelling," says M'Bride, " should suddenly sink and the acrid humor " appear to strike in, oppression or anxiety come on, and the pulse grow " weak, then we must blister, give wine with freedom, and the confec- " tio cardiaca or volatile alkaline salt and spirit, according to the exigen- " cy of the case."

of these contents may still remain, by the use of acids or absorbents, according as bile or an acid prevails.

Erysipelatous fevers often terminate by sweat ; mild diaphoretics with dilution therefore form an useful addition to the treatment ; and when a diaphoresis of the inflamed part appears, it
has been found useful to support it by gentle warmth.

The semicupium and sinapisms, applied to the feet, have been
particularly recommended in cases of erysipelas of the face attended with coma ; but these, and other parts of the treatment, will be considered under the heads phlogosis and phrenitis.

It has been observed, that the erysipelatous eruption sometimes
shews itself after the typhus is completely formed, or even far
advanced. The combination is then of a very different nature
from that we have been considering ; the inflammation being incapable of changing the nature of the fever, partakes of it. Instead of the full florid appearance it assumes in synocha, the parts
affected become flaccid and livid.

It seldom appears in typhus in this country, unless as the consequence of injury applied to the part, from the patient being allowed to lie too long in the same posture, &c. " We have hith-
" erto," Dr. Cullen observes, " considered erysipelas as in a
" great measure of a phlegmonic nature, and agreeably to that
" opinion we have proposed our method of cure   But it is pro-
" bable that an erysipelas is sometimes attended with, or is a
" symptom of, a putrid fever ; and in such cases the evacuations
" proposed above may be improper, and the use of the Peruvian
" bark may be necessary. But I cannot be explicit upon this
" subject, as such putrid cases have not come under my own ob-
" servation." In other countries however, erysipelas often shews
itself in malignant fevers, independently of any injury of the
part, spreading rapidly and quickly running to gangrene.*

As the appearance of the erysipelatous eruption in synocha
renders the antiphlogistic mode of treatment more indispensible ; so, on the other hand, its appearance in the typhus gravior,
makes it necessary to push the invigorating plan to the utmost.
Bark and wine are still the remedies chiefly to be depended on,
and, in such cases, must be given in very large doses.

Virginian snakeroot, camphire, scordium, and vitriolic acid,
are recommended by foreign writers. The vitriolic acid and
alum are particularly indicated when the malignant erysipelas,
as often happens, is accompanied with a tendency to the worst
kinds of hemorrhagy. In other cases perhaps their refrigerant

* See an Account of the Malignant Erysipelas in the works of foreign
writers, Burserius, Quarin, &c.

property more than counterbalances any advantage to be expected from them.

Although when the fever becomes malignant, the bark and wine are the remedies on which we chiefly rely, we must be cautious not to exhibit them too early in erysipelatous fever, while there is still present any degree of synocha, by which Dr. Smith observes he has often seen gangrene induced instead of prevented. The typhus must be formed, and the florid appearance of the inflammation beginning to be changed to a purple, before the bark can be safely exhibited in large doses.

With regard to the treatment of the erysipelas infantum, which is evidently a phlegmasia, it will be considered under phlogosis.

BOOK III

OF THE EXANTHEMATA.

THE class of idiopathic fevers was divided into three orders, intermitting and remitting fevers, continued fevers, and the exanthemata. The two first of these orders have been considered; we are now to consider the exanthemata.

It appears from what was said in the Introduction, that the fever in this order of diseases is as truly idiopathic as in either of the foregoing. The exanthemata indeed are constantly attended by a local affection, an eruption on the skin, but this appears a considerable time after the commencement of the fever, and cannot therefore be regarded as its cause; besides, the degree of fever is not at all proportioned to that of the local affection, in some of the exanthemata so much the contrary, that the more severe the local affection, the milder is the fever. This is often the case in the plague, and almost always in the scarlet fever; nay where certain causes conspire to prevent the fever, the local affection of the exanthemata is often present and that to a considerable degree without fever; this frequently happens in the plague and small-pox. We shall find also that in the exanthemata, the fever with all its peculiar symptoms has often appeared without any eruption; this is true of the plague, small-pox, and measles, and probably of the other exanthemata. So far indeed is the local affection in these complaints from occasioning the fever, that the latter generally suffers an abatement, and is sometimes wholly removed, on the appearance of the eruption.

In the exanthemata then, the fever is as truly an idiopathic affection as in fevers properly so called, and in laying down the practice in the exanthemata we shall find it treated as such.

Among the orders of idiopathic fevers we readily perceive a striking analogy. Between remitting and continued fevers it is impossible to draw the line of distinction, and the exanthemata we shall find bear a strong resemblance to the eruptive fevers we have been considering. The whole forms evidently a natural class of diseases, of which the arrangement that has been followed points out the different gradations.

The exanthemata were defined in the Introduction, contagious diseases beginning with an idiopathic fever, at a certain period of which, pustules, often in considerable number, appear on the skin.

---

* See the Introduction.

This order comprehends six species : Small-pox, Chicken-pox, Measles, Scarlet Fever, Plague, and Nettle-rash.

CHAP. I.

Of the Small-Pox -

THE Small-Pox is defined by Dr Cullen, " Synocha conta-
" giosa, cum vomitu et ex epigastrio presso, dolore. Tertio die
" incipit, et quinto finitur, eruptio papularum phlegmonodea-
" rum ; quæ spatio octo dierum, in suppurationem, et in crustas
" demum abeunt, sæpe cicatrices depressas sive foveolas in cute
" relinquentes."

Such are the distinguishing marks of the disease as it most
commonly appears, but we constantly meet with cases to which
this definition will not apply. We shall find that the eruption does
not uniformly appear on the third day, nor does it always cease on
the fifth, and in many cases the matter of the pustules remains so
crude, that they can hardly be said to have undergone suppuration.
Even the pain of the stomach increased on pressure, and vomiting
are not constantly present in the eruptive fever. Nay, in certain cases, there has been no eruptive fever at all, the pustules
appearing without any previous complaint. But the definition
just quoted, marking the common course of the disease, is perhaps the best that can be given.

The small-pox has been long divided into distinct and confluent. The former is defined by Dr. Cullen,

" Variola, pustulis paucis, discretis, circumscriptione circular-
" ibus, turgidis, febre, eruptione facta, protinus cessante."

The distinct small-pox occasionally varies from that described
in the foregoing definitions.

Sometimes the matter of the pustules, instead of being purulent, appears a colourless fluid. This variety is termed Variola
Discreta Crystallina.

It sometimes happens in all forms of the small-pox, but more
rarely in the distinct, that small vesicles appear in the interstices
of the pustules. This variety has been termed Variola Discreta
Vesicularis.

Sometimes small empty vesicles appear among the pustules,
or the matter of the pustules themselves disappears leaving them
empty. When this happens the disease is termed Variola Discreta Siliquosa.

* The small-pox is termed by medical writers, Variola or Febris Variolides.

The pustules have sometimes been observed solid throughout; these solid pustules either appearing alone, or being interspersed with others of a more common appearance. This is a rare form of the disease. It has been termed the Warty Small-Pox, or Variola Verrucosa.[*]

When the pustules are of the common appearance but very numerous, yet upon the whole distinct and unattended by any of the symptoms just mentioned, the disease has been called Variola Adjuncta; and this may be regarded as the connecting link between the distinct and confluent small-pox.

All these varieties are attended with more danger than the simple distinct kind, where the pustules suppurate favourably, and are few in number. The empty vesicles indeed sometimes appear in very mild cases.

Many more varieties of distinct small-pox are enumerated by authors. Sauvages,[†] for instance, enumerates twelve species, but many of them are marked by symptoms which cannot be regarded as sufficient to characterize different species of the disease.

Dr. Cullen defines the confluent small-pox,

" Variola, pustulis numerosis, confluentibus, circumscriptione " irregularibus, flaccidis, parum elevatis, febre post eruptionem " perstante."

Although, as expressed in this definition, the number of pustules in the confluent, is generally much greater than in the distinct, small-pox, yet it sometimes happens that, though numerous, the pustules remain distinct; and, on the other hand, but more rarely, that, though few, they appear in clusters and run together.

The nature of the disease is best known, and consequently the names should be determined, from observing the state of the face. The danger is better ascertained by the number and appearance of the pustules there, than on any other part of the body If they be distinct and few in number on the face, even although they are in some degree confluent elsewhere, the disease is termed the distinct small-pox, and the danger is inconsiderable. If, on the other hand, there be a load of pustules on the face, if they run into each other so that the face appears uniformly of a whitish colour, as if, to use Sydenham's expression, it were covered with parchment, whatever appearance the eruption may have on other parts of the body, the complaint is termed confluent, and the danger is considerable.

[*] See Cleghorn's Diseases of Minorca, Burserius's Institut. Med. Prac. Mead De Variolis, Friend's Epistola de quibusdam Variolarum Generibus, &c.

[†] See the Nosologia Methodica of Sauvages.

Dr. Sims, in his Account of Epidemical Diseases, even observes, that the danger was not to be estimated so much from the number of small-pox on the whole face, as from that on the upper part of the forehead, about the junction of the hairy-scalp with the smooth skin. If any were distinct there, and filled properly, little was to be apprehended.

It is evident, from what has been said, that we can draw no line of distinction between the distinct and confluent small-pox. They insensibly run into each other. In the worst kinds of the confluent, there are generally some distinct pustules. In cases which deserve the name of distinct, we often observe two or more pustules running together. Concerning this division therefore it is proper to observe, that where the greater number of pustules are evidently confluent, the complaint has received the one appellation; when the greater number are distinct, the other.

The appearance of the pustules also, as appears from the foregoing definitions, as well as their number and degree of confluence, forms a striking mark of distinction between the benign and confluent small-pox.

The confluent small-pox varies in the same manner as the distinct; hence the names variola confluens crystallina, vesicularis, siliquosa, verrucosa, &c all which varieties are attended with great danger. Most of the symptoms expressed by these terms are more apt to attend the confluent than the distinct small-pox.

In the confluent the pustules sometimes appear almost black from a degree of mortification taking place, and blood being mixed with the matter they contain; hence one variety is termed Variola Confluens Nigra.

When blood is effused into the cavities of the pustules without giving them a perfectly black appearance, the complaint has been termed Variola Sanguinea.

When the pustules are here and there collected together in clusters, with few in the intermediate spaces, the complaint has been termed Variola Confluens Corymbosa.

When petechiæ appear between the pustules, it is called Variola Confluens Petechialis, or Maligna.

After laying before the reader the symptoms of the distinct and confluent small-pox, it will be necessary to take notice of some of the principal varieties of this complaint, which may properly enough be termed anomalous.

In detailing the symptoms of small-pox, it is unnecessary to consider separately what has been termed the simple distinct, and contiguous distinct, the simple confluent and putrid confluent, as some have done. The two former I shall comprehend under the term distinct, and the two latter under that of confluent. The contiguous are only the worst kind of the distinct ; and the putrid the worst form of the confluent.

- It will be necessary to point out the symptoms which indicate most danger. Those indicating most danger in the distinct small-pox, belong to that called contiguous distinct ; those indicating most danger in the confluent, to that called putrid. These divisions 'are of no use ; it is only necessary to take notice of them, because they have been adopted by authors.

SECT. I.

Of the Symptoms of the Small-Pox.

IN order to avoid confusion, it will be proper to consider the symptoms of the distinct and confluent small-pox separately.

1. Of the Symptoms of the Distinct Small-Pox.

Small-Pox attacks in a manner similar to the fevers we have been considering.

The patient sometimes complains of sickness for several days before the fever is distinctly form ed ; this however is not very often observed. The fever generally comes on about mid-day, with the symptoms of a cold stage, often attended with a considerable degree of drowsiness.

If the patient is old enough to give an account of his feelings, he complains of languor and listlessness, with the other uneasy sensations that attend the commencement of synochus These symptoms are soon followed by considerable heat, thirst, and the other symptoms which characterize those fevers in which the synocha prevails.

The skin and fauces are parched, the body costive, the urine at first pale, afterwards more scanty and high coloured, and hemorrhagies are frequent, particularly from the nose. When the small-pox is of the distinct kind, the fever which precedes the eruption, and on that account termed the eruptive fever, is always a synocha, and the more moderate the symptoms of excitement are, the more favourable is the prognosis.

Such are the symptoms which the eruptive fever of small-pox has in common with many other febrile diseases, but certain symptoms generally attend, by which the disease may be known before the eruption makes its appearance.

It has been observed, that pains of the back, limbs, and loins, are more common and severe than in most other febrile complaints. The patient also sometimes complains of pains in the breast and fauces, and coma is apt to supervene.* All these symptoms afford an unfavourable prognosis.

In adults particularly, when the eruption is about to be numerous, there is often uncommon tendency to sweat, which recurs as often as the patient goes to bed.+ A coldness of the extremities is often present during almost the whole course of the disease, especially in children even where the danger is not considerable, and has been regarded as one of the best diagnostic symptoms of the eruptive fever ‡ But the most unequivocal are those mentioned by Dr Cullen in the foregoing definition, the vomiting and pain of the stomach increased on pressure. Even these however, like the other diagnostic symptoms of this fever, are not universally present.||

The vomiting is generally bilious,§ and then there is often present at the same time a degree of bilious diarrhœa.

A little before the appearance of the eruption, some change in the state of the symptoms generally takes place. Children are subject to starting during sleep from the commencement of the complaint. On the night before the eruption they are often seized with an epileptic fit. If it only occur once or twice. it is hardly to be regarded as unfavourable, and has even been believed to afford a favourable prognosis.¶ If the child has already teethed, this symptom may always be regarded as the forerunner of the pustules.

Instead of the fit, children sometimes have a grinding of the teeth, and convulsive twitching about the mouth often spreading to other parts of the face, and these symptoms in many cases precede the fit.

At the same period the fever often suffers an exacerbation, the lips are frequently edged round with inflammation, the eyes are glaring and cannot endure the light, the face glows, there is a considerable increase of temperature, the skin and fauces become parched. and coma, although it had not shewed itself at an ear-

* Bang observes, that coma is most apt to supervene in this complaint in the vigour of life See Acta Societ .Med. Hafn.

† Sydenham says, he never observed this symptom in children either before or after the appearance of the pustules.

‡ See Dr. Walker's Treatise on the Small-Pox.

|| See the observations of Van Swieten in his Commentaries, and others, on the diagnosis of this fever.

§ It is, difficult to say on what foundation Dr. Thompson has asserted that the vomiting is most frequently bilious in women and children. See Dr. Thompson's Treatise on the Small-Pox.

¶ Epileptic fits have sometimes though rarely occurred at a late period of the distinct small-pox. The son of Lord Sunderland, inoculated by Mr. Maitland soon after the introduction of inoculation into England, died of an eleptic fit after the greater part of the pustules were dried off. See Woodville's History of Inoculation.

 tter period, often supervenes. The patient is sometimes troubled with cramps in the legs, and a severe pain in the back now
and then comes on a short time before the appearance of the pustules. Few of these symptoms however are observable in mild
cases; the coma and cramps of the legs generally forebode a copious eruption.

The period at which the eruption appears is not exactly the
same in all cases; generally towards the end of the third day, or
the beginning of the fourth, counting from the commencement
of the febrile symptoms. Sydenham observes, that in the distinct
small-pox the eruption generally happens on the fourth day, including the day on which the fever commences, sometimes rather later, but rarely before this period. Dr. Cullen makes the
time of its appearance about the end of the third day. If we
class together all kinds of smal-pox, we shall perhaps find the
third day the mean time of its appearance.* It is to be observed
that the later the eruption the more favourable is the prognosis.

The pustules on their coming out are small red points, appearing first on the face and hairy scalp, then on the neck, gradually
spreading over the whole body. It frequently happens that as
soon as the pustules make their appearance the patient is affected
with sneezing, which continues to recur while they are coming
out. The interruption of this symptom has been regarded as a
sign of the eruption being finished.

About the fifth or sixth day, counting from the commencement
of the fever, that is, the second or third of the eruption, a little vesicle, which appears depressed in the middle, is seen on the top of
each pustule, containing a matter nearly colourless. For two or
three days the vesicles increase in breadth, the matter gradually
assuming the appearance of pus. About the eighth day of the
increase they become spherical, and the pustules are completely formed; being then very itchy, hard, and prominent, and
appearing almost terminated in a point.

When the pustules are more numerous, although benign, they
neither rise so high nor are so much pointed, as when fewer in
number; but are then often rather flat on the top.

* Nothing can be more vague than the manner of ascertaining the period of the eruption. The eruption is said to happen on the second, third,
fourth, &c. day, whether it occurs in the morning or evening of these
days, and whether the accession of the fever has been in the morning or
evening. Great accuracy in this respect however would not be of much
consequence.

It has been proposed to make every day consist of 24 hours in compu-
ting the appearance of the eruption, so that were the fever to attack to-day
at one, and the eruption to appear to-morrow at twelve, it should be regarded as appearing on the first day. If it appears between one of the
second day and the same hour of the following it should be regarded as
appearing on the second day, and so on. See Dr. Thompson's Treatise
on Small-pox.

In the most benign small-pox, from their first appearance the pustules are surrounded with a perfectly circular inflamed margin. When the pustules are more numerous, though still of a favourable kind, the margin is less exactly circular. These margins coalescing in places where the pustules are crowded, give a red colour to the skin lying between them, which is always a favourable appearance.

In the mildest cases, no more pustules appear after the end of the first day of the eruption, or the second at furthest. In cases where they are about to be numerous, they often continue to make their appearance a day or two longer.

About the eighth day, when the pustules are pretty numerous, the face swells and is often affected with lancinating pains. The swelling sometimes extends to the whole head, the eye-lids seem as if distended with a fluid, and are often so much enlarged as entirely to close the eyes.

When the eyes are much affected from the beginning, the sight is sometimes lost, generally in consequence of one or more pustules forming on the cornea. This indeed is a rare occurrence. Pustules are rather more apt to appear on the sclerotica, and there their consequences are less to be dreaded.

When the tumefaction of the face begins to subside, which happens about the tenth or eleventh day, the hands and feet swell, which in the space of some days subside in like manner.

All these are symptoms not very remarkable in mild cases: at the same time it is not to be overlooked, that when the other syptoms are severe, these swellings, if not in excess, are to be regarded as favourable appearances.

As the disease advances, the matter of the pustules becomes by degree more opaque, thick, whitish, and at length yellow. When the pustules are very numerous, the matter is thinner and not so yellow as in the most benign forms of the disease.

About the eleventh or twelfth day, still counting from the commencement of the fever, the pustules have gained their full size, which differs a little in different epidemics, but is generally about that of a pea. A dark spot now appears on each. From being soft and smooth, they become rough and throw out a yellow matter. The pustules now begin to shrink, and the matter drying forms a small crust over each of them. Sometimes only part of the matter is thrown out, which, together with that remaining, hardens; and, in a few days, falls off, leaving the skin in the places which it covered of a dark brown colour, that often remains for a long time after the patient is well.

While this takes place, the swelling of the face and other parts gradually subsides. But the foregoing process does not go on at the same time on every part of the body. The pustules in those places on which they first appear first arrive at maturation. They generally remain longest on the hands. The sooner the pustules become dry and fall off, the better in general is the prognosis.

It often happens in cases where the pustules have been more numerous on the face, continued for a longer time, and been filled with a matter less thick and benign than usual, that after they fall off, the parts which they covered suffer desquamation, so that small pits are formed, for the pustules do not on falling off leave pits; they are formed by a succeeding operation. Pits are seldom the consequence of the distinct small-pox, unless the pustules are very numerous.*

It sometimes happens that the matter of the pustules, particularly on the arms and hands, is either absorbed, or, as Dr. Walker alleges, transudes through the cuticle, so that they appear empty vesicles, giving rise to the variety termed siliquosa. Lobb† observes, that he has seen these empty vesicles filled with a well conditioned matter, which is a favourable symptom. It is not uncommon indeed, when the strength is considerably reduced, for the pustules on every part of the body to appear rather flat; the tumor of their base subsides, and the matter seems in part either to have been absorbed, or to have transuded‡ through the cuticle; and on the exhibition of any remedy which renews the strength, walking for instance in cool air, or in certain circumstances using the cold bath, the pustules again swell and become turgid with matter.

While these symptoms proceed, others at the same time demand attention.

On the coming out of the pustules, the fever suffers a remission, and in the mildest cases disappears entirely about the fifth day, at which time the eruption is completed.|| About the sixth or seventh day, when the pustules are numerous some uneasiness of the throat comes on, with an increased secretion of saliva, the voice at the same time often becoming hoarse. A considerable degree of any of those symptoms tends to afford an unfavorable prognosis.

As the disease proceeds, the secretion from the mouth and throat often becomes thick, and is not easily spit out, sometimes

---

* Sydenham remarks, that when pitting follows the distinct small-pox, it is generally the consequence of several pustules having run together, which usually happens, he observes, in the last six months of the year. He generally found the small-pox milder in the spring than in the autumn.

† See his Practice of Physic.

‡ See Walker's Treatise on the Small-Pox.

|| When the tendency to sweating has occurred, it has been observed, notwithstanding the abatement of the fever, to continue nearly to the time of maturation.

occasioning such difficulty of swallowing, that liquids taken into the mouth are spit out again, or rejected by the nose. The swelling or parched state of the fauces also sometimes considerably affects the breathing, and deafness is now and then a symptom at the same period, from a pustulary affection of the meatus auditorius externus. These symptoms however, in the distinct small-pox, are generally of little consequence ; they all wear away as the more essential symptoms decline.

When the pustules are numerous some return of fever generally happens about the eleventh day, a period we shall find much dreaded in some forms of the disease ; but for the most part it disappears in a few days, and in this kind of small-pox is seldom attended with much uneasiness, and less frequently with danger.

But even in the distinct small-pox, when the pustules are numerous, a train of symptoms indicating more danger now and then supervenes at an earlier period, about the seventh or eighth day. This train of symptoms has been called the secondary fever.

It sometimes happens at this period, after the patient has appeared almost well, the pulse having returned to its natural frequency, that symptoms of fever more or less gradually, in some cases very suddenly, return, and in the space of a few hours the pulse becomes more frequent, and the other symptoms of fever more severe, than at any former period But when this fever occurs in the distinct small-pox, it is attended with less danger than in the confluent. In the former it seldom appears when the pustules are of a benign kind, and almost never when the patient has received the disease by inoculation and been properly treated.

When the pustules are numerous they must, in many places, run together. When the greater number run together, the disease is termed the Confluent Small-Pox. The symptoms peculiar to this form of the disease we are now to consider.

2. Of the Symptoms of the Confluent Small-Pox.

Although there is much similarity in the eruptive fever of the distinct and confluent small-pox, yet, even from the commencement, in some respects they differ essentially. The symptoms common to both, the sensation of cold, the anxiety, sickness, vomiting, &c. more uniformly attend and are experienced to a greater degree in the confluent than in the distinct form of the disease.

The pains of the back and limbs in particular, which are only sometimes troublesome in the distinct small-pox, very generally precede the confluent eruption. Van Swieten observes, that when the complaint comes on with a severe lumbago, so that the patient can hardly move his limbs, he always suspects danger. Even although the fever be slight, he adds, these symptoms always afford an unfavourable prognosis ; and Morton remarks, that he always found coma and a severe pain of the loins to be dangerous symptoms in the eruptive fever of small-pox. There are few authors indeed who treat particularly of the small-pox without making similar observations.

The most striking difference however between the eruptive fever of the distinct and confluent forms of the disease, is, that in the distinct it is synocha, never shewing a tendency to typhus, while in the confluent, although at the beginning synocha, it is apt to be changed into typhus by any error in the treatment, or even without any evident cause. In the most alarming cases indeed the fever is a typhus almost from the beginning ; petechiæ, and sometimes hemorrhagies of a bad kind, appearing at a very early period.

Epileptic fits now and then occur during the first days of the fever, and have even proved fatal before the eruption appeared ; at other times they continue to recur after the eruption is out, and sometimes through the whole course of the disease.

The tendency to sweat is not common in this kind of small-pox ; but a diarrhœa often precedes the eruption, and continues for a day or two after its appearance, which Sydenham declares he never saw happen in the distinct small-pox. If the stools are unusually fetid, the prognosis is very bad.

This diarrhœa is generally confined to children ; in adults an affection of the fauces, often amounting to a salivation, attends, instead of the diarrhœa.* It was observed, that at a later period, even of the distinct small-pox, there is sometimes an increased secretion of thin saliva.

The eruption in the confluent, generally appears earlier than in the distinct, small-pox, seldom later than about the beginning of the third day, and often on the second ; in some cases even before the expiration of the first twenty-four hours ; and fresh pustules continue to come out for the space of three or four days. The period of the eruption is more uncertain than in the distinct small-pox ; for although generally earlier than in mild forms of the disease, it has been delayed by the appearance of inflammatory symptoms to the fourth or even to the fifth day. An acute pain of the loins resembling a fit of the gravel, in the side like that attending pleurisy, in the limbs resembling rheumatism, or in the stomach accompanied with sickness and vomiting, are enumerated by Sydenham as symptoms which he has known to have the effect of delaying the eruption in confluent small-pox.

* The salivation sometimes, though rarely, appears in children. Tissot says, he has seen several, scarcely four years of age, seized with the salivation, while the bowels remained costive. See Tissot's Treatise on the Small-Pox, Apoplexy, and Dropsy.

VOL. I. X x

On the second day of the fever an erythematic inflammation often appears on the face, and soon spreads over the neck and breast, and in some cases over the whole body. This is the fore-runner of pustules, which begin to emerge from it in the form of small red points, many of which soon coalesce. They sometimes appear in clusters, the intermediate spaces being free from them; at other times many parts, and particularly the face, seem almost covered with them.

The eruption in the confluent small-pox on its first appearance is sometimes so like that of the measles, that they can only be distinguished by the accompanying symptoms.

The pustules form matter sooner in the confluent than in the distinct small-pox; they are not much raised above the surround-ing parts, nor do they retain the circular form, but even in places where they are not confluent they become of an irregular shape; nor are they surrounded with an inflamed margin as in the distinct small-pox; the spaces between the pustules are pale and flaccid, and the pustules themselves, about the time of maturation, often appear like thin pellicles fixed upon the skin.* On the face, where they are generally most numerous and confluent, they often so run into each other, that almost the whole seems one large ve-sicle, the surface being perfectly smooth.

The matter becomes whitish, brown, or almost black, but never thick and yellow like that of the distinct small-pox. The lighter coloured the matter, the better is the prognosis. When the pus-tules are of a black colour, the danger is very great. The same may be said of those cases where extravasated blood is mixed with the matter, giving it the appearance of a bloody sanies.

The matter of the confluent small-pox has sometimes been so virulent as not only to destroy many of the soft, but even the bony parts of the face. The nose, cheek bones, palate, fauces, velum pendulum palati, and uvula, have been wholly destroyed by it, and the jaw-bones so much affected that the teeth have fallen from their sockets.†

The swelling of the face, which only now and then occurs in the distinct small-pox, is a constant symptom of the confluent; and in this form of the disease it both appears earlier and rises to a greater height.

About the ninth day of the eruption, that is, about the eleventh of the disease, the pustules begin to pour out their matter, which hardens on the surface, forming crusts of a brown or black colour, that do not fall off for many days; and are almost always on the face followed by a desquamation which leaves pits. The more

---

* This flat appearance of the pustules in the confluent small-pox has been termed Sessile. By some writers the confluent small-pox is termed Variola Sessilis.

† See Burserius's Inst. Med. Pract. and other works on this disease.

numerous and confluent the pustules are, and the darker their colour, the longer they are in disappearing ; and the desquamation is sometimes protracted beyond the twentieth day.

It often happens, that although the pustules are crowded on the face, they are few, and even distinct, on every other part of the body. But while the face is loaded with those of the confluent kind, the pustules on other parts never have a benign appearance ; they are never circular, raised, nor filled with a well conditioned matter, but in this respect resemble those on the face. In all cases of the confluent small-pox however, the pustules on the trunk and extremities are generally rather larger, and more prominent, than those on the face.

Although the fever in the confluent small-pox often becomes more moderate on the appearance of the eruption, yet it never wholly ceases. This remission generally continues till about the sixth or seventh day, that is, from soon after the period of eruption till near that of maturation, when it suffers a remarkable exacerbation, the commencement of the secondary fever, which often appears with more alarming symptoms than any that preceded it. If coma does not supervene, the patient is distressed with head-ach and obstinate watchfulness, often the forerunners of delirium. The inflammatory affection of the fauces, with hoarseness and dyspnœa, increases, and in many cases all the worst symptoms of typhus supervene, and the patient is carried off on the eleventh day from the commencement of the disease including that on which it made its attack. The eleventh day the reader will find frequently mentioned by Sydenham, and other writers, as the most fatal in the small-pox.

Such are the appearances of the regular distinct and confluent small-pox. It will be proper to recapitulate the circumstances in which they differ, and point out the manner in which they insensibly run into each other, that the means of collecting the prognosis may be placed in a clearer point of view.

3. Parallel of the Symptoms of the Distinct and Confluent Small-Pox.

The eruptive fever in most cases at its commencement differs only in degree. It is generally accompanied with those symptoms which characterize synocha, but in the confluent they are more severe than in the distinct, and the pain and confusion of the head more frequently rise to delirium.

In the distinct small-pox we often observe in adults a tendency to sweating. In proportion as the succeeding eruption is about to be numerous, this tendency begins to disappear, and that to purging, particularly in children, to shew itself. When the eruption is about to be confluent, the purging is generally considerable; and in the worst cases, the stools are unusually fetid and sometimes mixed with blood ; hence it is, that Sydenham justly considers a tendency to sweating a favourable, and to purging an unfavourable, symptom.

In the most benign small-pox there is little affection of the fauces and no salivation When the eruption is numerous, yet distinct, the affection of the fauces is evident, and often attended with a spitting of thin saliva. In the confluent small-pox the salivation, particularly in adults, comes on early and is generally considerable.

In the mildest form of the disease, the eruption seldom appears before the fourth day. If the pustules are about to be numerous, it generally shews itself about the end of the third, if about to be confluent, often on the second, and in the worst cases, even on the first day. The eruption in the confluent however is sometimes, though rarely, delayed to the fourth or even to the fifth day ; so that the period of eruption here is less certain than in the distinct small-pox.

In the mildest cases, the first appearance of the eruption is that of small red points. In cases where the pustules are about to be numerous, and still more if they are about to be confluent, they are often preceded by a rash on the face, neck, and breast, sometimes spreading over the whole body.

In the mildest form of small-pox the pustules appear few and distinct ; in more severe cases they are more numerous, and often here and there, particularly on the face, in small clusters. In the confluent small-pox they are still more numerous, and more frequently appear in this way.

In the mildest cases the pustules are considerably raised above the surrounding parts, and are terminated by a point ; they are quite circular at their base, and surrounded by a florid margin, which is also bounded by a very exact circle. In cases where the pustules are more numerous, they are less raised and the circular appearance is not so exact and uniform. In proportion as the number of pustules increase, their elevation is less, and the circumference of the base and margin become more irregular. When they are confluent, particularly in the worst cases, the pustules are almost flat, and the circular shape and florid margin nearly or altogether lost.

In the most favorable cases, although the matter at first appears colourless, it soon becomes thick, white, opaque, and at length yellow. Where the pustules are numerous, it continues colourless longer, becomes however opaque and thick, though not so much so as in the mildest cases, and whitish ; but seldom assumes the proper yellow colour. In the confluent small-pox it never becomes thick, but changes to a brownish white colour ; and in the worst kinds, it is mixed with blood or becomes almost black.

In the mildest kind of small-pox, pustules cease to come out about two days after the commencement of the eruption. When they are about to be more numerous, they generally continue to make their appearance for a longer time ; and in some cases of the confluent, for three or four days.

b. In the distinct small-pox, matter is seldom observed in the pustules before the fifth day of the complaint. In the confluent, it generally appears earlier. In the former, a dark spot, appears on the pustules, they become rough, and pour out part of their matter, very uniformly about the eleventh day. In the confluent, although this frequently happens about the same period, yet the pustules sometimes continue fresh as it is termed for a much longer time. Dr. Cleghorn* observes, that it was often the fourteenth or fifteenth day before the confluent small-pox in Minorca became rough on the face ; and on the legs and arms it frequently continued fresh till near the thirtieth day. So that the period of exsiccation, like that of eruption, is less certain in the confluent, than in the distinct, small-pox.

In mild cases the pustules fall off about the twelfth or fourteenth day, and are not followed by pitting ; when they are more numerous, they adhere longer, and pitting generally follows. When they are confluent, they are still longer in falling, and pitting almost uniformly succeeds them.

In the most favourable forms of small-pox, the fever almost entirely leaves the patient soon after the pustules make their appearance. Where the pustules are more numerous, a considerable remission takes place, but seldom complete apyrexia. In the confluent the remission is less considerable, and in the worst cases hardly to be perceived.

In the mildest small-pox the patient experiences no return of fever about the seventh or eighth day. Where the pustules are more numerous, he is attacked, about the latter of those days, with the secondary fever ; when they are confluent, this fever generally makes its appearance a day or two sooner, and all its symptoms are more alarming.

In the mildest small-pox there is little or no degree of fever on the eleventh day. When the pustules are numerous, there is generally on this day a considerable exacerbation of the febrile symptoms ; where they are confluent, such an exacerbation takes place on this day, that it frequently terminates life.

In the more favourable cases, the secondary fever is a well-marked synocha, slowly assuming the form of typhus. In the confluent small-pox, the fever is sooner changed to typhus ; and in the worst kinds of the confluent, the secondary fever is a typhus almost from the beginning.

* See his Treatise on the Diseases of Minorca.

The most benign small-pox is accompanied with little or no swelling of the face. When the pustules are numerous, but distinct, this happens on or about the eighth day ; when they are confluent, the swelling of the face comes on sooner, and rises to a greater height ; the same may be said of the swelling of the hands and feet.

Upon the whole, the more any kind of small-pox differs from the simple benign form of the disease, the periods are less certain, the various symptoms generally appear earlier, rise to a greater height, are protracted for a longer time, and attended with greater danger.

From what has been said it appears, that we may often, before the appearance of the eruption, determine of what kind it will be, since many of the symptoms, characterising the distinct and confluent small-pox, precede the eruption. The following, as appears from the foregoing parallel of the symptoms of distinct and confluent small-pox, are the principal circumstances which enable us to predict of what nature the eruption will be.

When the symptoms of the eruptive fever are moderate and readily relieved on exposure to cold, the eruption will almost always be distinct. When the excitement is more considerable and less readily relieved ; when the patient is harrassed with pains of the back, limbs, and loins ; when there is much coma, or any degree of delirium, especially if the fever in other respects also shew a tendency to typhus, we may expect a confluent eruption. A tendency to sweat in the eruptive fever generally precedes the distinct ; a tendency to purging, the confluent. If the affection of the fauces is either not perceived at an early period, or is present only in a slight degree, the eruption will probably be distinct. When this affection is considerable and accompanied by salivation, a confluent eruption may be expected.

The method I have followed in detailing the symptoms of regular small-pox, has occasioned some repetition. This appeared to me admissible, in order to place the prognosis, in so important a disease, in a clear point of view, which cannot, for reasons mentioned in the Introduction, be done without some repetition.

4. Of the Symptoms of Anomalous Small-Pox.

It will be sufficient to point out the circumstances in which some of the most remarkable forms of anomalous, differ from the regular distinct and confluent, small-pox.

One of the most common of the irregular forms of small-pox is that termed crystalline, from the appearance of the pustules.

At first view it may appear wrong to regard the putrid as a regular, and the crystalline as an anomalous, form of the dis-

ease. When we recollect however that the putrid small-pox, as
it has been termed, only differs in degree from the common confluent, which from improper treatment, or peculiarity of constitution, every day assumes this appearance; and that neither the
distinct nor confluent small-pox are apt to degenerate into the
crystalline; the propriety of this mode of arrangement is sufficiently apparent. Besides, the crystalline small-pox is often
epidemic, while other forms of the disease hardly shew themselves.* It is more common however for a few cases of crystalline to appear while the greatest number of patients labour under the regular small-pox.

Dr. Rogers divides the crystalline small-pox, in the same
way in which the regular has been divided, into distinct, contiguous, and confluent. But here there is not the same room for
such a division; for although in some instances the pustules are
fewer and more distinct than in others; yet the state of the matter, as well as the appearance of the pustules themselves, does
not vary much in different cases; and in all, the danger is considerable.

The crystalline small-pox makes its attack, like other forms
of the disease, with the common symptoms of fever.

The vomiting, pain at the pit of the stomach increased on
pressure, and coldness of the feet and hands, are still the diagnostic symptoms of the eruptive fever.

It is more apt than the regular small-pox to be attended with
those symptoms which indicate danger, coma, delirium, prostration of strength, petechiæ, hemorrhagies, &c.; for although the
fever, as in the regular small-pox, is synocha at the commencement; the typhus more frequently shews itself at an early period.

The eruption on its first appearance frequently looks well,
and even continues to do so for one or two days. The pustules
are of a good colour and distinct, producing a considerable remission of the febrile symptoms. About the third day of the
eruption, however, there generally appears a numerous crop of
pustules; which, although in general distinct, are of an irregular
shape, seldom appearing circular as in the distinct form of regular small-pox.

After the eruption is finished, a considerable remission of the
fever takes place, but never complete apyrexia; and the urine
generally remains limpid throughout the whole complaint. The
distinguishing symptom is the appearance of the matter, which
is a colourless fluid that rarely acquires any degree of the purulent appearance.

As in the regular small-pox, there are now and then intersper-

* See an Account of the Epidemic Small-Pox of Cork, in Dr. Rogers's
Essay on Epidemic Diseases.

sed among the pustules some which are empty, or clear and dense having no cavity.

Whatever be the appearance of the pustules on their first coming out, they soon become pale. They are never indeed surrounded with the well-defined florid margin of the regular distinct small-pox, and the interstices have the flaccid appearance observed in the confluent.

The period at which the face and head swell is more uncertain than in the regular small-pox, and the swelling in a day or two after its appearance is often suddenly translated to the hands or feet. When this happens it has been observed that no salivation takes place.

If the eruptive fever runs high, it is often followed by a confluent eruption, and then the danger, which is at all times considerable in the crystalline small-pox, is very great, few escaping from this form of the disease ; in which the fever generally soon becomes a malignant typhus.

In the worst cases, the face and head either do not swell at all, or only in a slight degree, but instead of the swelling, there is generally inflammation about the eye-lids, lips, or some neighbouring part.* The inflammation sometimes seizes on the encephalon, occasioning violent head-ach and delirium. In the latter cases traces of inflammation of the brain and its membranes are generally apparent after death. Even abscesses form in different parts of the head, and matter is sometimes discharged by the ears.† The strong pulse at the temples, while that at the wrist is feeble, mentioned among the symptoms of synochus as denoting a tendency to phrenitis, is a frequent symptom in the crystalline small-pox, and there affords the same inference.‡

The crystalline small-pox sometimes proves suddenly fatal before the eruption appears ; more frequently however death is delayed to the seventh day ; sometimes to the fourteenth, seventeenth, or even longer.‖

---

* Soreness of the mouth and throat, instead of the swelling of the face, attended a malignant small-pox, described by Dr. Cleghorn in his account of the Diseases of Minorca. Solid and empty pustules frequently appeared in this epidemic, which was one of the most fatal of which we have any account.

† In the irregular forms of small-pox it is not uncommon for abscesses to form in different parts of the body, and recovery seems often to depend on the pus being discharged Abscesses, Rosen observes, are often favourable if the latter is properly discharged. Haller's Disp. ad Hist. et Cur. Morb. Pert.

‡ The inference from this symptom is the same in all cases of fever. In nervous complaints, unattended by fever, the pulse is often strong and full at the temples, while it is weak at the wrist, the face at the same time appearing flushed, and the eyes frequently inflamed, without denoting any tendency to inflammation of the encephalon.

‖ See Dr. Walker's Treatise on the Small-pox.

A remarkable form of the anomalous small-pox is that which it sometimes assumes when influenced by the measles appearing at the same time, illustrating an observation made when speaking of contagion, namely, that during a contagious epidemic, almost every disease which appears is sometimes more or less influenced by it.

We have an instance of this form of small-pox in the epidemic described by Sydenham, which raged in London in 1670, 1671, and 1672. It appeared while the measles were prevalent, and continued for sometime after they had ceased, gradually becoming milder and more regular till the year 1674, when the measles again became epidemic, and the small-pox as irregular and fatal as before.

Every case was attended with danger, although the pustules were not always confluent. But even where these were distinct, the complaint was attended with many symptoms which in the regular small-pox belong to the confluent form of the disease. The eruption appeared on the third day, the pustules were never spherical, and became black sometime before their separation. In some cases, although the pustules were distinct, salivation came on, from which, Sydenham observes, we must infer, that notwithstanding the pustules being distinct, the disease partook more of the confluent than of the distinct small-pox.

In confluent cases this epidemic differed more essentially from the regular small-pox. On many places, particularly on the thighs, there appeared among the pustules small vesicles filled with a colourless fluid. When the pellicle forming these was broken, the serum ran out, and the parts beneath appeared black and gangrenous.* All died in whom the blisters became gangrenous.

On the eleventh day a white shining pellicle covered the face, which threw out a matter that soon formed a crust, neither yellow like that of the distinct, nor brown like that of the confluent, small-pox; but resembling concreted blood, which during the maturation of the pustules grew darker, till at last the whole face became almost black; from which the disease was termed, the black small-pox.

The eleventh day was less to be dreaded than in the regular forms of the disease; in the greater number of cases the patient surviving to the fourteenth and sometimes to the seventeenth day; if he escaped during these periods, his chance of recovery was better. Those in whom the blisters appeared, generally died within a few days after the eruption.

* Such cases are to be regarded as a combination of small-pox with the symptomatic eruption which characterizes the vesicular fever.

The symptoms upon the whole were more severe than in the regular confluent small-pox, and the eruption on its first coming out had more of the appearance of the erysipelas or measles, so that at an early period, it was only known to be small-pox by attending to the diagnostic symptoms of the eruptive fever.   The discolouration of the skin also remained longer, and the face was deformed with deeper pits.

It is remarkable and farther illustrates an observation just made, that towards the end of the epidemic, at which time the dysentery raged, the small-pox was apt to assume the form of this complaint. " Operæ pretium est et illud adjungere, quod, durante hac " omni constitutione qua tam epidemice seviebant dysenteriæ; " variolæ regimine justo calidiore provocatæ, per dysenteriam " nonnunquam viam sibi facerent ; quod ne semel accidisse hac- " tenus quidem animadverteram."*

We cannot here help remarking the concurrence of the measles, and the unusual fatality of the small-pox, which has been observed in other instances.

It is an observation even among the vulgar that the small-pox is apt to appear immediately before or after the prevalence of the measles.   In such cases however it is not always of a remarkably malignant kind as Sydenham found it.†

Another curious observation has been made relating to the symptoms of these complaints, namely, that if, while a patient labours under the small-pox, he is seized with the measles, the course of the former is interrupted till the eruption of measles is finished.‡ 'The measles appear, for instance, on the second day of the eruption of small-pox, the progress of the small-pox ceases till the measles terminate desquamation, and then goes on in the usual way ; and the time from the first appearance of the eruption of small-pox to its termination, is found longer than it ought to be, by the time during which the measles were present.   In the third volume of the Medical Commentaries, however, cases are related by Dr. Rainey, in which a concurrence of the small-pox and measles took place without the progress of the former being retarded || Analogous to the foregoing fact, is one mentioned by Dr. Heberden, in Dr. Kirkpatrick's Analysis of Inoculation, namely, that when the small-pox appeared during an epidemic intermittent, if any la-

* Sydenhami Opera, sect. iii. cap. 6.   De Variol. Anomal.

† See the 134th and following pages of Sim's Treatise on Epidemic Disorders.

‡ See the first volume of Dr. Duncan's Medical Commentaries, &c.

|| Cases of this kind I have known.   Several are related in the Medical and Physical Journal.   Pechlinus, Vogel observes, saw a case in which small-pox appeared on the right side of the body, and at the same time measles on the left, the line of division being a perpendicular drawn through the middle of the body.   This case is too extraordinary to gain implicit credit.

bouring under the fever were seized with the small-pox, the former ceased till the small-pox had run its usual course, and then went on as before.

We meet with similar facts relating to other erupti e diseases. Thus Dr. Jenner, in the Continuation of his Observations relating to the Cow-pox, relates a case in which the scarlatina was interrupted by the appearance of this disease. " But the most re- " markable part of this history is, that on the fourth day after- " wards, as soon as the efflorescence of the cow-pox began to die " away upon the arm, and the pustules to dry up, the scarlatina " again appeared, her throat became sore, and the rash spread all " over her. She went fairly through the disease with its com- " mon symptoms."

To return from this digression; there is still another form of the anomalous small-pox which deserves to be mentioned. It is met with only in children, and seems to be merely the regular confluent small-pox considerably modified by peculiarity of constitution, those only of a debilitated habit of body being subject to it.

The patient is attacked with langour and oppression, that continue for some days without considerably affecting the pulse, which is seldom much more frequent than in health, and the temperature is not above the healthy degree, sometimes below it. As the symptoms advance, the patient loses his appetite, is troubled with nausea and insatiable thirst, becomes drowsy and often comatose. On the third day a few pustules generally come out, but they soon disappear, and the coma increasing terminates life in a few days.

There is still another set of symptoms which deserve the name of anomalous, yet do not constitute a distinct form of the disease. They are apt to occur when the course of the disease is disturbed by improper treatment or any other cause.

When the sweating becomes profuse, the swelling of the face either does not appear, or only in a slight degree, the skin remaining flaccid and the interstices of the pustules pale, although the eruption is distinct ; and had not the sweat been profuse, the complaint would have proved mild. In such cases indeed, the pustules themselves generally look well, are red and raised, and even remain so after death.

It now and then happens that the sweat, after flowing freely for some time, suddenly ceases, which is also a very dangerous accident. In many cases neither cordials, external warmth, nor any other means, are capable of recalling it. The patient is seized with sickness, anxiety, extreme restlessness, often delirium, passing the urine frequently and in small quantity, and sometimes expires in the space of a few hours.

It now and then happens in like manner in the confluent small-pox, that the salivation suddenly ceases ; and unless this acci-dent is immediately followed by the swelling of the face and hands, the patient generally dies. In the confluent small-pox, Sydenham remarks, both the salivation and swelling are necessa-ry ; if either fails, the patient is in danger. Where the salvation does not wholly cease, but the saliva becomes so thick that it cannot be spit out, the patient is sometimes threatened with suf-focation ; and the deglutition is often so impeded that a liquid taken into the mouth is apt to fall into the trachea, and is thrown out by the nose with much coughing. When a thickening of the saliva is attended with coma, the patient generally dies on the eleventh day. This state of the saliva however may be present in some degree without indicating much danger.

A total suppression of urine sometimes comes on about the height of the disease, even in the distinct small-pox, especially if the habit be full and the patient in the vigour of life.

Although a diarrhœa is to be regarded as a favourable symp-tom in the confluent small-pox, yet it sometimes becomes so pro-fuse as considerably to modify the disease and add to the unfa-vourable prognosis. Where this or other debilitating causes, such as sudden exposure to cold after the hot regimen has been employed, unseasonable blood-letting, &c. have existed ; it some-time happens that the eruption, or swelling of the face and hands, or both, recede ; and then the danger is very great.*

It sometimes happens that after the exsiccation of the pustules, a new crop shews itself ; and, on the other hand, that the fever with all its peculiar symptoms appears without any eruption at all. It is asserted by Frank, Burserius, and others, that in the latter case the patient is as secure against a second attack of the disease, as if the eruption had made its appearance. There are some observations however which contradict this opinion. In the fourth volume of the Memoirs of the Medical Society of London, Mr. Kite relates two cases in which inoculation produced the usual suppuration in the part inoculated, and at the usual time the patient sickened, but no variolus eruption followed. Both pa-tients were again inoculated fourteen days after the first inocula-tion. One of them had the disease in the usual way and in a mild form ; the other remained unaffected.

I shall have occasion to mention many of the more remarka-ble deviations from the ordinary course of the disease, in speak-of the means to be employed when such accidents occur.

The small-pox, especially the confluent and irregular forms of the disease, is apt to leave behind it a variety of troublesome consequences. Most of those who survived the irregular small-

* See Sydenham's chapter entitled, Variolæ Regulares, p. 140.

pox of Minorca, Dr. Cleghorn informs us, remained blind, con.
sumptive, or lame with caries of the bones, ulcers, &c. Some.
times a grangrenous erysipelas of the limbs, or apoplexy, has su.
pervened and proved fatal. Blindness from a pustulary affection
of the cornea is not uncommon, more rarely the hearing is de.
stroyed, and the voice is sometimes lost. The palpebræ, the sides
of the nares, and even those of the throat,* have grown together.

All kinds of small-pox leave behind them a predisposition to
inflammatory complaints, particularly to rheumatism, ophthalmia
and visceral inflammations. On this part of the subject.the reader may consult the 582d and following pages of the fifth vol. of
Haller's Disput. ad Hist. et Cur. Morh. Pertinentes, and the third
vol. of Frank's Epitome de Curand. Hom. Morb.

SECT. II.

Of the Causes of the Small-pox.

THIS is one of the diseases which have only made their appearance in Europe in modern times. There is no mention in
the writings of the Greek or Roman physicians of any disease
which can be supposed to have been the small-pox ; and we are
unable to determine how long this disease has been known in
other parts of the world, or where it first made its appearance.

The Arabian writers are the earliest we are acquainted with,
who mention it. Both Rhazes and Avicenna treat of the small-
pox. Of these, Rhazes is the oldest. The oldest writer on the
small-pox mentioned by Rhazes [Aahron] resided at Alexandria
when it was besieged by the Saracens in 640 of the Christian
æra. There is no distinct mention of the small-pox earlier than
this.

The most prevalent opinion is that it was brought to Alexandria from the East, having been known in many parts of Asia,
particularly in China, from much earlier times. Many circumstances however tend to contradict this opinion. There is reason
to believe that it raged among the Abysinians, when they besieged Mecca in the year 569 ;† from whence it probably travelled
into Egypt with the Mahometans, spread with them along the
northern parts of Africa, and accompanied them when they passed over into Europe.‡

The opinion that the small-pox was first brought into Europe
by the crusaders is unfounded, as Dr. Woodville has met with it,
under the name Variolæ, in manuscripts of the Harlean and

* See Vogel De Cog. et Curand. Morb.
† See Dr. Woodville's History of Inoculation.
‡ See Friend's History of Medicine from the days of Galen, to the be-
ginning of the 16th century.

Cottonian Collections in the British Museum, which bear evidence of having been written before the year 900. There can be little doubt however, that by means of the crusaders the small-pox was more generally disseminated throughout Europe.* It is mentioned by British writers as early as the 13th century, but at what time it was introduced into this island is not known. In America it was unknown till carried thither by the Europeans.

This imperfect history of the small-pox, although there were no other facts on the subject, is sufficient to prove, that it arises from a peculiar contagion, the presence of which, or of the concurrence of causes which first gave it birth, is necessary for the production of the disease.

An opinion has prevailed indeed respecting the small-pox, as well as most other contagious diseases, that besides the presence of the contagion, a certain state of the air, which authors term an epidemic constitution of the atmosphere, is necessary to render the complaint prevalent ; an hypothesis, once maintained by the best writers, but now so obsolete as hardly to deserve discussion ; which I had occasion to consider when speaking of contagion. The only fact which tends to support the opinion is, that the small-pox and other contagious diseases often cease to rage while there is reason to believe clothes, furniture, &c. to be still impregnated with the contagion, and while many still remain capable of receiving the disease. Why this should happen it is impossible to say in the present state of knowledge ; if we are however to frame an hypothesis to explain it, it must be one more consistent with other facts than the theory of the epidemic constitution of the atmosphere.

The fatality of the small-pox soon led to the employment of a variety of means with a view to obviate its effects. It is computed that one of six dies who receive the small-pox in the natural way, and that about the eighth part, and in some places many more, of the people of a country where the casual small-pox is prevalent, fall a sacrifice to the disease. " The celebrated M. " De La Condamine computes that in France one in ten of all who " are born dies of the small-pox. Dr. Rosenstein, who wrote an " excellent Treatise on the Diseases of Children, shews, that " every tenth boy and every ninth girl dies of it in Sweden, according to the accurate reports of the commissioners appointed " to make the inquiry. In London, the births are to the deaths " by the small-pox, as six and a fourth to one ; in Manchester, as " six and a half to one ; in Liverpool, as five and a half to one ; " in Chester, as six and two thirds to one."†

* In some of the northern parts of Europe, which have little intercourse with the rest, the small pox was not known, it is said, before the beginning of the present century.

† See the Introduction to Dr. Haygarth's Sketch of a Plan to exterminate the casual Small-pox, &c.

At certain times the Small-pox proves much more fatal. Of thirty-seven ill of the worst kind of small-pox, attended by Baron Dimsdale while in Russia, thirty-five died.

One of the most evident and earliest means adopted to moderate the fatality of small-pox, was removing the sick from all intercourse with the healthy. A convenient place was appointed for the reception of the former, who were not again admitted into society till they had been well for some time.* In the Highlands of Scotland, when a child is seized with a very mild kind of small-pox, those in the neighbourhood expose their children to be infected by it. We now know, that the nature of the small-pox depends less than might a priori be expected on its being received from the mild or confluent forms of the disease, so that little advantage can accrue from the practice.

They practice another method however, which must be attended with better success. Worsted threads wet with matter are tied round the wrists, by which the disease is frequently induced. Dr. Rush observes indeed, that he could not induce the small-pox by rubbing the matter on the entire skin, from which it is probable, that the practice of the Highlanders only proves sucessful when the wet worsted threads produce a degree of excoriation. Such is the rudest mode of inoculation, the most effectual of all the means which have been devised for preventing the mortality of the small-pox.

The prejudice against inoculation among the lower ranks has hitherto in a great measure prevented the beneficial effects which it is calculated to produce ; for the inoculation of a single child often infects a whole neighbourhood ; so that it is alleged, and in many places even appears from the bills of mortality, that upon the whole the deaths by this disorder have rather been increased than diminished since the introduction of inoculation.

This has induced some to propose rejecting the operation, and endeavouring entirely to prevent the disorder, by the means employed for checking the progress of contagious diseases. This plan however promises but little. It is impossible that such a disease as the small-pox can be entirely eradicated from so immense and populous a country as Europe ; and who would propose to banish it from this island while it raged on the Continent, with which we every day have the freest intercourse? nay, were it

---

* The Calmucks, who first received this disease from the Russians, have the practice of carrying those seized with it into the woods and leaving them in huts with some provisions. Those who survive are not permitted to have intercourse with the other inhabitants, till they have been washed, and have remained well for a considerable length of time. The Hottentots, who it is said first received the disease from some Dutch sailors, set guards around the place where it appears, and every person who attempts to escape is immediately shot.

even possible at once to extirpate it from Europe, would it not be immediately received from the Asiatics? Intercourse among nations is now more frequent than in ancient times. It would be impossible to exclude so infectious a disease from Europe, if it raged on the coasts of the Levant and other western parts of Asia. Unless therefore we can extirpate the disease, from the whole world, plans of extirpation are vain.

It is urged indeed that the plague has been banished from most countries of Europe, and that were the proper means employed, we might in like manner banish the small-pox.* But can the circumstances of the two complaints be compared? Was the plague ever so general throughout Europe as the small-pox? The former is confined to a few spots. The whole world know when it shews itself, and avoid communication with the places where it rages. It visits chiefly large and populous cities, and is for the most part effectually banished by the removal of crowded and dirty streets, and by having a cautious intercourse with the few places which it still visits, and from which, were the proper means employed, it is more than probable it might also be banished.

Others assert, that it is better to suffer the returns of the small-pox, such as it appeared before the introduction of inoculation, than thus constantly to preserve it amongst us. To this it may be answered, that admitting that the deaths by the small-pox have not been lessened by the introduction of inoculation, it is evident that this is owing to the operation not being sufficiently general.

What have been the effects of inoculation, under proper regulations? At Chester it is found, that the mean number of deaths by the small-pox are 14 annually. Before the institution of a society there for promoting inoculation, the mean number of deaths were 63 annually. It is probable indeed that the time is not very distant, when, in many places at least, inoculation will be general, and then comparatively the small-pox will hardly deserve the name of a disease; for by a moderate computation, of those who have been inoculated while in health, properly treated, and in whom no other complaint supervened, not above one in 150 died.† According indeed to many, particularly late, observations, the proportion of deaths is much less. It has been computed that at Chester only one in 208 died of the inoculated small-pox. Of 416 patients inoculated at Liverpool, one only died. In the

* See Vogel's Prælect, Acad. De Cog. et Cur. Morh.

† See the accounts of Drs. Jurin, Monro, and Dimsdale. Dr. Monro's Treatise in particular deserves attention. It contains an answer to certain questions put to him by the delegates of the faculty of medicine at Paris, concerning the inoculation of small-pox. It is entitled an Account of the Inoculation of Small-Pox in Scotland, by Alexander Monro senior.

London Small-pox and Inoculation Hospital, of the last 5000, only one in 600 died of the inoculated small-pox.*

Reflecting on these circumstances, instead of endeavouring to eradicate the small-pox,† it should be the aim of physicians to render inoculation and the proper treatment as general as possible. They will thus most effectually check the fatality which has hitherto attended this disease. It is of great consequence therefore to be well acquainted with the practice of inoculation.

The circumstances respecting inoculation which demand attention may be arranged under three heads.

1. The choice of proper matter, and the mode of performing the operation. Inoculation should be made as effectual and at the same time as easy for the patient as possible. When the operation is more severe than necessary, we deter people from submitting their children to it. When done carelessly and too slightly, it often fails of producing the disease, which both puts the patient to unnecessary trouble and destroys his confidence in the operator.

2. The state of the patient at the time he is inoculated, and his treatment before and after the operation till the commencement of the eruptive fever. They must be such as afford the best chance of the complaint appearing in the mildest form.

3. Cautions to prevent the introduction of the casual small-pox.

In the first place, of the operation, and the choice of proper matter.

The mode of performing the operation at present generally adopted is extremely simple. A pustule is opened, and the point of a lancet dipped in the matter. This may either be used immediately when received from the pustule, or it may be allowed to dry, and when about to be used, moistened with warm water.

The matter may be kept for a number of years without losing its power. It is the custom in some parts of the East to keep it for a great length of time, where inoculators often boast of using matter collected by their grand-fathers. Nor does it seem necessary to be particularly careful in defending it from the air. Some experiments have been made to determine whether or not exposure to the air is capable of so altering the properties of variolous matter, as to prevent its producing the disease. " It has not been

* See Dr. Woodville's reports respecting the inoculation of the Variolæ Vaccinæ.

† See the observations on the Cow-Pox at the end of this section.

" in my power," Dr. Currie observes in Dr. Haygarth's Sketch
of a Plan to exterminate the casual Small-Pox, " to attend to the
" experiments you suggested, but I have tried whether variolous
" matter exposed to the air, and indeed to the wind, for thirty
" days, can communicate the disease by inoculation, and the re-
" sult has been as I expected ; the disease was communicated
" with the usual certainty and success.   I inoculated three pa-
" tients at the same time ; in one the eruptive fever appeared on
" the fifth day ; in another on the seventh ; and in the third on
" the ninth....My opinion is, that I shall be able to inoculate with
" the same matter, diluted in the same way, many months or
" perhaps years hence.   The reason why variolous matter long
" kept has sometimes failed in producing the disease, I apprehend
" to have been that the dried matter was not previously reduced
" to a state of fluidity."   Many practitioners however prefer recent fluid matter.*   It appears from some trials, that matter
which has been long kept may produce inflammation and general derangement of the system, and yet fail in producing the
small-pox.

  The point of the lancet armed with the matter is introduced
obliquely beneath the cuticle, so as to wound very slightly, and
occasion little or no flow of blood.†   In withdrawing the point of
the lancet, it is proper to press the wound with the finger, that
the parts in contact with the matter may wipe it off the lancet,
and thus secure the success of the operation.   The wound is so
slight that bandages, or plasters of any kind are unnecessary.

  Such is at present the most approved and simple mode of performing inoculation.   Others have been practised, which put
the patient to much uneasiness without answering the purpose
any better.‡   Some do not introduce the lancet, but only scratch
the skin ; and Mr. Mudge has proposed a method, which he
thinks succeeds with more certainty than that generally in use,
namely scratching the skin, and rubbing it with a bit of spunge
which has absorbed some variolous matter.‖   With this part of
the subject, which rather comes under the province of surgery, I
shall not detain the reader.

  Although it belongs to surgeons to settle all disputes concerning the best modes of performing operations, in some circum-

  * See the observations of Baron Dimsdale and others.

  † It is of consequence to guard against a considerable flow of blood, as
this often washes out the matter, and thus prevents the success of the
operation.

  ‡ See an account of the old modes of inoculating by large incisions, and
by vesication, in Dr. Kirkpatrick's Analysis of Inoculation.

  ‖ The reader will find an account of this method, and the instrument
with which he performs the operation, in his Treatise on the Inoculation
of Small-Pox.

stances it is the physician's part to determine when it is proper to recommend them. It is therefore necessary for him to be acquainted with what has been determined respecting the preference to be given to particular kinds of matter, that he may not find himself at a loss when all kinds, or only one kind, of matter can be procured.

Many prefer the matter in a crude state, that is, before it assumes the purulent appearance ; and the success which attended the practice of Sutton, a celebrated inoculator in Essex, was by some ascribed to his using the matter in a crude state.* Dr. Dimsdale preferred the matter taken from the inoculated part during the eruptive fever; and some inoculators prefer it at a still earlier period, supposing that the more crude the matter is, it will produce the disease with the greater certainty.† From the following experiment however it would appear, that matter in a very crude state will sometimes fail to produce the disease.— " Messrs. Langworthy and Arscot, surgeons at Plimpton, in the " spring of 1776, inoculated forty patients, of which number thir- " ty were inoculated with crude matter from the arm of a young " woman, five days after she herself had been inoculated with " concocted matter, which produced in her pretty smart fever, " and a sufficient number of pustules ; the other ten were ino- " culated with matter of another kind, which I procured in " a concocted form from a pustule of the natural small-pox. " The arms of all the forty patients took the infection, and the " latter ten, after the eruptive fever, had the small-pox in the " usual way." Of the other thirty, though the infection took " place on their arms, so as to inflame them considerably, and to " produce a very large prominent pustule with matter in it on each " of them ; yet not one had any eruptive fever, or a single subse- " quent pustule on any part of the body ; but about the eighth, in " some the ninth, and in others the tenth, day, the inflammation " began to disappear ; and about the twelfth or thirteenth, the " pustules on their arms scabbed off. It is to be remarked too, " that the matter which was in those pustules, having been used " to inoculate others, produced on them exactly the same appear- " ances, unattended also with either fever or small-pox."

" It was thought worth while to inoculate all those patients " with well concocted matter, in order to see whether or not the " effects of the crude matter had so altered their constitutions as " to render them incapable of afterwards having the small-pox. " The whole were inoculated with well-formed matter, and all of " them had the small-pox in the common form."

In the malignant kinds of small-pox the matter always has a

---

* See Mr. Chandler's Treatise on Inoculation.

† A surgeon informed me, he had known the crude matter succeed where the maturated had failed to produce the disease.

crude appearance. It is found however as certainly to produce
the disease as the matter of the most benign; and, what is remarkable, generally at least, produces it in as mild a form; the
mildness or malignity of the small-pox seeming, little if at, all to
depend on the state of the inoculating matter. From the worst
kinds of matter, the most favourable forms of the disease have been
produced, and from the best matter, the most malignant. The
choice of what is termed good matter, therefore, is not of such
consequence as at first sight it may appear. Even the daring experiment of inoculating with matter taken from a dead body,*
has been practised with safety.

I But although we were better convinced than we are of the
safety of inoculating with bad matter, yet the general prejudice
against it would make a prudent practitioner choose that of a benign kind. Where this cannot be procured, and the patient is evidently in danger of the casual small-pox, we should not hesitate a
moment in recommending inoculation from any kind of matter
that can be procured.

Nor does the quantity of matter introduced seem to have much,
if any, effect in determining the mildness or severity of the disease; an hypothesis on which some attempt to explain the benefit derived from inoculation; the disease, as has been observed
a thousand times, proving equally benign or otherwise whether
a larger or smaller quantity be introduced. Some practitioners
indeed, Burserius, Dr. Fordyce, and others maintain an opposite opinion, and consider the quanty of matter employed in inoculation a point of much consequence. Burserius observes, that
those inoculated by many incisions have the disease in a worse
form than those who have it from 'one' incision. And Dr. Underwood in his Treatise on the Diseases of Children says, he has
observed that when several inoculations have failed, in which
case we may also suppose a greater than usual quantity of variolous matter introduced, the disease proves more severe than in
other cases.

How far such observations are accurate, it is difficult to say.
It is certain that different modes of inoculation have been practised, in which very different quantities of matter were introduced,
and all have produced an equally benign form of the disease.
" In the case of small-pox," Dr. Cullen observes, " a considera-
" ble difference in the quantity of contagious matter introduced
" has not discovered any effect in modifying the disease."

* See an Essay by Mr. Chandler. Mr. Keate also inoculated with
matter from a dead body, but from an accident no inference respecting
its safety can be drawn from his experiment. See Dr. Pearson's observations in the 19th volume of the Medical Commentaries.

† Many experienced practitioners maintain that the choice of good
matter, though not of such importance as once supposed, has some effect in insuring the mildness of the disease.

When inoculation fails in producing the disease, the inoculated part nevertheless sometimes inflames and suppurates, as in cases where the disease is about to follow; and it is remarkable that the matter produced in such cases is as fit for inoculation, as that taken from a person actually labouring under the disease. It has even been found, that if a person, who has already had the small-pox, be inoculated and the wound suppurates, the matter it produces is capable of giving the disease.†

Although it sometimes happens, that in those who have not had the small-pox the inoculated part inflames and suppurates without producing the disease, yet this is comparatively rare. When the part inflames and small pustules are seen surrounding the incision, we may, with great certainty, expect the disease.

A considerable and early inflammation in the part inoculated is favourable; paleness and flaccidity the reverse; and Dr. Dimsdale even observes, that he has found some degree of stiffness and pain in the axilla to foretel a favourable disease.

The matter of small-pox must be applied to a wound in order to induce the complaint. It was observed above, that Dr. Rush could not induce the small-pox by rubbing the matter on the entire skin; and Dr. Cowel, the same author informs us, gave a negro girl some variolous matter mixed with a dose of physic which produced no sensible effect.

2. Of the state of body in which inoculation has proved most successful; and the treatment of the patient before and after the operation, till the appearance of the eruptive fever.

It has always been considered one of the chief advantages of inoculation, that by means of it we are enabled to induce the small-pox at a proper age, at a time when the patient is not labouring under any other disease, and after the body has been prepared for receiving it in the mildest form. The subject therefore divides itself into two parts: the state of the person about to be inoculated with respect to age and habit; and the preparation necessary, by exercise, diet, or medicines, before and after the operation.

As the view of inoculation is to prevent the casual small-pox, it should be performed early in life. But the tender constitution of infants, for some time after birth, renders the slightest complaints dangerous. Many have therefore laid it down as a rule, that children ought not to be inoculated under two years of age. Very

* Mr. Davidson, in the third volume of the Medical Transactions, mentions two instances of children in whom the disease did not appear till after the second inoculation, the first inoculation only producing inflammation and suppuration of the part; from which however matter was taken that produced all the usual symptoms of small-pox.

† This, we are informed by Dr. Rush, Dr. Way ascertained by an experiment made on himself.

young children sometimes in the inoculated, much more frequently in the casual, small-pox, are carried off by epileptic fits.
It is chiefly on this account that most practitioners make it a rule
to delay inoculation, at least till the first dentition is over. Another reason for delaying inoculation till children are taken from
the breast, is the injury done in this disease by external warmth.
Dr. Underwood remarks, that when the mother suckled only
with one breast, he has observed the side of the child which lay
next her loaded with pustules.

Delaying inoculation however for so long a time as two years
is often attended with considerable risque, and it is now generally
admitted, that when the patient is in danger of the casual small-
pox, inoculation may be recommended at a much earlier period.
Dr. Dimsdale observes, that although he is still of opinion that
inoculation under two years of age is objectionable, yet he has
nevertheless had repeated occasion to inoculate many under that
age without a single instance of any fatal consequence. The
reader will find in the proceedings of the society of Chester for
promoting inoculation, and in other publications, that children
have been inoculated within the first month with the best effects.
When we are at liberty however to choose the period for inoculation, it is certainly proper that the constitution should have acquired some degree of strength, before we induce any disease
however mild.

Dr. Fordyce says, that of children he has known die of the
small-pox, more than two-thirds were under nine months. He
therefore considers it improper to inoculate before this period.
When the child runs no risque of the casual small-pox, it may be
proper to delay it even longer. Dr. Percival thinks the best age
for inducing the small-pox is between two and four in stout healthy
children, and between three and six in delicate children.

There is perhaps no period of life but that of infancy in which
inoculation may not be performed with safety. It is a general
opinion that the small-pox is frequently severe in those advanced
in life. Boerhaave observes, that the more age has dissipated the
fluids and condensed the solids, the more violent is this disease;
on this account, he adds, it proves favourable in children, women,
and others of a lax habit of body, and the reverse to persons hardened by labour, to men, and old people.

By others however the justness of the observation has been
called in question, and it is asserted that the small-pox is least severe in young and old people, and most so in those in the vigour
of life; and from tables in the second volume of Dr. Percival's
Essays, it appears, that the small-pox, in the instances which he
gives, was more fatal to females than males. Some imagine that
the age of puberty is particularly unfavourable for inoculation.

Whatever the time of life be, we should if possible avoid inoculating those labouring under other diseases. Dentition, especially if attended with troublesome symptoms, is a sufficient reason to delay inoculation, when it can be delayed with safety.

Children with large heads, particularly those who have been threatened with water in the head, generally have the small-pox in a dangerous form, and are consequently bad subjects for inoculation. Dr. Dimsdale mentions two cases of this kind, in which, although the eruption was favourable, coma supervened and both patients died. A similar accident happened under the management of Mr. Charles Maitland, on the introduction of inoculation into Scotland, which procured the operation a very bad reception in that part of the island. In short, inoculation should be performed while the subject is in all respects in good health.

There are some diseases however which shew little or no tendency to increase the severity of the small-pox. A tendency to scrophula, or even its presence, is not found to increase the danger of the small-pox. Dr. Heberden, in Dr. Kirkpatrick's Analysis of Inoculation, mentions the case of a boy dying of scrophula, who had the small-pox in a very mild form. Dr. Cullen remarks, that several diseases of the skin are equally innocent when complicated with small-pox; and justly observes, "They are the diseases " of the febrile kind, or those ready to induce or aggravate a febrile " state, that especially give the concurrence that is most dangerous " with the small-pox." Dr. Dimsdale did not wish to inoculate those labouring under any acute disease, or much debility, and he avoided inoculation when any epidemic prevailed.

It may be observed upon the whole however, that the habits of body in which the small-pox is most apt to prove unfavourable are far from being thoroughly ascertained. The sum of all that we know with certainty seems to be, that the disease is apt to be severe in the debilitated, the plethoric, and those labouring under febrile diseases. In some families it is particularly unfavourable, instances of which I know, where it is impossible to detect the cause of this peculiarity.

Pregnant women are bad subjects for inoculation, for although the disease generally appears in them in as mild a form as in others, it is apt to be followed by miscarriage. This may sometimes be owing to the foetus receiving the disease from the mother, of which there are many well-authenticated instances; and it has sometimes happened, that where the mother had but a very few pustules, the child has been found almost covered with them. When the mother is near her time before she is seized with the small-pox, as in a case mentioned in the 13th volume of the Medical Commentaries, the eruptive fever sometimes appears in the child a day or two after birth. The reader will find cases supporting these observations in the 19th volume of the Medical Commentaries, in the 155th and following pages of the 2d volume of Burserius's Institut. Med. Pract. and other works on this disease. Burserius mentions cases from different authors, in which the fœtus had the disease, from the mother being exposed to its contagion, although, it did not produce the small-pox in her; Vogel also observes, that the fœtus may be infected with the small-pox without the mother having it; so that there may be some danger in pregnant women exposing themselves to the contagion of small-pox, although they have had the disease. It is almost unnecessary to observe, that the patient is as secure from a second attack of the disease by having it before, as he is by having it after, birth.

Dr. Pearson says, that inoculating about the sixth month of pregnancy is seldom fatal to the mother, but often kills the fœtus. In about twenty cases of the casual small-pox in the last months of pregnancy, it proved fatal to above three-fourths of the women, and a still larger proportion of the fœtuses.

The occurrence of the menses during the small-pox has been regarded as dangerous, but many observations, as Camper* observes, prove this opinion to be unfounded. A difficult or very profuse menstruation is certainly unfavourable.

Some constitutions are incapable of having the disease in any form. It is even said that there is a whole family at Geneva† who are incapable of having the small-pox.

Others do not receive the disease at one time, however freely exposed to its contagion, even though repeatedly inoculated, and yet afterwards receive it merely perhaps from approaching those labouring under it. " I know an old nurse," Dr. Huxham‡ observes, " and one apothecary, who for many years attended per-" sons and a great number too in the small-pox, and yet never had " them; nay many that have industriously endeavored to catch " the infection by frequenting the chambers of the sick, have done " it without effect, and yet some of these persons some months or " years after have been seized with the small-pox." It has been computed that only one of 38 escape the small-pox when properly inoculated or otherwise fairly exposed to the contagion.

It has long been a prevalent opinion that a certain regimen previous to inoculation and even medicines are indispensible.

The person to be inoculated is put on a spare diet, desired to use regular exercise, and to take various medicines, generally mercurial or antimonial, for some days before the operation, and

* See a Treatise by Camper, entitled, Les Avantages de l'Inoculation, et la meillure Methode de l'administrer.

† See Dr. Haygarth's Sketch, &c.

‡ See Huxham's Treatise en Pevers, Small-Pox, and Peripneumony.

till the commencement of the eruptive fever. That these precautions by their antiphlogistic tendency are sometimes of use,
and that it may be proper to delay feeding children with animal
food till after they have had the small-pox, as Dr. Cullen recommends, we have every reason to believe. Many are of opinion
however that when the patient is in perfect health, and when the
only tendency of a change in diet and a course of medicines is
that of inducing a state in some measure different from health,
they are not only useless, but hurtful. " Gatti," Dr. Baker*
observes, " who was sometime ago much employed in inocula-
" tion at Paris, declares himself an enemy to any general plan
" of preparation. In all the Levant," he continues, " where
" the natural small-pox is as fatal as elsewhere, and where, you
" may find old women who have inoculated 10,000 without an
" accident, the only inquiry is, whether or not a person is pre-
" pared by nature. All that is considered is, whether the breath
" be sweet, the skin soft, and whether a little wound in it heals
" easily."

It is improper however in all cases to neglect every means of
preparation. In full habits the eruptive fever often runs high,
although this consequence is not so certain as some have supposed it. The reader will find cases, (a very striking one is
related by Mr. Mudge) in which patients of the most plethoric
habit paid no attention whatever to regimen, either before or
after inoculation, and yet had the disease in a very mild form.
He will even find in Dr. Percival's Essays, that the bark, so
generally allowed to increase the inflammatory diathesis, has
been given, between inoculation and the eruptive fever, to remove an intermittent, without any bad consequences. From a
few facts however no general conclusion can be drawn. We
should endeavour to observe a proper medium, neither reducing
the strength by unseasonable evacuations, nor inducing the disease on the plethoric, without using precautions to moderate the
ensuing fever.

The preparation recommended by Dr. Rush* can never prove
hurtful. It consists merely in the use of mild cathartics and a
vegetable diet. He reprobates the use of mercurials, to which
he attributes the glandular swellings, loss of teeth, and weak
habit, which often succeed the small-pox.

We are led to believe however, from a great variety of observations, that a prudent use of antimonial and mercurial preparations, previous to inoculation, tends to insure the mildness of the
disease. For a proof of this the reader may consult Dr. Gale's
Dissertation on the Inoculation of Small-Pox in America, Dr.
Andrews's Treatise entitled The Practice of Inoculation impar-

* See Dr. now Sir George Baker's Treatise on the Inoculation of
Small-Pox.

† See his Medical Inquiries and Observations.

tially considered, &c. Dr. Baker's Account of the Suttonian Mode of Inoculation, Mr. Chandler's Treatise on the same subject, and Baron Dimsdale's Treatise entitled The present Mode of Inoculating the Small-Pox.

The following was the mode of preparation which Dr. Dimsdale thought most successful. If the patient was debilitated, he endeavoured to restore the strength; if plethoric, to correct this habit He made it a rule to clear the stomach and intestines, and generally confined the patient to a milk and vegetable diet for nine days before inoculation, during which he purged with Glauber's salt; the night before each purge he gave a dose of calomel, and a small quantity of tartar emetic. The exhibition of the powder and cathartic was generally repeated three times, but the treatment was varied according to the state of the patient. After inoculation, when the inoculated part remained pale, which gave reason to dread a severe disease, he gave the mercurial and antimonial powder every night; and, if it did not prove cathartic, joined with it Glauber's salt or an infusion of senna with manna and tincture of jalap.

It is to be recollected, that the habit of body may be considerably affected by particular states of the weather: that in which rheumatic and other inflammatory diseases are epidemic, and that in which complaints of a contrary tendency, malignant fevers, &c. prevail. In the one case, evacuations will be more frequently serviceable; in the other, more generally pernicious.

In choosing the season for inoculation, the spring is generally preferred, in order to avoid the extremes of heat and cold, and because the epidemic small-pox is generally mildest in this season. It is also observed, that the casual small-pox is milder about the vernal equinox, than when it appears earlier.* Dr. Dimsdale, although he preferred the spring, thought there was little objection to inoculating either in summer or winter, provided the patient was protected from the extremes of heat† and cold. The autumn he thought the most exceptionable, on account of the putrid small-pox being most common at this season. Attention to the time of year however, provided there be no malignant epidemic raging, is not of much consequence, since the inoculated small-pox, with proper treatment, is a mild disease at all seasons.

Situation seems often to have more effect in modifying the small-pox. At a distance from large towns it is less apt to appear of the putrid and anomalous kinds, and the more crowded and dirty a city is, the more apt the small-pox is to prove unfavoura-

* See the 5th vol. of Medical Observations and Inquiries.

† Dr. Cleghorn remarks, that he has observed the virulence of the small-pox increase with the heat of the weather.

ble. Dr. Walker* ascribes the unusual severity of the small-pox in the city of Cork to the following circumstances. " In the city " of Cork, from its situation upon the edge of the great Atlantic " Ocean, the winds three parts of the year blow from west and " south west, and drench the inhabitants in the warm and watery " vapours detached from the surface of that wide extended sea. " The city is situated in a deep valley, built on islands, and sur- " rounded by branches of the river Lee. There are considerable " marshes to the east and west of it. Quantities of animal offals " occupy the streets, and particularly the close confined alleys " and lanes. At the season endemical diseases rage most, there " are a great number of slaughter-houses in the north and south " suburbs ; vast pits containing putrifying blood and ordure, " which even corrupt the northern blasts which blow down upon " the city ; vast quantities of animal offals used by the common " people in the slaughtering seasons, rendered more pernicious " by the quick transition from diet of another kind and different " nature."†

We cannot doubt that inoculation, by enabling us to induce the small-pox at a time when the state of body is most favourable, is alone a matter of considerable importance ; yet we cannot agree with those who, believing that all the advantages of inocula- tion may be attributed to this, subscribe to the opinion of Dr. Huxam when he observes, " I am persuaded if persons regular- " ly prepared were to receive the variolus contagion in the natu- " ral way far the greater part would have them in a mild man- " ner."

It appears, from a variety of facts, that the advantages of inoc- ulation are owing neither to the preparation of the patient, nor any other circumstance which we can detect, but to some pecu- liar disposition in the animal economy, which will ever perhaps re- main a secret ; for what has been said of the casual small-pox be- ing received by the lungs, and on this account proving more dan- gerous, is merely hypothetical.‡ The other opinions on the sub- ject rest, if possible, on a still worse foundation. It appears, from what was said above, that none of the advantages of in- oculation is to be ascribed to the quantity or quality of the matter employed, as some have thought ; and with regard to the opinion of the body being peculiarly disposed to the disease when the small-pox is taken in the natural way, and the poison on this ac- count operating more violently, a moment's reflection shews its invalidity, since very few who have not had the complaint will at

* See his Treatise on the Small-Pox.
† The malignant small-pox is frequently observed to precede the plague. See Haller's Disput. ad Hist. et Cur. Mob. Pert. vol. v. p. 557.

‡ This opinion seems to receive some support from the practice of the Chinese, who inoculate by putting the dry scales of the small-pox into the nose, and among whom the disease is far from being favourable.

any time escape it if freely exposed to its contagion. It is un, necessary even to recapitulate the different opinions on this subject. The reader will find another, though not a mo,e success-ful attempt, in the 2d vol. of the Collect. Soc. Hafn. Obs. 9th,

With respect to the treatment of the patient after the operation till the commencement of the eruptive fever, it is similar to the treatment previous to the operation, and may easily be collect-ed from what has been said. Animal food and fermented liquors should be avoided, unless there is much debility. Cold, fatigue, and every other cause of fever is highly pernicious. Gentle lax-atives are to be continued as the state of the body requires, which should be open; and the continued exhibition of small doses of mercurials and antimonials tends to ensure the mildness of the dis-ease, although they are certainly far from being necessary in the generality of cases. Where there is any thing unfavourable, such as a plethoric habit, an unusual deficiency of inflammation in the inoculated part, &c. they ought never to be neglected.

Dr. Dimsdale believed the excellence of the Suttonian mode of inoculation to consist in the three following circumstances: the last of which we shall presently have occasion to consider at length. 1. The preparation by antimonials and mercurials. 2. Inoculat-ing with recent fluid matter. 3. The free exposure to cold and the laxative course in the eruptive fever.

The most important part of the subject remains to be consi-dered.

3. The cautions to be employed in the practice of inoculation, have been too much neglected; to which alone. we owe the me-lancholy reflection, that the fatality of the small-pox has hitherto been little, if at all, diminished by the introduction of inoculation into Britain.

When any one is about to be inoculated, where the small-pox is not already prevalent, all who are accustomed to come to the house, or live near it, should be made acquainted with it, that those who have not had the disease may either be inoculated, or avoid intercourse with the patient and his attendants. It is the duty of the inoculator to insist on this alternative, and to offer inoculation gratis to the poor.

Various plans have been proposed with a view wholly to banish the casual small-pox. Dr. Dimsdale inoculated all the inhabit-ants of a village who had not had the small-pox in one day, having previously removed those who from bad health, or other causes,* were improper subjects for inoculation. And when this can be done, he thinks it should be repeated every five or six years.

This plan however is but ill calculated to banish the casual

* See what has been said respecting the habit, age, &c. proper for inoculation.

small-pox. It would be impossible to secure the inhabitants against its introduction during the intervals of inoculation.

No writer has bestowed so much attention on this subject as Dr. Haygarth.* The following are his regulations for preventing the casual small-pox ; and from his own observations as well as those of his correspondents, there is reason to believe, that could they be enforced, they would be found sufficient for the purpose. It is the opinion of Dr. Haygarth, and most of his correspondents, that clothes, furniture, &c. cannot imbibe the contagion of small-pox from an infected atmosphere, and therefore only communicate the disease when the matter adheres to them. Should future experience contradict this opinion, some addition to the following precautions will be necessary. There is also reason to hope, on the other hand, that experience may prove some of them to be superfluous ; if this should not be the case, it is to be feared that they are too various and troublesome to be generally adopted.

" 1. Suffer no person who has not had the small-pox to come into
" the infectious house. No visitor, who has any communication
" with persons liable to the distemper, should touch or sit down
" on any thing infectious.

" 2. No patient after the pox have appeared† must be suffered
" to go into the street or other frequented place. Fresh air must
" be constantly admitted by doors and windows into the sick
" chamber.

" 3. The utmost attention to cleanliness is absolutely necessa-
" ry : during and after the distemper, no person, clothes, food,
" furniture, dog, cat, money, medicines, or any other thing that
" is known or suspected to be bedaubed with matter, spittle, or
" other infectious discharges of the patient, should go, or be car-
" ried, out of the house till they be washed, and till they be suffi-
" ciently exposed to the fresh air. No foul linen or any thing
" else that can retain the poison should be folded up, or put into
" drawers, boxes, or be otherwise shut up from the air, but must
" be immediately thrown into water and kept there till washed.
" No attendants should touch what is to go into another family
" till their hands are washed. When a patient dies of the small-
" pox, particular care should be taken that nothing infectious be
" taken out of the house, so as to do mischief.

" 4. The patient must not be allowed to approach any person
" liable to the distemper till every scab has dropped off; till all
" the clothes, furniture, food, and all other things touched by the
" patient during the distemper, till the floor of the sick chamber,

* See his Treatise, entitled A Sketch of a Plan to exterminate the casual Small-Pox from Great-Britain, &c.

† Should it not be, after the appearance of the eruptive fever, since the disease is infectious from its commencement?

" and till the hair, face, and hands, have been carefully washed.
" After every thing has been made perfectly clean, the doors,
" windows, drawers, boxes, and all other places that can retain in-
" fectious air, should be kept open, till it be cleared out of the
" house."

When the casual small-pox has actually appeared, then the various means for checking the progress of contagious diseases,
enumerated when speaking of typhus, must be had recourse to.
The separation of the sick from the healthy is particularly to be
attended to, for which purpose a proper place* should be appointed at a small distance from towns for the reception of the poor,
who are seized with the disease. Care should be taken to bury
the dead privately, and to use proper means to free from the contagion those who recover before they are permitted to return to
their houses.

Many have placed confidence in some of the medicines mentioned when speaking of the means of checking contagious diseases, for defending against the contagion of small-pox. Mercury
and musk have been particularly recommended, but nothing of
this kind is to be depended on. The various means belonging
to this head are to be regarded as less efficacious in defending
against the contagion of small-pox, than that of typhus. General
inoculation will be found the best means of preventing the spreading of the small-pox. It would be fortunate if we could discover as
easy and effectual a method of cutting short the progress of other
malignant fevers. By taking care that none should be exposed to
its contagion but those who have had the disease or submitted to
inoculation,† we place an almost insuperable barrier to the pro-
ress of the small-pox ;‡ nor is it necessary that those who have

* There should be a permanent building for this purpose in the neighbourhood of every considerable town, without which it is almost impossible
to prevent the casual small-pox among the lower ranks, on account of
their refusing to have their children inoculated.

† A proposal has lately been made in Scotland to render inoculation
general, by publishing a set of simple regulations respecting inoculation,
and the treatment of inoculated small-pox, and endeavouring, with the
assistance of the clergy, to induce parents to inoculate their own children.
The inoculated small-pox is generally so mild a disease, and the proper
mode of treatment in it so simple, that the danger of constantly introducing
the casual small-pox appears to be the principal objection to this plan.
If the cow-pox, a disease we shall presently have occasion to consider
more particularly, be found, as we have reason at present to believe, capable of securing the constitution against the attack of small-pox, there
will not be the same objection against inoculating for it in this way, as it is
not contagious. It is even a milder disease than the inoculated small-pox.

‡ Well authenticated cases indeed are on record of the small-pox having attacked the same person a second time or oftener ; such cases however are rare. There are instances in Burserius's Inst. Med. Pract. at-
tested by the best authority, of the small-pox having appeared a second
or even a third time in the same person. In the 2d vol. of the Collect. Soc.

not had the disease should remain at a considerable distance from the infected; it is sufficient that they remain at the distance of a few feet, and be careful not to touch any thing which has been in contact with the sick, or is besmeared with any secretion from their bodies.

. It, is even the opinion of some, that the contagion of small-pox cannot be applied through the medium of the air, and although it appears from a variety of facts that this opinion is erroneous, it is certain that it is very rarely conveyed by the air to the distance once supposed. The reader will find sufficient proofs of this in the experiments of Dr. Ryan.*

¶ The small-pox, contrary to an opinion once prevalant, is infectious from the first attack of the eruptive fever. It has already been hinted, that it has not been accurately ascertained when a person, who has laboured under this disease, is perfectly free of the contagion. It is asserted by Burserius, that if the disease runs its ordinary course, the patient is incapable of communicating it forty days after inoculation, that is, rather more than thirty days after the commencement of the eruptive fever.

· The eruptive fever generally makes its appearance at some period from the seventh or eighth to the tenth or eleventh day after inoculation. In 810 inoculated patients 519 became feverish before the ninth day, 291 on or after the ninth day, that is, the fever in the proportion of more than five to three comes on before the ninth day. It is observed of the inoculated small-pox, that the earlier the eruptive fever appears after inoculation, the more favourable is the disease.† In the casual small-pox the fever seldom appears before the ninth day after infection. It is allowed that the fever never appears earlier than the fifth day, whether from in-

Hafn. there is a well-attested case of the same kind; and a very extraordinary one, quoted from Borellius by Rosen, in the 5th vol. of Haller's Disp. ad Hist. et Cur. Morb. Pert. A woman had the small-pox seven times, and died of it at the age of 118. Mr. Kite, in the 4th vol. of the Mem. of the Medical Society of London, relates several cases, in which there could be no doubt of the small-pox appearing for a second time; and Mr. Withers, in the same vol. mentions an instance of a person labouring under the small-pox, who many years before had had his face deeply pitted and seamed by it. In Dr. Jenner's Continuation of Facts relative to the Variol. Vaccinæ, Dr. Mills relates his own case. He laboured under the small-pox a second time from inoculation.

* See Dissertations sur les Fievres Infectieuses et Contagieuses, par M. O'Ryan, D. M. de l'Universitc de Montpelier, &c. There is an account of his experiments in Dr. Haygarth's Sketch, &c. It has been observed, that infants in particular are less liable to the casual small-pox than has been supposed. Dr. Underwood, in his Account of the Diseases of Children, says, that infants in particular are not apt to have the disease in the natural way, and that he has known them sleep in the same cradle with those under it without being infected by them.

† See Dr. Dimsdale's Treatise.

oculation or not. It has been known to be as late of appearing as the 16th, 17th, or even 23d day.[†]

It is a fact of importance, which has been ascertained by a great variety of observations, that after the commencement of the eruptive fever, whether the complaint be the inoculated or casual small-pox, there is no danger of increasing its severity by the freest exposure to a second infection. It even appears, that the patient might be exposed without danger to the contagion of small-pox as soon as inoculated, provided we could be certain that the inoculation was about to prove successful; the presence of the complaint in consequence of the first application of the contagion, obviating any consequence to be apprehended from a succeeding infection.

In the transactions of a society for the improvement of medical and surgical knowledge, among other observations Dr. Fordyce remarks, that if a person be successfully inoculated, and a few days after again inoculated, the fever will appear when the wound from the first inoculation suppurates, and will not be increased when that from the second does so. There is reason to believe indeed, that were a person inoculated immediately after being infected in the natural way, the appearance of the inoculated would prevent that of the casual small-pox; and that the patient, having been infected in the natural way previous to inoculation, would not even increase the severity of the disease. The reader will find a variety of observations in the works which have been mentioned, in confirmation of these remarks, particularly in the different accounts of the Suttonian method of inoculating. Mr. Sutton did not hesitate to expose his patients in the freest manner to the contagion from the moment they were inoculated.

Such are the principal circumstances to be attended to in the practice of inoculation. We probably owe this, like many other useful inventions, to chance. It has been ascribed to the Circassians, and was first employed by them, it is said, as a means of preserving the beauty of their women. From other observations it would appear, that inoculation originated in Africa. Mr. Colden, in his Letter to Dr. Fothergill on the Malignant Sore Throat, says, that he found, from conversing with several Negroes from Guinea, that inoculation had been long practised in their country, nearly in the same manner and at the same time of life as in Europe; and Mr. Mungo Park, in his travels into the interior of Africa, found it so.

But the truth is that inoculation has been practised not only in various parts of Asia and Africa, but even in some parts of Europe, for an unknown length of time; nay it is even certain,

† See the conclusion of Dr. Haygarth's Sketch, &c. page 539, 548, and 549.

that it was, long known in the Highlands of Scotland, and in Wales, before its introduction into England, so that it is probable, that accident suggested the expedient in most places where the small-pox had been long known, independently of any intercourse they had with each other ; and what adds to the probability of this opinion is, that in most places where inoculation can be traced back for a considerable length of time, it seems to have been practised chiefly by old women before it was adopted by regular practitioners. Had it been imported from a distance, those who were best informed would have been soonest acquainted with it, as happened in England ; but being suggested by accident, it would probably originate among the most numerous, that is the more ignorant, classes of society, and be only gradually adopted by the better informed ; as seems to have been equally the case in Africa, Asia, and Europe.

It was first introduced into England in April 1721, at which time Mr. Charles Maitland inoculated the daughter of Lady Mary Wortley Montague ; and soon after, some successful trials having been made on criminals, the children of the Royal Family were inoculated in London in 1726. Mr. Maitland also introduced inoculation into the Lowlands of Scotland, where he met with difficulties owing to an accident mentioned above. Since his time, from a variety of misrepresentations, it has occasionally met with much opposition, and once or twice has nearly fallen into neglect. Dumfries was one of the first places where it became common. It was introduced there in 1733, and as the casual small-pox often appeared in this place in a very bad form, the great advantage derived from inoculation soon rendered it pretty general.

There is no difference in the mildest kind of small-pox whether received in the natural way, or by inoculation. The great difference between the casual and inoculated small-pox is, that the former, although sometimes very mild, is much more generally of a worse kind, nor is it possible to insure its being mild by any precaution hitherto discovered ; while the inoculated small-pox on the contrary, is almost always favourable, unless the patient is injured by improper treatment. We often indeed meet with physicians of extensive practice who declare they never saw the secondary fever supervene in the inoculated small-pox. At the same time it must be confessed, that a practitioner may be deceived if, with every attention to the preparation and mode of treatment, he expects never to see a troublesome, or even a fatal, case of inoculated small-pox.

Inoculation also has the advantage of enabling us to practice with more certainty in the eruptive fever, in which the diagnostic symptoms are sometimes so obscure, that when the disease is taken in the natural way we cannot positively determine whether it is the small-pox or not, till the eruption appears. When the eruptive fever appears at the usual time after inoculation, there can be no doubt respecting its nature.

The circumstances which have tended chiefly to prevent inoculation becoming general, are certain religious opinions, and the fear of communicating other diseases along with the small-pox. Many conceive that they are not justified in inducing disease on their children, at a time when in the natural course of things they might escape it; and it is only in late times that this mode of reasoning has been confined to the uninformed. In some places they have reasoned in a different way, and conceived it culpable to neglect so simple a means of converting a very dreadful disease, which sooner or later in all probability their children would labour under, into one so mild as hardly to deserve the name. According as one or other of these opinions has prevailed, inoculation has become more or less general.* The one is often adduced with success against the other; against the former it has also been frequently and very justly urged, that by the same mode of reasoning we must lay aside the whole practice of medicine. Are not vomiting, purging, sweating, blistering, &c. so many means of inducing slight diseases, in order to avoid or remove more dangerous ones?

With respect to the opinion that other diseases may be communicated along with the small-pox, it is now generally regarded as unfounded. Scrophula is the disease which has been chiefly dreaded; but notwithstanding matter is every day taken from scrophulous patients, I have not met with, either in reading, or conversing with those extensively engaged in the practice of inoculation, one unequivocal instance of this disease being communicated along with the small-pox. The reader will find in a treatise entitled an account of the Preparation and Management necessary to Inoculation, by Mr. Burgess, an account of three persons inoculated from a patient labouring under syphilis, all of whom had the small-pox in a very mild form, and grew up perfectly healthy. Dr. Kirkpatrick in his Analysis of Inoculation mentions a similar instance in which the event was the same. I have been informed on respectable authority, of several cases in which a cutaneous disease seems to have been communicated along with the small-pox. These cases are the same which Dr. Jenner mentions in one of his publications on the variolæ vaccinæ.

From what has been said of inoculation it appears, that the chief circumstance which has prevented the salutary effects, that under proper management it is certainly calculated to produce, is, that the inoculated, like the casual small-pox, is contagious; so that both are generally introduced at the same time, and with all the care that can be taken there will always be considerable risk.

* See Dr. Monro's Treatise on Inoculation.

of this. Were the inoculated small-pox not contagious, or could we induce any other disease equally mild and equally, a preservative against the small-pox, which could only be communicated by inoculation, we might hope that the casual small-pox would in a short time be wholly banished. Such a disease has lately engaged much of the attention of medical men.

The Cow-Pox has been long known in some parts of England, and even known as a preventive against the small-pox, but Dr. Jenner first called the attention of the public to it in a treatise enentitled, ".An Inquiry into the Causes and Effects of the Variolæ Vaccinæ, &c."

Cows are subject to an affection of the teats which appears in irregular pustules of a blueish or livid colour, surrounded by an erysipelatous inflammation. These if neglected often degenerate into troublesome eating sores, the animals seem indisposed, and the secretion of milk is lessened.

Inflamed spots often appear on the hands and wrists of those employed in milking such cows, at first assuming the appearance of small vesications, similar to those produced by scalds ; they quickly however run to suppuration, the edges of the suppurating parts, which are generally circular, being raised and of a blueish colour. Tumors appear in the axillæ, and all the usual symptoms of fever with more or less severity frequently supervene, occasionally attended with pains in the limbs and loins, vomiting, head-ach, and even though very rarely delirium.

These symptoms continue from one to three or four days, leaving troublesome sores on the hands, sometimes becoming phagedenic. The lips, nostrils, eye-lids, &c. are also sometimes affected with ulceration, but this seems to proceed from the patient touching those parts with the hands, for where eruptions appear in the cow-pox they are not apt to degenerate into sores.

In some parts of England the oldest farmers remember this complaint from their youngest days ; and had always considered it as a preservative against the small-pox. This induced Dr. Jenner to inoculate with the matter of cow-pox, in order to determine whether or not the disease possessed this property. And we have now reason to believe, from a very large body of evidence afforded by the experience of Dr. Jenner, his correspondents, and others, that those who have laboured under this disease are incapable of having the small-pox.

Dr. Woodville among others inoculated 400 patients for the small-pox, who had formerly laboured under the cow-pox without being able to induce the former disease in any of them. " Upwads of 6000 persons," Dr. Jenner observes in his continuation of Facts and Observations relative to the Cow-Pox, " have now " been inoculated with the virus of cow-pox, and the far greater

" part of them have since been inoculated with that of small-pox,
" and exposed to its infection in every rational way that could be
" devised, without effect." See also the Medical and Physical
" Journal for July 1800, p. 22 and 23.

Some have doubted whether the security against attacks of
small-pox from having had cow-pox, will be permanent. Dr.
Jenner among others mentions one case in which the constitution resisted the small-pox 53 years after the patient had had the
cow-pox.

It is true indeed that cases have been adduced by Dr. Beddoes
in his Medical Contributions, Dr. Sims in the Medical and Physical Journal, and others, in which those supposed to have had
the cow-pox were still found liable to the small-pox. Such patients however, Dr. Jenner alleges, had not laboured under the
true cow-pox, but a disease similar to it, to which cows are also
subject, and which, he thinks, may be distinguished from the
true cow-pox, by being a milder disease, having no blue tint, nor
erysipelatous margin, creating no general derangement, and by
quickly terminating in a scab. Many cases however of the true
cow-pox are attended with little or no derangement of the system ; the blue tint is sometimes not to be perceived,* and it is
not uncommon for a scab to be formed ; so that the foregoing diagnosis will not enable us with any certainty to distinguish the
true and spurious form of the disease ; this point therefore remains to be determined.

Dr. Jenner also gives other reasons for believing that some
similar diseases may have been mistaken for the cow-pox. Variolous matter, he observes, may by keeping undergo such a
change, either from putrefaction or some other cause, as not to
be capable of communicating the small-pox, yet it still produces
inflammation and matter in the part, swelling of the axillary
glands, general indisposition, and eruptions. Dr. Jenner thinks,
the matter of the cow-pox may undergo a similar change.† He
also thinks it probable, that the matter of the cow-pox when it
has degenerated into ulcers, may not produce the disease, but a
train of symptoms resembling it. Lastly, he remarks, the disease produced immediately from the horse may be different
from the cow-pox.

Concerning the origin of the cow-pox there is some difference
of opinion. Horses are subject to inflammation and swelling in
the heel, which farriers term the grease. It is the opinion of
some that the cow-pox derives its origin from this complaint,

* Several engaged in the inoculation of cow-pox have assured me that
they often could perceive neither the general derangement nor blue tint.

† Mr. Kelson's observations in the Medical and Physical Journal tend
to confirm this supposition.

Those employed in dressing the heels of such horses, and afterwards in milking cows, it is said, communicate the complaint to the latter. It throws some obscurity on this part of the subject however, that the matter of the horse should produce the cow-pox in the cow, and not in the human body, which appears equally susceptible of it; for it is admitted that a horse rarely infects his dresser; and Dr. Woodville, in his Reports of a Series of Inoculations for the Variolæ Vaccinæ, &c. relates experiments in which the matter produced by the grease in horses, taken in its various stages, did not produce the cow-pox by inoculation in cows, neither did this or other morbid matter from horses produce any effect on the human body. "If the thing could have been procured from greasy-heeled horses," Mr. Kelson observes, in the Medical and Physical Journal for July 1800, "I should have had "the means of propagating the disease some months sooner." "I left no experiment untried upon my poor cows to procure it." It would appear, on the contrary, from some other observations, that not only the matter produced by the heel, but that produced by other parts of the horse, is capable of occasioning the disease in cows.*

Another circumstance which has occasioned much difference of opinion respecting this disease, is, that in some cases it has been attended with eruptions. Dr. Woodville says, that about three-fifths of his patients had pustules on different parts of the body, resembling those of the small-pox. The appearance of pustules Dr. Jenner is inclined to attribute to the small-pox matter having been used instead of, or mixed with, that of the cow-pox; and observes, that all his correspondents who met with small-pox-like pustules, had the cow-pox matter from the Small-pox Inoculation Hospital in London.

There are several circumstances however which lead us to question the justness of this opinion. Dr. Woodville, in order to determine the effects of mixing the two matters, made the following experiment : " Twenty-eight patients were on the "same day inoculated with the matter of cow-pox and that of "small-pox mixed together in equal quantities, in order to try "which would prevail, or if it were possible to produce a hybrid "disease by an union of both. The result was, that in more "than one-half of the patients thus inoculated, the local affection "distinctly assumed the characters of the cow-pox. In the oth-"ers it more resembled the small-pox, but in none of them was "there much indisposition or many pustules.

"At the request of Dr. Jenner, I transmitted to him in Glouces-"tershire, some of the cow-pox matter from the patients then "under my care, which he used for the purpose of inoculation. "After a trial of it he informed me, that the rise, progress, and

* See Dr. Jenner's first publication above alluded to.

" termination of the pustule created by this virus on the arm,
" was exactly that of the true uncontaminated cow-pox. The
" matter sent was taken from the arm of Ann Bumpus, who had
" 310 pustules, all of which suppurated, yet with the matter of
" this stock Dr. Jenner inoculated twenty, and another gentleman
" in the same county 140 persons without producing any pustules
" which maturated.

" This fact would appear to confirm an opinion entertained by
" Dr. Jenner in his second publication on the variolæ vaccinæ.
" He seems disposed to attribute the pustules which so often at-
" tended this disease in London and its vicinity to some peculiar
" influence of the town air. But of the cases which I have stated,
" several were those of patients who were inoculated eight miles
" distance from London, yet these patients in the proportion of
" about one in five, had an eruption. And at 'a small village still
" further from London, eighteen persons were inoculated' with
" similar matter, in all of whom it produced pustules."

There are also some other facts which would induce us to believe, that the eruption is not the consequence of any admixture
of variolous matter, but peculiar to the cow-pox, for even those
pustules which maturate do not run the same course with the pustules of small-pox. Mr. Jukes, surgeon at Stourport, who has
been extensively engaged in the inoculation of cow-pox, has fa-
voured me with some very pertinent remarks, which his accuracy of observation permits me to quote with confidence. The
matter he used was procured from Dr. Woodville. With respect to the eruption, he observes, " Several of my patients this
" spring have had pustules, few of which have come to suppura-
" tion; those that did, and which were well characterised, were
" of shorter duration than the small-pox pustules." From this it
appears, that pustules occasionally appear in other parts of the
country as well as in the neighbourhood of London, but that
their duration, if it be found uniformly such as in Mr. Jukes's patients, will be a sufficient diagnostic between them and small-pox
pustules. At other times, Mr. Jukes, although inoculating with
the matter originally from the small-pox hospital, has not met
with pustules in any of his patients. " I inoculated eleven children," he observes, " twelve months ago, none of whom had pustules."

Comparing these different observations, we should be inclined
to believe, that a peculiar eruption belongs to the cow-pox, the
appearance of which is determined by some peculiarity in the situation or season, which we cannot at present detect. Future observations however must determine respecting the nature of this
eruption.

The great point being admitted, that the cow-pox secures the
constitution against the small-pox, the next questions of impor-

tance respect the prognosis and the contagious nature of the cow-pox. On these heads there is less difference of opinion.

Respecting the prognosis, Dr. Jenner observes that the cow-pox is never fatal ; and the experience of all, (with the exception of, Dr. Woodville) who have written on the disease, in this respect agrees with Dr. Jenner's. Dr. Woodville, in his reports of a Series of Inoculations for the Var. Vacc. mentions the case of an infant at the breast, in whom the disease proved fatal ; it had about 80 or 100 pustules ; the eruption came out on the seventh, and it died on the eleventh day after inoculation. It was carried off by epileptic fits, which first appeared on the seventh day.

The cow-pox does not appear to be attended with any particular danger in pregnant women.* Dr. Woodville found, from an experiment made on a large scale, that in cow-pox, the matter from the mildest cases, upon the whole, produces the mildest disease ; and the result of this experiment is confirmed by other observations.†

Dr. Woodville is also the only writer, who considers the cow-pox as ever contagious. When the disease produces pustules, he observes, it may be taken by infection ; he saw two cases in which the disease was received in this way ; in one the eruption was confluent and the disease severe ; in the other it was mild.

It is certainly very rarely contagious. Dr. Jenner observes, that it is not even communicated by sleeping with those labouring under it. Dr. Pearson‡ and others make similar observations. Mr. Kelson, in the paper just alluded to, observes, " I selected " about forty people in our work-house, and inoculated half of " them, some in both arms, and fixed them to sleep with those " who had not had it ; but in no instance was it communicated to " the others. I broke the pustules and frequently made them " smell the parts, but to no effect."

It is probable that the matter of cow-pox may undergo such a change by keeping that it shall be incapable of exciting the disease, but it appears from a variety of observations that it is not changed by passing through different constitutions. Whether the matter is taken from the cow, or from the human subject inoculated from the cow, or has passed through a variety of constitutions, the disease is still the same.‖

* See Dr. Marshall's observations in Dr. Jenner's Continuation, &c.

† See the observations of Mr. Kelson in the Medical and Physical Journal. In the different numbers of this work the reader will find a variety of papers containing much information respecting the cow-pox ; which is the more valuable, as it comes from different quarters and from people wholly unconnected with each other.

‡ See Dr. Pearson's Inquiry concerning the History of the Cow-Pox, &c.

‖ See Dr. Jenner's Continuation, &c.

Inoculation for the cow-pox, as far as I can learn from those
employed in this practice, more frequently fails than that for
small-pox, and more frequently the inoculated part produces a
troublesome ulceration.   Dr. Woodville remarks that he never
saw the part ulcerate.   With most inoculators this has been a frequent accident, and the treatment of the inoculated part therefore has demanded some attention.   In Dr. Jenner's first publication, he advises us, after the constitution is affected, to destroy the
pustules with unguentum hydrargiri nitrati, or a more speedy
caustic.   But in his last publication he observes, " In the early
" part of this enquiry, I felt far more anxious respecting the in-
" flammation of the inoculated part than at present ; yet that this
" affection will go on to a greater extent than could be wished, is
" a circumstance sometimes to be expected.   As this can be
" checked or even entirely subdued by very simple means, I see
" no reason why the patient should feel an uneasy hour, because
" an application, may not be absolutely necessary.   About the
" tenth or eleventh day, if the pustule has proceeded regularly,
" the appearance of the arm will almost to a certainty indicate
" whether this is to be expected or not.   Should it happen, noth-
" ing more need be done than to apply a single drop of the aqua
" lythargyr, acetati upon the pustule, and having suffered it to
" remain two or three minutes to cover the efflorescence sur-
" rounding the pustule with a piece of linen dipped in the aqua
" lythargyr. compos.   The former may be repeated twice or
" thrice during the day, the latter as often as it may feel agree-
" able to the patient."   ,

    As far as we are acquainted with the cow-pox, we have reason
to believe that there is no danger of communicating other diseases along with it.   And with respect to preparation Mr. Kelson
observes, " I never thought it necessary to give a dose of physic
" either after or before inoculation."

    The small-pox is not always a security against the cow-pox.
" Although," Dr. Jenner observes,* " the susceptibility of the
" virus of the cow-pox is for the most part lost in those who have
" had the small-pox, yet in some constitutions it is only partially
" destroyed, and in others it does not appear to be in the least di-
" minished."   The matter of the cow-pox from the human subject produces the disease in cows.   The variolous matter does
not produce the small-pox in them.

    * See his Continuation, &c.

SECT. III.

Of the Morbid Appearances on Dissection in those who die of the Small-Pox.

IN those who have died under a load of pustules, the nares and inside of the cheeks are often found covered with them, and the teeth are besmeared with a thick viscid saliva. Pustules are frequently observed on the upper, very rarely on the under, part of the tongue, which is better moistened with saliva ; the palate is often covered with them ; they also frequently occupy the more external, very rarely the internal, parts of the meatus auditorius.

The maxillary, frontal, and other sinuses of the face are free from any morbid appearance. The cellular substance of the face, as well as of other parts of the body, especially where the swelling is most considerable, is distended with a serous fluid as in anasarca.

On removing the cranium the dura matter appears perfectly sound, but the vessels of the brain, as in most other cases where coma is a frequent symptom, appear more turgid and filled with a darker coloured blood than usual, and a greater quantity of serous fluid is found, particularly towards the base of the brain, " Circa infundibulum, integra illa arachnoideæ vagina quæ nervos " tertii paris, adsitasque partes concludit, saccum aqua plenum " referebat."* In other respects the brain is generally sound.

On examining the parts situated in the neck, the œsophagus is found free of pustules, even where the pharynx is loaded with them ; or if any be observed in it, they are towards the upper part. The state of the larynx and trachea is often very different. These with the bronchiæ as far as their third division are sometimes more or less loaded with pustules, from which, and the state of the nares, we readily account for the dyspnœa and cough which frequently attend this disease. It sometimes happens however even in the worst forms of the disease that the wind-pipe is free from pustules. Tissot says he has dissected some so covered with pustules that there was scarcely room for one more, without finding any pustules in the larynx or trachea. The trachea is sometimes lined with a whitish crust which is easily separated, and the secretion from the bronchiæ is now and then tinged with blood.

The fluid of the pericardium is also sometimes tinged with blood, and small particles like coagulated blood broken down now and then appear floating in it. The surface of the heart has been found rougher than usual, and polypi are sometimes found in its cavities. It is doubtful if any of these appearances be essentially

* See Cottunnius de Sede Variolarum, p. 22.

connected with the disease. With respect to the last, it is a common appearance after death, whatever be the complaint of which the patient dies. The lungs have often a darker appearance, and their moisture is more copious than usual. When no inflammatory affection has supervened, they are in other respects sound. The form of the thorax has been observed considerably affected by enlargement of some of the abdominal viscera; this seems to be merely accidental.

The various parts, as the mouth, pharynx, larynx, trachea, &c. which are sometimes covered with pustules, are now and then in the worst cases affected with gangrene.

There are but few morbid appearances in the abdomen. In the stomach there is sometimes found a thick whitish matter, which also frequently besmears the œsophagus, but this is a common appearance of mucus when it has lain in these cavities for a considerable length of time. In examining bodies we often meet with morbid appearances which cannot be regarded as connected with the disease of which the patient died, as they are not observed in perhaps one of 50 cases. Thus in those who die of the small-pox, the liver is sometimes enlarged, sometimes soft, at other times hard and gritty, now and then hydatids are found in it. The state of the bowels also varies; worms, for example, or traces of inflammation, are sometimes found in the stomach and intestines. None of these appearances throw any light on the ratio symptomatum, nor indeed seem at all connected with the disease.

What principally demands our attention in the abdomen is, that pustules are never found on any of its viscera. Some have asserted the contrary, but it appears probable from the observations of Cottunnius that they had mistaken small lymphatic glands for pustules. He dissected forty bodies in the presence of several people, without observing any pustules on the stomach or intestines. " Did variolous pustules," Dr. Walker remarks, " invest the external membrane of the lungs, liver, stomach or " intestines, and pass through the common stages of inflammation and suppuration, we might expect a regular course of " complaints more urgent and distressing, than what occurs on " the surface of the body; but we never find this to be the case."

It appears then that variolous pustules never attack the cavities of the body, except those to which the air has free access; as the nose, mouth, trachea, the larger branches of the bronchiæ, and the outermost part of the meatus auditorius. It has also been observed in cases of prolapsus ani, that pustules very frequently attack that part of the gut which is exposed to the air.

Cottunnius alleges that pustules appear only on those parts which are exposed to the air, because moisture prevents their appear-

ance ; and in confirmation of this opinion, he observes that if
the eye-lids be kept moist by wet bread from the first attack of
the disease, pustules never appear upon them, and by the same
means, he alleges, pustules may be prevented on other parts.
This opinion however is invalidated by the fœtus in utero being
subject to the variolous eruption.

The seat of the pustules is neither the true skin nor the cuticle,
but the mucus which lies between them. The author just mentioned made frequent dissections in order to determine this point.
" Quoties pustulam incipientem dissecui, vidi cuticulam eleva-
" tam ad pustulæ formam, cutis corpore, intacto, et tumoris im-
" muni."* The seat of the pustules, a question at one time
much agitated, is thus very accurately ascertained ; but this
knowledge has not hitherto improved the treatment of the disease.

SECT. IV.

Of the Treatment of Small-Pox.

FOR the sake of perspicuity I shall divide the treatment of
small-pox into that of the Distinct and that of the Confluent forms
of the disease ; or rather, I shall consider at length the mode of
treatment in the former, and afterwards point out the circumstances in which the treatment of the Confluent differs from that of
the Distinct. And farther, to avoid confusion I shall refer to
the end of this section, for the means to be employed when those
symptoms which have been termed anomalous appear, which will
prevent interruption in laying down the general plan of treatment.

1. Of the treatment of the Distinct Small-Pox.

It was soon observed that the appearance of the eruption in
small-pox generally brings relief, and from this circumstance very
unwarrantable inferences were drawn, which for a long time influenced the practice in this complaint, and, it cannot be denied,
greatly increased its fatality.

Because the eruption was generally attended with a remission
of the symptoms, it was inferred, that the more copious the
eruption, the more relief it would bring. Every means tending
to promote the eruption were therefore employed, and whatever
tended to check it was deemed pernicious. By external warmth
and stimulating medicines, physicians endeavoured to support the
fever ; while evacuations and whatever else tended to moderate
excitement, was carefully shunned.

A very extensive experience has now unfolded the tendency of

* Cuttunnius de Sede Var. p. 202.

these maxims ; and established in their stead others of a very different nature. So far from the most copious eruption bringing most relief, the relief is always most complete, when the eruption is most scanty ; so that instead of supporting the excitement, that the eruption may be copious ; the indication in the eruptive fever, which in the distinct small-pox is always a synocha, is to moderate excitement, that the pustules may be as few as possible. All that was said of this indication in speaking of the treatment of synocha, is nearly applicable to the case before us.

The chief difference between the treatment of the eruptive fever of the distinct small-pox and the treatment of synocha arising from other causes, is, that in the former, the means for diminishing excitement must be more vigorous in proportion to the excitement, than in the latter. In common synocha, which is succeeded by typhus, a liberal use of antiphlogistic measures is seldom warrantable. In the eruptive fever of the distinct small-pox, on the contrary, where the synocha is not succeeded by typhus but terminated by the appearance of the eruption, the same degree of excitement warrants more vigorous antiphlogistic measures.

Besides in synocha, it is not only dangerous, but no advantage is to be expected from reducing the excitement, unless very considerable. In the eruptive fever of the distinct small-pox, and we shall afterwards find in most cases of the confluent also, it is not merely safe, but the best effects are to be expected from it, the severity of the ensuing disease being generally proportioned to the degree of excitement which prevails in the eruptive fever. " The good or bad management of the eruptive fever," Dr. Nisbet* justly observes, " in most habits, stamps the ex-
" tent and future progress of the disease, perhaps I may venture
" to say the very nature of the pock." " It is probable," says Dr.
Cullen, " that the measures taken for moderating the eruptive fe-
" ver and inflammatory state of the skin afford the greatest im-
" provement which has been made in the practice of inocula-
" tion."

Nay the very effects which we dread from evacuations in the common synocha, may be the consequence of avoiding them in the eruptive fever of small-pox ; for wherever the eruptive fever runs high, the secondary fever is apt to supervene ; and this in spite of all we can do often degenerates into an alarming typhus.

It is not to be inferred however from what has been said that the use of antiphlogistic measures and particularly evacuations cannot be too free. Here, as in all other cases of increased excitement, we are not to overlook one of the most valuable max-
ims in medicine, that the excitement is to be diminished with as little expense of strength as possible.

* See the Transactions of the Newhaven Society.

Such are the principles afforded by experience for conducting the treatment of the eruptive fever of small-pox when it is a synocha. It will be necessary to take a more particular view of the several means employed at this period.

In the practice of inoculation, it appears from what was said, above, a light diet for sometime previous to the appearance of the eruptive fever is proper, except in very debilitated habits. After the commencement of this fever such a diet becomes still more indispensible. It should be as diluent and cooling as possible. Some advise abstaining from all aliment but fresh acessent fruits, at this period, if the excitement be considerable. Whey mixed with acids has been regarded as the best drink, milk has also been warmly recommended by Rhazes and others. M. De Lassone bestows the most extravagant encomiums on it. He particularly recommends it in the confluent small-pox with a decoction of parsley roots, which he thinks the only articles of diet necessary. Milk he found particularly serviceable when the diarrhœa was profuse, and for moderating the pustulary affection of the fauces We must always make a large allowance in reading the encomiums bestowed on a favourite remedy. On comparing together the observations of a variety of writers we shall find reason to believe that provided the diet in this case be mucilaginous, diluent, and refrigerant, it is of little consequence what articles compose it. To such a diet it is proper in almost all cases to add other means of diminishing excitement.

Few medicines tend more to diminish excitement in idiopathic fevers than emetics. When the symptoms are at all considerable, they are particularly useful in the eruptive fever of small-pox, especially when the stomach is loaded, as often happens in this complaint. At the commencement of the eruptive fever, emetics, Rosen* remarks, are recommended by all. They are never to be omitted, he observes in another place, unless contraindicated by the presence of gastritis. An emetic has been regarded as particularly useful at the commencement of the casual small-pox, from the opinion that the contagion is received by the stomach. It is too severe a remedy to be generally employed in so mild a disease as the inoculated small-pox.

The class of medicines which have been termed refrigerant are of more general use. Of these, nitre and saline draughts given in the state of effervescence, are esteemed the best ; but the most useful of the neutral salts in the eruptive fever of small-pox are those best calculated to produce a cathartic effect.

I shall afterwards have occasion to speak more at length of the use of cathartics in the small-pox ; it is enough at present to observe, that the sulphate of soda or any other cathartic salt, re-

* Haller's Disput. ad Hist. et Cur. Morb. Fert. vol. v.

peated at intervals, so as to support a moderate catharsis, forms an essential part of the treatment of the eruptive fever. The bowels are apt to be costive, and costiveness is particularly unfavourable in the small-pox, and especially in the eruptive fever.

Much purging however is not necessary but hurtful in mild cases; which is admitted by Dr. Walker and others, who make a very liberal use of cathartics in the most alarming forms of the disease. In the distinct small-pox the repetition of cathartics is to be regulated by the degree and obstinacy of the symptoms of increased excitement, particularly the strength and hardness of the pulse. This we shall find cannot be said of all cases of the confluent small-pox.

Boerhaave, Mead, Tennent, and others, have insisted on the advantage of mercurial cathartics in the small-pox. Dr. Fowler in particular, in his Inaugural Dissertation, which was written after he had been sometime engaged in practice, speaks in the highest terms of mercury in this complaint. When it is given so as gently to affect the mouth, the disease, he maintains, is as certainly rendered mild as when it produces catharsis. Mercury, he asserts, renders even the mildest cases more mild and of shorter duration. It often, according to Dr. Fowler, renders the casual small-pox as mild as the inoculated, and almost always milder than might have been expected. He confesses indeed, that the small-pox has sometimes proved severe in those under a course of mercury,* but observes, that a few cases cannot be adduced as an argument against a remedy generally successful. The acknowledged tendency of mercury to obviate the inflammatory diathesis is in favour of Dr. Fowler's observations.

Whatever cathartic we employ, the occasional use of cooling clysters is always useful when the excitement runs high.

It is remarkable that Sydenham made little use of cathartics in the small-pox, which tended to confirm a prejudice against them, at the commencement of the disease, that prevails in some places even to this day. Sydenham however very generally recommended another evacuation, the propriety of which is now called in question in 99 cases of a 100.

He made a very free use of the lancet, and in this practice many of his successors have persevered. " Si vel minime suspicari " liceat," says Sydenham, ", variolas mox erumpentes, e conflu- " entium genere futuras esse ; utile prorsus erit ut, non solum " sanguis quam primum mittatur, sed et emeticum propinetur ob " rationes alio in loco fuse dicendas." Huxham also frequently had recourse to venesection in the small-pox, although he admits the impropriety of recommending it in certain cases in which Sydenham believed it useful. These will afterwards be consider-

* Cases of this kind are mentioned by Dr. Fordyce.

ed ; in the mean time let us endeavour to ascertain when blood-letting is to be employed in the distinct small-pox.

It is an observation with a few exceptions universally applicable, that blood-letting is only to be recommended when the effects expected from it cannot be procured by other remedies. Of all the means employed by the physician it is the most dangerous. There is no disease which tends more directly to impair the powers of life ; and in the most dangerous cases it is often a doubtful point whether the disease, or the blood-letting which relieves it, is most to be dreaded.

It is true indeed, that in most cases of unimpaired vigour, a moderate loss of blood is not attended with danger. But in the strongest its frequent repetition is always to be feared, and a prudent physician, as he cannot with absolute certainty foresee the course of almost any disease, and still less what new diseases may supervene, will choose to reserve so powerful a remedy, in case symptoms should appear that render its exhibition necessary. One of the first maxims in the treatment of febrile diseases is to save the patient's strength as much as possible, that our practice may have sufficient latitude, if I may use the expression ; when it is cramped by a debilitated habit, the danger is always great. I shall have many opportunities of illustrating these observations. What practitioner has not seen cases prove fatal, because the patient was too weak to bear the loss of a few ounces of blood ?

In the present case then we are to enquire when advantage is to be expected from blood-letting, which cannot be procured by less debilitating means. The question is very easily answered, if it be admitted that diminution of excitement is the only effect to be expected from blood-letting in idiopathic fevers ; which is evident, as far as I can judge, from what was said of blood-letting when considering the treatment of intermitting and continued fever ; or if the reader does not deem this sufficient, let him take the trouble to compare together the facts there alluded to, or to be found in the various works on the disease we are considering. This is not one of the many points in medicine concerning which, facts are wanting ; it has been sufficiently ascertained by a very ample and fatal experience.

If then the diminution of excitement is the only object we have in view, shall we unnecessarily reduce the strength by blood-letting, while safer measures will produce this effect ? If exposure to cool air or a mild cathartic will sufficiently diminish the excitement, what need is there for venesection ? We are not, says Burserius, from the appearance of one or two symptoms indicating blood-letting, at once and without consideration to have recourse to this remedy in the small-pox, unless such symptoms be constant and vehement, and such as leave no room to doubt of the propriety of blood-letting; for blood-letting may often be deferred or omitted without running any risk.

When the increased excitement resists the gentler means, as it is of the greatest consequence that it should be reduced at an early period, we must have recourse to venesection; and here the following remark of Sydenham is fully warranted by expe-rience, " Vulgare illud atque tralatitium argumentum, quo ad-versus phlebotomiam aliasque evacuationes utuntur, nempe, quod non liceat a circumferentia ad centrum movere humores, cum natura in hoc morbo contrarium adfectare videatur, nulla-rum plane virium est."

Where blood-letting is improper before the eruption, it must be still more so after it, when the fever either becomes milder or wholly disappears. Even in the distinct small-pox indeed, the secondary fever sometimes supervenes. At its commencement it is a synocha, and we must again have recourse to blood-letting if the symptoms resist other means, remembering however that now the fever will not be relieved by the appearance of an erup-tion, but will suddenly assume the form of typhus if the anti-phlogistic plan be pushed too far.

Some authors, and those of the highest authority, have recom-mended blood-letting at the very termination of the complaint, or rather after every symptom had disappeared. " Die decimo-quarto," Sydenham observes, " ægrum e lecto surgere permi-si, vicesimo primo sanguinem e brachio educendum curavi." " Superest ut dicam," says Dr. Mead,* " nullam febrem magis requirere, ut morbi reliquiæ e corpore exterminentur, sanguis igitur, si vires adhuc constent, convalescente jam ægro detra-hendus est."

This practice is now very generally abandoned, unless symp-toms demanding blood-letting supervene. It was not however the mere offspring of hypothesis. The small-pox, like some of the other exanthemata, it was observed above, often leaves be-hind it a predisposition to inflammatory complaints; but it is sufficient to have recourse to blood-letting when the presence of these renders it necessary. The reader may consult what was said in the first volume, of blood-letting during the apyrexia of intermittents, which is altogether applicable to the case before us; in which indeed there is an additional argument for not let-ting blood till the symptoms we dread shew themselves; namely, that there is much less chance of their appearance, than of the recurrence of the paroxysm of an intermittent.

Local blood-letting by scarification of the temples or leeches, is a valuable remedy where the coma or inflammation of the eyes is considerable.

* Monita et Præcepta Medica cum Notis Wintringhami.

Although I had not arrived at the period of eruption when I had occasion to mention blood-letting, it appeared a more distinct plan to collect in one place the remarks to be made upon it, than repeatedly to mention it in speaking of the different stages of the disease. To return to the treatment of the eruptive fever.

Of all the means employed for moderating the excitement during this fever, none has proved so generally beneficial as the application of cold. Sydenham* was the first who in this country introduced the cool regimen in small-pox. It is one of his greatest improvements in medicine. The injury done by a high temperature, and the advantage of a free admission of cool air, in continued fever, have been pointed out. Both are still more remarkable in the treatment of small-pox. There is perhaps no other disease in which cold is now applied so freely and with so much advantage.

This practice has been long known in the East ; it is only in late times however that it has been introduced into Europe, for even the authority of Sydenham could not for a long time render the cool regimen in the small-pox prevalent. In this country it is now practised to a greater extent than he ventured to recommend.

The patient is at no period of the disease confined to the house, whatever be the season, unless the fever be such as confines him to bed. When an exacerbation comes on he is taken to a cooler place, which generally relieves it. It is proper to keep his bedroom cool. For this purpose it will often be necessary to exclude the light as much as possible, and to promote a free circulation of air ; and, as Tissot recommends, frequently to sprinkle the walls and floor with water.†

The patient should lie with few bed-clothes and on a mattress ; a feather bed always occasioning too great an accumulation of heat. A crouded room is particularly hurtful, the heat thus occasioned being the most pernicious of any. A free use of cold drink is equally grateful and salutary.

It is almost unnecessary to observe, that our directions respecting the temperature must be regulated by the state of the weather, and the severity of the symptoms. The free admission of the external air will be more necessary in warm than in cold weather ; when the excitement runs high than when it is moderate. The temperature should always be such that the patient may experience no disagreeable degree of heat, but rather sen-

* See his chapters De Variol. Regular. An. 1667, 1668, 1669 ; and De Variol. Anomal. An. 1670, 1671, 1672.

† See what was said of diminishing the temperature of the patient's bed-room, in the treatment of continued fever.

sation of cold; except indeed he complains of being cold we need not be afraid of carrying the cool regimen too far.

There is no part of this regimen more beneficial than frequently changing the linen of the sick, which should be dry but cool. The patient should be shifted at least twice a day.

There can be no doubt however, that the cool regimen, like every other mode of treatment, may be pushed too far. Dr. Makittrick Adair,* in a letter to Dr. Duncan, makes some observations on the Suttonian plan of treatment; that is, the very low diet and free exposure to cold; and alleges that it often does harm, especially when carried so far as entirely to prevent the eruption. This however rarely happens, and although Dr. Adair's observations certainly demand attention, on comparing them with those of other writers, as well as with what we every day see in practice, it will appear that he endeavours to restrict us too much in the employment of the cool regimen.

Such are the means to be employed in the eruptive fever of the distinct small-pox. And many have advised us to continue the exhibition of cathartics and the cool regimen in its full extent after the eruption is finished, and even in cases where the fever has almost or wholly disappeared. But if our view in the employment of these means, is to moderate excitement, of what service can they be when the excitement has returned to the healthy degree? The truth is that in such cases a perseverance in these measures is found to do harm. "After the eruption," Dr. Cullen observes, " when a few pimples have appeared on the face, " the continuing the application of cold air, and the employment. " of purgatives, have indeed been the practice of many inocu- " lators; but I think these practices cannot be said to give any " particular advantages to inoculation; for when the state of the " eruption is determined, when the number of pustules is very " small, and the fever has entirely ceased, I hold the safety of " the disease to be absolutely ascertained, and the farther use of " remedies superfluous. In such cases I judge the use of purga- " tives to be not only unnecessary, but that they may be often "hurtful."

At the same time we must be careful to avoid the opposite and more dangerous extreme of relaxing too suddenly in the employment of the cool regimen, which has often been attended with alarming consequences.† The use of gentle laxatives, as far as is necessary to prevent costiveness, is to be continued; and with regard to the application of cold, it should at this period be regulated by the patient's feelings.

* See the 8th vol. of the Medical Commentaries.

† A very striking instance of the injury done by an unguarded relaxation of the cold regimen is related by Mr. Perkins, in the 3d vol. of the Medical Observations and Inquiries.

If on the other hand the febrile symptoms continue considerable, notwithstanding the appearance of the eruption the plan of treatment must not be relaxed. The continued use of cathartics and the cool regimen is then necessary; and as at an early period they are the best means of moderating the eruptive fever, they are now the most effectual for preventing the appearance of the secondary ; which is always to be feared where the remission on the completion of the eruption is inconsiderable. The Indians, Dr. Rush informs us, plunge themselves in cold water as soon as they perceive the eruption of small-pox ; which is found to moderate the disease. Cold bathing in the small-pox is also practised by Europeans in sultry climates. A person who had spent many years in the East-Indies informed me, that when the pustules have a flaccid unfavourable appearance, on the use of the cold bath they become in the space of a few minutes well filled and more prominent. If it be improper to persevere in the liberal use of cathartics when the appearance of the eruption has nearly or altogether removed the febrile symptoms, what shall we say of this practice after every symptom of the complaint has disappeared ? " After having conducted patients through the " small-pox," Dr. Brocklesby* observes, " physicians have gen-" erally supposed purgatives necessary, in order as they say to " carry off the dregs of this disease. I must own I have been " so far from placing confidence in the supposed advantage of ",this practice, that I have been convinced that it tends too much " to weaken the body, already relaxed and broken by the prece-" ding disease."

Notwithstanding what is here said, this practice is not wholly unfounded, but rests on the same foundation with that of blood-letting at the same period.; and, when carried to the extent that some have recommended, is nearly as objectionable. But as the small-pox leaves behind it a predisposition to inflammatory complaints, it is of great consequence for some time after this disease to guard against any accumulation of irritating matter in the bowels, which may be the means of inducing such complaints, as I have known it to be, and the patient thus nearly destroyed by an inflammation of the intestines.

There is for the most part some foundation for modes of practice which have been generally prevalent ; and we should be cautious in wholly abandoning them. It will often be found that their pernicious effects are owing to physicians having lost sight of the circumstances which first suggested them. Guarding against the accumulation of irritating matter in the primæ viæ at this period must have always been found useful ; but when physicians began to talk of draining off the dregs of the disease, and employed the same practice in all cases, we cannot be surprised that it was often hurtful.

* See his work on the Diseases of the Army.

When the fever continues after the eruption, we must expect a considerable exacerbation about the seventh or eighth day. Means for moderating the febrile symptoms are therefore particularly necessary at this period.

Blisters have been thought useful, and some have advised a succession of them for some days after this exacerbation; that is, after the commencement of the secondary fever. Blistering is certainly prejudicial when the synocha runs high, by increasing the excitement, which is admitted by Tissot, who is a strong advocate for their exhibition after the typhus has appeared. Blisters, like opium, he observes, recruit the strength, check the diarrhœa, and determine to the surface. It will be found however on comparing different writers, that the observations made on blistering when considering the treatment of synochus are applicable to all idiopathic fevers.*

Except when local affections are present, little is to be expected from them. I shall have occasion to speak of their use in considering the treatment of certain symptoms which do not come under the general plan of cure. When blisters are used, the proper place for their application is to be chosen, without regard to its being covered with pustules.

Although, where coma is not considerable, the sleep is often much disturbed, opiates are a doubtful remedy, particularly in the eruptive fever, and at other periods, if the excitement is considerable. Some also dread their tendency to induce coma.

Paracelsus was the first who gave opium to a considerable extent in the small-pox ; and Sydenham, although he neglected the general plan of treatment adopted by Paracelsus and his followers, considered opium a valuable medicine in this disease. Some late writers defend this practice ; while others go so far to the opposite extreme as to condemn the use of opium in almost every case of small-pox.

The result of all that has been said on the subject appears to be, that if opium be given when the excitement or coma is considerable, or if it be found to induce coma, it is hurtful ; but in all other cases, especially where the watchfulness is obstinate, a quantity sufficient to allay restlessness, provided proper care be taken to prevent its constipating effects, is beneficial.

Opium, upon the whole, is better adapted to the confluent than distinct forms of the disease. Bursérius frequently employed it to relieve the acute pains of the back and limbs which frequently attend the former. The reader will find some good observations on the use of opium in the small-pox, in Tissot's Letter to Haller on this disease.

* See the observations of Dr. Browne Langrish on Blisters in his Treatise on the Small-Pox.

Although the eruptive fever in the distinct small-pox is always a synocha; yet towards the end of the disease, if the fever has continued after the eruption, and especially if the secondary fever has supervened, a greater or less degree of typhus always shews itself; and then the mode of treatment is the same as in typhus from other causes.

2. Of the Treatment of Confluent Small-Pox.

The more alarming the eruptive fever is, the more assiduous must be our attention to every part of the cool regimen. On this head there is little to be added to what has already been said.

It cannot be denied that an alarming train of symptoms have sometimes been induced by sudden and imprudent exposure to cold. The eruption recedes, the patient falls into syncope* or convulsions which sometimes terminate fatally; and it is in the confluent forms of the disease that this accident is most to be dreaded; and there, it appears from the observations of authors, chiefly at the time of maturation. It will be found however on reviewing the history of such cases, that previous to the exposure to cold the patient had generally been debilitated by the hot regimen, or other improper modes of practice. When the disease has been properly treated from the commencement, such a train of symptoms is a very rare occurrence.

Instances of this kind ought not to deter us from the cautious application of cold even where the hot regimen has been employed at an early period. The immediate and sudden application of cool air has often snatched the patient from death.† Caution however is requisite.

There is but one form of small-pox, in which the good effects of the cool regimen have been called in question, namely, the crystalline. Dr. Rogers of Cork, who had extensive opportunities of treating this form of the disease, declares that he has not there found the cool regimen produce its usual good effects.‡

In the confluent small-pox, where the fever is always considerable, every kind of irritation or exertion is injurious. The patient should neither attempt to walk about nor even sit up, as in the milder forms of the disease; and all the directions respecting the management of the natural agents laid down in the treatment of synocha, are to be strictly followed.

No part of the treatment of confluent small-pox demands more attention than the employment of cathartics. Whatever opinion

* See the observations of Dr. Dimsdale and others.

† See the observations of Sydenham, and Sir George Baker in his Treatise on this disease.

‡ It is unnecessary to make a separate division for the few observations which apply exclusively to the anomalous small-pox.

we might form of them, where the excitement is above the healthy degree; we should, a priori, in all cases where it falls below this degree, be inclined to dissuade from their exhibition, except as far as it was necessary to prevent costiveness. A very extensive experience however has contradicted this inference.

Practitioners were first led to recommend catharsis in confluent small-pox from having observed that when a spontaneous diarrhœa occurred, especially if it appeared early in the disease, the pustules were less numerous, the fever more moderate, and the swelling of the head less considerble. " A spontaneous diar- " rhœa," Dr. Cleghorn observes,* " often occurred with the best " effects, particularly moderating the symptoms of the eruptive " fever ; from whence we learn," he adds, " how reasonable it " is to give purgatives in this stage of the disease according to " the rules laid down by Drs. Friend and Mead." " If an, ap- " prehension," says Dr. Walker,† " of weakening the vital pow- " ers in this species of small-pox," viz. the putrid, " when nei- " ther diarrhœa nor any other apparent evacuation occurs, ex- " cepting what is discharged by the salivary glands, induce us " to suspend purging altogether or even delay it long, the prog- " nosis, in every case of this sort, must be desperate." In another place the same author observes, " Purging is much more " necessary in the confluent than in the distinct small-pox. But " farther," says Huxham,‡ " if nature neither by her own ef- " fort, nor the help of art, is capable of keeping the morbific " humor from falling on the more vital parts, but from an un- " fortunate translation of it is like to sink under its weight ; as " upon a sudden retrocession of the humor of the face and hands, " a premature suppression of the saliva, and the like ; doth it " not seem necessary to carry off the offending matter by some " other out-let, as particularly by the guts, which are much " more easily and certainly solicited to discharge than the pores " of the skin, the urinary passages, or the salivary ducts." The reader will find cases to prove the benefit of purging in the confluent small-pox in Dr. Walker's Treatise just alluded to, and in a Treatise by Dr. Friend entitled " De Purgantibus in Secunda " Variolarum confluentium Febre adhibendis." " Vides ut aliis," Dr. Friend remarking on these cases observes, "inopinatam " præsentissimamque opem attulerit purgatio ; ut aliis paulisper " subvenerit cunctatius per vices repetita."*

* Account of the Diseases of Minorca.
† Treatise on Small Pox.
‡ Treatise on Fevers, Small-Pox, &c.

* Dr. Friend even relates one case, in which the gangrenous blisters mentioned by Sydenham, and which he always found a fatal symptom, appeared ; which treated with mild cathartics terminated favourably. There are some good observations on purging in small-pox by Dr. Simson, Professor of Medicine at St. Andrew's. In the works of Hoffman, Mead, and Wintringham, this practice is also warmly recommended.

It is observed that the good effects of purging are not so soon observed where the excitement is considerable, and that in these instances their frequent repetition is most necessary.

Upon the whole it appears, that cathartics are useful at all periods of small-pox, and particularly during the eruptive fever, and at the time the secondary fever is expected, unless a diarrhoea has supervened : and that they are the more indispensable the more severe the disease. They are necessary when the typhus shews itself, still more when the excitement is considerable.

Two circumstances in their exhibition always demand attention : that the mildest cathartics are the best, drastic purgatives being only necessary where there is an unusual difficulty in moving the bowels ; and that wherever there is much debility we must during their employment support the strength by cordials. If this caution be neglected, particularly in the worst forms of the disease, the danger may rather be increased than diminished by cathartics.

It is the opinion of some that purging has been carried too far by many practitioners, particularly in the secondary fever. If we find the patient's strength sinking, notwithstanding the use of cordials and tonic medicines, it is necessary to discontinue the cathartics or to employ only gently cathartic clysters.

To what the benefit derived from cathartics in the small-pox is to be attributed, has not yet been determined. With regard to the hypothesis of the variolous matter being discharged in this way, to the confinement of which the danger of the small-pox has been attributed, it deserves little attention. Nor can it well be supposed that the advantages derived from purging, are to be altogether attributed to its expelling irritating matter which is apt to accumulate in the intestines in this disease. If future observation should determine this to be the only use of cathartics in the small-pox, it will considerably modify the treatment ; at present we have reason to believe that they are serviceable in some other way.

It has long been a practice in eastern countries, and it is recommended by some late European writers, Tissot, Burserius, and others, to discharge the matter of the pustules by piercing them with fine needles, which occasions a copious secretion by the skin, for the pustules soon fill again, and are again opened, which is always done by making a very small aperture.* By this means it is thought the accession of the secondary fever is often prevented.

There is certainly a striking analogy between the prevention of the secondary fever in this way and by the use of cathartics, there being much similarity between the office of the skin and that of

* It has been considered as dangerous to admit air into their cavities.

the intestines ; but how an increased secretion either by the one or the other, acts in preventing the secondary fever, is impossible to say ; it is in vain to attribute their action to the evacuation of variolous matter, which has no existence till it is formed in the skin.''

In the confluent as in the distinct small-pox emetics are useful at the commencement. They are also recommended about the seventh or eighth day if the strength is not much impaired, and, seem often to moderate the symptoms of the secondary fever. They are particularly indicated when the stomach is loaded. Less however is then to be expected from them, than at an earlier period ; and if any degree of typhus has shewn itself, they are generally hurtful.

'Such are the observations which apply to the treatment of confluent small-pox in general. What remains to be said may be divided into the treatment peculiar to the confluent small-pox, while attended by synocha ; and that peculiar to the worst forms of the disease, in which a confluent eruption is attended with typhus.

On the former of these heads little remains to be said. While the fever is a synocha, the treatment of the confluent small-pox differs from that of the distinct in little more than degree. The means pointed out in the treatment of distinct small-pox are to be proportioned to the violence of the excitement.

It is to the confluent small-pox attended with synocha that nauseating doses of emetics are best adapted, and here they often form the best cathartics we can employ. In the distinct small-pox they are too severe a remedy, and in the confluent attended with typhus are too debilitating.

More harm may be done by incautious blood-letting in the confluent, than in the distinct, small-pox, and it is more difficult to determine when it should be employed. The confluent small-pox often shews a tendency to visceral inflammations, and the fever itself at an early period is often characterised by great excitement, accompanied with violent pains of the back, breast, and head ; so that an inexperienced practitioner would judge very copious evacuation necessary. One acquainted with the disease however would recollect, that these symptoms are the forerunners of a confluent eruption, which is sooner or later attended with typhus, which will very suddenly supervene if debilitating measures are pushed far.

The pernicious effects of such measures, which at first seem to promise much, are soon apparent. The pustules assume a more unfavourable character, black spots often appear on them, and the patient sinks under that train of symptoms which has been termed putrescent, enumerated in the preceding volume. The reader will find these observations illustrated in a striking manner, in

Dr. Cleghorn's Account of a Malignant Small-Pox which raged
in Minorca.

With respect to the treatment peculiar, to cases in which typhus has supervened, almost all that was said of the treatment of
typhus, properly so called, is applicable here. The typhus may
either, as in the worst cases, shew itself in the eruptive, or what
is more common, sooner or later in the secondary, fever. In the
regular small-pox, typhus never precedes a distinct eruption, nor
is such an eruption often followed by any considerable degree of
this fever. In anomalous cases, it often precedes, and more frequently follows a distinct eruption; and to such cases the observations about to be made are as applicable as to the confluent
forms of the regular small-pox. It is only necessary indeed to
make these observations, in order to shew that the treatment of
idiopathic typhus is still the same.

The earlier the typhus shews itself the greater is the danger,
and the more assiduous therefore we ought to be in the exhibition
of proper remedies. The diet, instead of being refrigerant and
diluent, must here be stimulating, and as nourishing as the state
of the stomach admits of. Wine we still find the article on which
experience teaches us to rely. It must be given alone or diluted
according to the urgency of the symptoms, always in sufficient
quantity to increase the strength and fullness of the pulse and to
remove or diminish the delirium; for such in all cases of idiopathic typhus are the effects of wine; and except in extreme cases,
where the digestive powers are wholly suspended, these effects
are increased by the addition of some farinaceous matter properly
prepared.*

It was observed in detailing the symptoms of typhus that the
delirium is sometimes, though rarely, of the furious kind. It appeared however, that notwithstanding the presence of this species
of delirium, wine was the most successful remedy. "There is
"something very singular and deceitful in the common typhus,"
Dr. Walker† observes, " in which the patient in the most violent
"delirium, tossing about his arms, speaking loud, and shewing
"every instance of the greatest vigour, with a galloping hard
"pulse, shall be instantly composed and his pulse at the same
"time brought down, upon getting him to swallow a draught of
" wine; when therefore small-pox is complicated with a disease
" of this kind, it always produces a dangerous complaint, requir-
" ing as much light support as the patient can receive, and wine
" to be given frequently, not only when he is in a low and de-
" pressed state, but when high and the delirium fierce."

Dr. Walker relates a case which shews in a striking manner
the similarity of the effects of opium and wine in such fevers.
They are not however to be used indiscriminately, as appears

* See the observations on diet in typhus in the first volume.
† See his Treatise on the Small-Pox.

from the observations made on their exhibition in typhus; from which and what was said of the use of opium in the distinct small-pox, the reader will readily perceive when and how this medicine is to be employed in the various forms of the disease.

The advantage of conjoining with wine the Peruvian bark in confluent small-pox, is generally acknowledged. Morton was among the earliest practitioners who employed the bark in the confluent small-pox. Succeeding practitioners adopted the practice, but the late Dr. Alexander Monro was the first who gave it freely in this complaint. It is now employed with the same freedom as in common typhus.

By the use of the bark, Dr. Monro observes, empty vesicles were filled with matter; watery sanies changed into white, thick pus; while petechiæ became paler and at last disappeared.

Whatever restores vigour, changes at the same time the state of the matter, from which in most cases the prognosis may with great certainty be collected.

In many cases other astringents are employed with advantage. Alum mixed with Peruvian bark, Vogel* observes, is the best of all medicines when the pustules are bloody. Dr. Wall† also insists on the advantage of alum in such cases. The sulphuric acid‡ has also been celebrated in the confluent small-pox. Its acidity as well as astringency may be useful.

Acids§ of all kinds have been much employed in this form of the disease. Dr. William Wright‖ particularly recommends a mixture of vegetable acids and common salt in all those diseases called putrid.

The various medicines which have been termed tonic and antispasmodic have been occasionally employed. On the use of these there is nothing to be added to what was said of them when speaking of typhus, except what comes under that part of the treatment in small-pox which still remains to be considered : the means to be employed when certain symptoms shew themselves, the treatment of which does not come under the general plan of cure.

These I shall consider the more at length, as the same observations apply to the other exanthemata when similar symptoms appear in them.

* Prælect. Acad. &c.

† Philosophical Transactions, No. 484, §. 4.

‡ Dr. Brocklesby mentions an instance in which recovery seemed owing to the exhibition of large doses of this acid. The patient took no less than an ounce of the acid. vit. ten. daily.

§ I am induced by long and repeated experience, says Tissot, to regard mineral acids as the most valuable remedy we have in the small-pox.

‖ See Dr. Wright's Letter to Dr. Morgan.

Inflammation of the brain is a more frequent accident in the crystalline than in other forms of small-pox. When the patient complains of an acute pain of the head, or is attacked with delirium ; when the eyes are inflamed, and incapable of bearing the light, the carotid and temporal arteries beating strongly while the pulse at the wrist is small and feeble, we have reason to dread an inflammation of the brain ; and it unfortunately often happens in such cases, that the patient is too weak to bear much general blood-letting. Local blood-letting therefore by scarification of the temples, or leeches, is what we chiefly trust to.

If general blood-letting be deemed admissible, the jugular should be opened in preference to any other vein, by which the general, serving at the same time the purpose of local, blood-letting, the symptoms will be relieved without pushing the evacuation so far as would otherwise be necessary.

Blisters applied to the head also make an essential part of the treatment. If the excitement be such as to warrant general blood-letting, the blister should be delayed till after the blood-letting.

Few remedies, we shall find, are better calculated to relieve inflammatory affections of the head, than a discharge by the intestines, and no cause more apt to increase such affections, than any accumulation of irritating matter there. Gentle cathartics therefore are doubly necessary, where any tendency to inflammation in the head appears.

For a similar reason, fomentation of the lower extremities is useful. " In some cases," Dr. Walker observes, " where the " delirium was obstinate, and there was reason to suspect too " great a determination of blood to the head, which is commonly " the case, I have found singular relief obtained, by a succes" sion of flannel clothes dipped in hot water, very well wrung " out, and applied to the legs, and continued for half an hour " or more at a time." Other writers make similar observations.

Inflammation is also apt to seize on other parts, particularly the lungs, occasioning much difficulty of breathing and cough. Here the same means must be had recourse to, the local remedies being applied to the chest instead of the head. But the treatment in such cases cannot be properly understood without being acquainted with the phlegmasiæ, which will form the subject of the two succeeding volumes.

Dyspnœa often supervenes in small-pox from other causes, a pustulary affection of the larynx, trachea, and larger branches of the bronchiæ, or an unusual degree of swelling in the fauces which also impedes deglutition. In such cases, large blisters applied as near the part affected as possible are the most successful remedy. The same may be said of difficulty of deglutition in consequence of the viscidity of the saliva.

In this case gargles, such as those recommended in the aphthæ infantum, must at the same time be employed. Huxham* recommends cyder and honey—or vinegar, water, and honey—or oxymel scilliticum with a little nitre or crude sal ammoniac. Bang recommends a gargle of oxymel of squils and water, and the application of sinapisms to the hands and feet, with gentle laxatives, and if the difficulty of breathing be great, the antimonium tarisatum. Dr. Brocklesby observes, that small doses of ipecacuanha tend to restore the salivation when it is either suppressed or too viscid, and to alleviate the dyspnœa which often attends this accident. When the state of the fever admits of full vomiting it is often the means of relieving the swelling of the fauces and promoting the secretion of saliva†. The dyspnœa which sometimes follows the sudden interruption of the salivation, seems frequently owing to a degree of pneumonia supervening.

In all these cases, when blisters and the other means which have been mentioned fail to bring relief, we must have recourse to local blood-letting, and in the last case general blood-letting is sometimes necessary. On the other hand, the salivation is sometimes so copious as to threaten suffocation from the fluid falling constantly into the trachea, especially where there is any degree of coma. In this case Vogel thinks cathartics the most successful remedy.

Profuse diarrhœa is a troublesome symptom in the confluent small-pox, particularly in children. Unless this symptom produces a dangerous degree of debility, we must be cautious how we endeavour to check it; and even when it does occasion much debility, the safest plan is to endeavour to moderate the discharge by tonic medicines. There is perhaps no instance, except towards the termination of the complaint, in which the diarrhœa can be safely stopped by opiates and astringents, and then it is to be done cautiously; and when these medicines produce too sudden an effect, it must be counteracted by gentle laxatives; the diarrhœa is sometimes, though rarely, rendered profuse by exposure to cold; some relaxation in the cold regimen is then proper.

Obstinate vomiting is a dangerous symptom, both by reducing the strength, and preventing the exhibition of medicines. If from the nature of what is evacuated, the vomiting appears to proceed from irritating matter collected in the stomach, we must

* On Fevers, Small-Pox, &c.

† Dr. Cameron dissuades from vomiting in this case, and alleges that it has sometimes occasioned suffocation. He strongly recommends breathing the steam of a decoction of marshmallows, myrrh, and honey in vinegar and water. See the 52d vol. of the Gentleman's Magazine.

in the first place by draughts of some diluting liquor, enable the stomach to free itself of its contents. • If they are bilious or acid, we must correct what may remain by acids or absorbents.

If the vomiting proceeds rather from the state of the stomach i itself than its contents, which may be known by the inoffensiveness of the matter rejected, we must have recourse to such medicines as tend to allay the tendency to contraction. . Few are more powerful than saline draughts given in a state of effervescence. If these fail, a few grains of camphire may succeed, or a dose of solid opium, or, what is perhaps the most powerful means, we possess in obstinate vomiting, a combination of the two last medicines. The extract of cascarilla given in some agreeable distilled water is often serviceable in allaying vomiting.*

The sweating is sometimes so profuse as considerably to reduce the strength. In the worst forms of the disease however, and in infants in any form of it, this symptom rarely appears, so that its excess is less to be dreaded. When it shews a tendency to become profuse, the patient should avoid being in bed in the day time, which, with the cool regimen and laxative plan, almost always sufficiently counteracts this tendency.

A suppression of urine sometimes comes on, particularly in the confluent and anomalous forms of the disease, and in some cases proves obstinate. People in the vigour of life, and particularly those accustomed to a free use of spirituous liquors, are most liable to this symptom. It seems generally to arise from neglecting evacuations at the commencement of the disease, or keeping the patient too warm.

If, as frequently happens, it be attended with costiveness, we must begin with an emollient and laxative clyster. When the hot regimen has been employed, Sydenham advises the patient to be supported by two assistants, and exposed in his shirt to a current of cool air. The same practice is recommended by Bang†. and others. Dr. Cameron of Worcester observes, in the 22d vol. of the Gentleman's Magazine, " To facilitate the discharge of " urine which is often difficult in the small-pox, Sydenham directs " us to get the patients up and lead them about the room, but I " would beg all young physicians to read Hoffman's Dissertation, " De Situ erecto, in Morbis periculosis valde noxio before, they " either advise or allow of this practice. I have known sudden and " fatal effects from it in very hopeful cases. I think there is no " need to make so hazardous an experiment while salt of amber " is to be had, for that will seldom fail to answer this intention." The former part of this observation however is chiefly, if not wholly, applicable when the debility is considerable. Where there is much excitement, the case in which suppression of urine

* See Vogel's Obs. on the treatment of Measles in his Prælect. Acad.
† Praxis Med. Systematice Exposita.

most frequently happens, although it may be proper in the first place to try the salt of amber, there is little hazard in adopting Sydenham's plan; and where the increase of temperature is steady and there is no moisture on the skin, if this plan fails it may be proper to dash cold water on the legs, as is sometimes practised to solicit the alvine discharge.

One or two epileptic fits, it was observed above, even in the mildest forms of the disease, frequently precede the eruption without being attended by danger. In the confluent and anomalous forms of the disease however, the fits are more frequent, and in proportion to their frequency more to be dreaded. This symptom is rare in adults, but in them it is most dangerous.

When from the nature of the disease, we have reason to dread the frequent recurrence of epileptic fits, or when they have repeatedly occurred in any form of the disease, we must endeavour to moderate their violence and prevent their return. Blood-letting was at one time very generally employed for this purpose, but practitioners now agree that it is seldom successful; and the operation of blisters, Dr. Cullen observes, comes too late.

As the violence and frequent repetition of the fits generally depend on the violence of the primary disease, the various means of moderating this, are among the best for moderating and preventing the fits. But of all the medicines which have been employed, none have been found so frequently successful as opium, on which Dr. Cullen chiefly depends, and advises us to throw it in per anum while the fit lasts.

Opium is not only useful as an antispasmodic, but also by promoting perspiration, one of the best means, it has been found, to prevent the return of the fit. Dr. Walker recommends for this purpose a preparation similar to the compound powder of ipecacuanha. Vogel with the same view recommends a mixture of cinnabar, the sulphur auratum antimonii, and musk. The last is also recommended by Dr. Brocklesby and Bang, who likewise employed some other of the medicines termed antispasmodic. There are none of these however much to be relied on. Cataplasms applied to the extremities are sometimes serviceable. Whatever other means are employed, gentle laxatives are not to be neglected, as the irritation of retained fæces might alone be capable of renewing the fits, especially in children.

The pustulary affection of the eyes is often very troublesome, and is sometimes followed by loss of sight. When the pustules are numerous on the face, the use of common mild and gently astringent collyria should never be neglected. M. De Lassone* recommends frequently wetting the eyes and eye-lids with rose-

* See Memoire sur quelques Moyens de remedier aux accidens graves dans les Petites Veroles, in the 3d vol. of the Histoire de la Société Royale de Médecine.

water, in order to prevent the appearance of pustules; or, if they
have appeared, to diminish inflammation. Burserius recommends
water, in which ignited iron has been quenched.

· It is of great consequence to prevent the eye-lids from growing
together, which, as Vogel observes, is often the source of all the
mischief, increasing the pustulary affection and preventing the
use of collyria. This accident may in general be easily prevented, by bathing the eyes from time to time with warm milk.

When the load of pustules on the face is very great, so that
there is reason to think the eyes in danger, it has been recommended to immerse the extremities in warm water, and apply
sinapisms to them, or even to scarify them.* Vogel condemns the
common practice of moistening the face with a view to prevent
or moderate the eruption there. When pustules have actually
appeared on the eyes, we must have recourse to emollient poultices and mild mucilaginous decoctions;† and fomentations are
useful when there is much swelling of the eye-lids.

. It has been observed above, that in small-pox, as in other eruptive fevers, a retrocession of the eruption sometimes happens, attended with an alarming train of symptoms.

' The means to be employed in such cases are in some measure
influenced by the causes which produce the retrocession. The
chief of these causes are, the sudden application of cold when
the hot regimen has been employed, particularly if the cold be
applied about the time of maturation and when the patient is much
debilitated; fatigue, from remaining too long out of bed or in the
erect posture; syncope; strong affections of the mind, particularly terror or grief; and above all, profuse evacuations.

' The remedies of most general application in such cases are
wine and opium. These, Rosen observes, are particularly indicated when the retrocession is the consequence of profuse evacuations. When it is the consequence of the sudden application
of cold, increasing the temperature and even the warm bath are
generally of service, and the application of sinapisms and blisters in this case is particularly recommended. Musk and camphire, as in other cases of repelled eruption, are very generally
employed. Vogel thinks the ammonia, the semicupium, and
blisters applied to the feet, the most successful remedies. If, as
sometimes happens, a diarrhœa supervenes on the retrocession
of the eruption, it is generally of service and should not be
checked. Some have recommended blood-letting on the sudden
retrocession of the eruption. But if, as Burserius justly observes,
whatever debilitates tends to occasion this accident, blood-letting

* Vogel De Cog. et Cur. Morb.

† See the observations of Burserius and Tissot.

is surely the last means we should think of employing in such a case.* , ,

When the swelling of the face subsides, especially if it subside suddenly, and is not followed by the swelling of the hands, Dr. Brocklesby recommends the application of blisters to the wrists and fore arms, which often excites the swelling of the hands, or if not, tends to obviate any consequences to be feared from its absence. When towards the period of maturation there is reason from the debilitated state of the system to apprehend that the swelling of the face may suddenly subside, Dr. Cameron, in a paper just alluded to, recommends the following plan, to which the author's extensive experience naturally calls our attention. "On " the day before the face is expected to sink," he observes, " I wrap " up the arms and legs lightly in a suppurating cerate ; the citrine, " for instance, spread on linen rollers and tacked together so as " to make one contiguous plaister.".........." I assure you, I have " known adults in the confluent small-pox in less than an hour " after the application of these plaisters, cry out with joy that " they were in heaven. I have seen the pustules as far as the " plaisters reached, ripen and fill even to bursting with laudable " pus, and this dargerous period pass without one alarming " symptom." About the same period the whole body has been anointed with mercurial ointment apparently with good effects.

Dr. Brocklesby also recommends blistering the wrists when the salivation suddenly ceases without any swelling of the hands.

When the swelling of the face and neck is excessive, bathing the lower extremities and applying sinapisms to them, often relieves it. For the same purpose Tissot recommends the warm bath.

When the eruption, Vogel observes, is delayed beyond the usual time, a single venesection, a dose of laudanum, or the tepid bath, seem frequently to promote its appearance. Of these means, opiates only are admissible when the fever is typhus. Although, as was observed above, the eruption is generally earlier in the confluent, than in the distinct, small-pox, yet in some cases it is much later.

When the pustules are longer of drying than usual, they should be opened ; and if the dried pustules adhere too long, fomentations are the best means to make them separate.

When the patient is plethoric we may let blood with a view to stop hemorrhagies ; in other cases we must trust chiefly to as-

* The reader who has sufficient knowledge of medicine to separate facts from theory, will find some excellent observations on blood-letting in this case, in Dr. Cameron's Paper in the 22d vol. of the Gentleman's Magazine.

stringents.* The serum lactis aluminosum has been particularly recommended, especially if the hemorrhagy be from the skin, tinging the matter of the pustules.†

When pustules appear in the nares and fauces, Tissot recommends washing them frequently by means of injections. This means is preferable to gargling, as the motion of the throat in gargling is apt to increase the pustulary affection of the fauces.

We have been advised to open the tumors, which sometimes appear after the small-pox, if they have suppurated ; if not, to apply poultices to promote the suppuration. The propriety of this mode of practice, particularly in scrophulous habits, is, doubtful. When the sore does not heal readily, the Peruvian bark is serviceable, provided there be no tendency to visceral inflammation.

When the inflammation of the inoculated part becomes troublesome, the remedies are the same as in cow-pox.‡ Dr. Rush recommends washing the part repeatedly with cold water, which never fails, he observes, to remove the inflammation.

When the pustules, it was observed above, have adhered for a longer time, and been filled with a matter less thick and benign than usual, after they fall, the parts which they occupied suffer a desqamation, and pits are formed. Various means have been proposed to prevent this consequence. Such attempts however do not seem to have answered the expectations of those who proposed them.

It is a prevalent opinion that exposure to the air is the cause of pitting from its not happening to parts which are covered. It has therefore been proposed to cover the face with something that shall exclude the air. The reader will find an account of this method, and arguments for having recourse to it, in Dr. Walker's Treatise on the Small-Pox. It would require an extensive experience to determine its success, as pits are not always the consequence of even a numerous eruption. Our faith in it is lessened by reflecting that the hands are often as much exposed to the air as the face, and that there is something in the disease which determines it to affect the face in preference to other parts. The pustules and swelling always appear first on the superior parts of the body, and the former are there most numerous, and in the more severe forms of the disease, of a less benign ap-

---

* See Burserius's Inst. Med. Pract. The various means both local and general to be employed in hemorrhagy will be considered in another part of the Treatise.

† See the foregoing observations on the use of alum and the bark.

‡ See what was said of moderating the inflammation of the inoculated part when speaking of cow-pox.

pearance. ; Besides, children have been born marked with the small-pox.

Other means have been proposed for preserving the face, but it is needless to give any account of them, since none have been found such, as would encourage us to recommend them. The best means to prevent pitting are inoculation and the cool regimen.

CHAP. II.

Of the Chicken-Pox.

THE Chicken-Pox is so mild a disease that it hardly ever requires the assistance of the physician. It is necessary however to be acquainted with it, that it may not be confounded with diseases of more importance.

It is readily distinguished from all other eruptive fevers, except the small-pox, for which there is reason to believe it is sometimes mistaken. A very little attention however enables us to distinguish the two complaints.

SECT. I.

Of the Symptoms of Chicken-Pox.

THE Chicken-Pox, or, as it is termed by medical writers, Varicella, is defined by Dr. Cullen,

" Synocha, papulæ post brevem febriculam erumpentes, in " pustulas variolæ similes, sed vix in suppurationem euntes, post " paucos dies in squamulas, nulla cicatrice relicta, desinentes."

In all, even the mildest, cases of small-pox, the complaint begins with more or less fever, on the third or fourth day of which the pustules appear. In the chicken-pox the eruption often appears without any previous sign of indisposition; in others, Dr. Heberden† remarks, the pocks are preceded by a little degree of chilliness, lassitude, cough, broken sleep, wandering pains, loss of appetite, and feverishness for three days.

On the first day of the eruption the pustules are similar to those of the small-pox; on the second day there is formed on each a small bladder which contains sometimes a colourless, sometimes a yellowish, fluid; " on the second, or at farthest on the third, " day from the beginning of the eruption, as many of these pocks

* See a paper by Detharding in the 5th vol. of Haller's Disp. ad Hist. et Cur. Morb. Pertinent.

† The Med. Transactions, vol. i.

" as are not broken seem arrived at their full maturity, and
" those which are fullest of that yellow liquor very much resemble
" what the genuine small-pox are on the fifth or sixth day, espe-
" cially, where there happens to be a larger space than ordinary
" occupied by the extravasated serum."* It often happens however, either by the rubbing of the clothes, or the patient's scratching to allay the itchiness which attends this eruption, that the vesicles are broken on the first or second day of their appearance.
When this happens, the pustules, previously more or less raised,
subside, and the matter forms a crust without having at all assumed the appearance of pus. Even in those pustules which escape being broken, it has very little if any of this appearance.
On the fifth day of the eruption all the pustules are dry and covered with crusts, which in the small-pox does not happen till the
eighth or ninth day of the eruption, that is, the eleventh or
twelfth of the disease. The pustules in chicken-pox are less inflamed and their size is sometimes less than those of small-pox,
but in the latter respect there is generally little difference.

The chicken-pox is never confluent or very numerous. The
greatest number which Dr. Heberden saw was about twelve on
the face and 200 on the rest of the body. The eruption sometimes makes its first appearance on the back. When this happens, it affords another mark of distinction, the eruption of small-
pox always first appearing about the face, neck, and breast.

The last circumstance mentioned in Dr. Cullen's definition
" nulla cicatrice relicta," assists but little in forming the diagnosis, the milder kinds of small-pox being rarely followed by pitting, and pitting having sometimes though rarely been the consequence of chicken-pox.

Upon the whole then, the small-pox and chicken-pox differ in
the eruption of the former being preceded by a fever of a certain duration, while that of the latter is either preceded by none
or one of uncertain duration ; in the vesicles and succeeding
scabs appearing much earlier in the chicken-pox than in the small-
pox ; in the matter of the former never acquiring the purulent
appearance, which it always does in the distinct small-pox, the
only form of the disease which can be confounded with chicken-
pox. This diagnosis is more important than at first it appears, as
it is of consequence to determine positively whether or not a person has had the small-pox.

With respect to the prognosis in chicken-pox, it is uniformly
good, so that medical assistance being seldom necessary, practitioners are less acquainted with this, than most other eruptive
fevers ; and we have reason to believe that it has not only been
mistaken for small-pox, but that its matter has been used for that
of small-pox in inoculation, to which we may ascribe many of

* Dr. Heberden's Obs. Med. Trans. vol. i.

the supposed cases of small-pox having appeared a second time in the same person.*

SECT. II.

Of the Causes of Chicken-Pox.

ON this subject there is little to be said. The chicken-pox like other exanthemata arises from a specific contagion, which seems to produce the disease about the same period after the infection with that of the small-pox. Dr. Heberden thinks that people are not liable to a second attack of chicken-pox. " I wetted a thread, " he observes, in the most concocted pus-like liquor of the chick- " en-pox which I could find, and after making a slight incision it " was confined on the arm of one who formerly had the disease, " the little wound healed up immediately, and shewed no signs " of any infection."

SECT. III.

Of the Treatment of Chicken-Pox.

THE treatment of chicken-pox is very simple, and differs in nothing from that of a gentle synocha. The mildness of the symptoms renders blood-letting and other powerful means unne-cessary. Cooling saline cathartics in sufficient quantity to keep the body open, with a mild and diluent diet, form the principal part of the treatment. With respect to temperature and exer-cise, they should be regulated by the patient's feelings.

CHAP. III.

Of the Measles.

THE Measles, or, as it is termed by medical writers, Rube-ola, Morbilli, or Febris Morbillosa, is defined by Dr. Cullen,

" Synocha contagiosa cum sternutatione epiphora et tussi sicca " rauca. Quarto die, vel paulo serius erumpunt papulæ, exiguæ,

---

* Dr. Heberden thinks the swine-pox the same with the chicken-pox. See also the 1263d and 1264th paragraphs of Lobb's Practice of Physic. . Dr. Heberden describes another disease which he believes to be only a more severe species of chicken-pox. In this form of the disease, the symp-toms of the eruptive fever are considerable and continue for three or four days before the eruption appears. Nor does the fever remit on the ap-pearance of the eruption even where there are but few pustules. The pustules are redder than in the common chicken-pox, spread wider, but hardly rise so high, and instead of one little vesicle, they have from four to ten or twelve. In other respects they resemble the common chicken-pox.

" conferta, vix eminentes, et post tres dies in squamulas furfura-
" ceas minimas abeuntes."

Dr. Cullen divides this disease into two species, the Rubeola
Vulgaris, and Rubeola Variolides.   The former he defines,

" Rubeola, papulis minimis confluentibus corymbosis, vix em-
" inentibus."

Under this species he ranks three varieties.

1. Rubeola Vulgaris, " Symptomatibus gravioribus et decursu
" minus regulari."

2. Rubeola Vulgaris, " Comitante cynanche."

3. Rubeola Vulgaris, " Comitante diathesi putrida."

His second species, the Rubeola Variolides, he defines,

" Rubeola papulis discretis eminentibus."

Although he mentions this species in compliment to Sauvages,
he does not regard it as properly belonging to measles.   " Sau-
" vagesium secutus, hunc morhum hic indicavi, etsi multum du-
" bito, an recte ad rubeolum referundus est, non solum enim for-
" ma pustularum plurimam .differt, sed, quod majoris momenti
" esse videtur, est plerumque absque symptomatibus catarr-
" halibus, rubeolæ adeo propriis."*   Matthiew is of the same
opinion, and observes, that this complaint is seldom met with unless the small-pox be prevalent at the same time with the measles.†

The following is the division of measles generally adopted by
authors.   It comprehends only the first species of Dr. Cullen,
and is similar to his division of this species.

1. Rubeola Vulgaris or Morbilli Regulares, the measles such
as they generally appear when their course is undisturbed by any
unusual symptom.

2. Rubeola Anomala, Morbilli Anomali, Morbilli Epidemici,‡
or, the putrid measles, comprehending those forms of the disease in which the usual course is disturbed.

3. Rubeola Anginosa, in which the affection of the fauces
makes a principal part of the disease.

The similarity of the measles and small-pox has induced Rhazes, Eller, and some other writers, to regard them as little more

* See Dr. Cullen's Syn. Nosologiæ Meth. p. 136.
† See Matthiew's Observations on this species of Measles in the 47th
and following pages of the 4th vol. of Baldinger's Sylloge Selectiorum
Opusculorum.
‡ Morton, Huxham, &c.

than varieties of the same complaint. The more nearly they resemble each other however, the more cautious we must be not to confound them, since the treatment in the two complaints in some respects differs very essentially.

In by far the majority of cases however, there is a well marked difference in the symptoms of the eruptive fever, and in all cases in the appearance of the eruption, at least after it has been out a day or two at most.

It was observed above, that when the symptoms of diseases run imperceptibly into each other, the same is true of the modes of practice suited to them. Thus we found that the symptoms of synocha imperceptibly run into those of typhus, and that between the modes of practice in these complaints, however opposite, no well marked line of distinction can be drawn. The same, it appeared, is the case with respect to intermitting and continued fever in general. The symptoms and treatment of the one run into those of the other. Did a perfect diagnosis between such cases exist, it would be useless. We may regard them as one complaint, and we feel no difficulty in suiting the practice to the symptoms. Should symptoms of increased excitement appear in typhus, that is, should the complaint suddenly become synocha, we know that the treatment of synocha is applicable. Should symptoms of debility supervene in synocha, that is, should the complaint suddenly become typhus, we are assured that we run no risque in adopting the treatment of typhus. But where states of the system, requiring very different modes of treatment, produce nearly the same symptoms, as happens in many instances which we shall have occasion to consider (in the complaints termed the convulsive asthma of children, and the croup, for example) however difficult it may be, it is necessary, to find a diagnosis.

The small-pox and measles resemble, but never run into, each other; and the same observation, we shall find, applies to their modes of treatment.

SECT. I.

Of the Symptoms of Measles.

It will be sufficient to divide the measles into the regular and irregular forms of the disease ; the characteristic symptoms of the rubeola anginosa not being of sufficient importance to constitute a separate division.

The division of measles into regular and irregular has not unaptly been compared to that of small-pox into distinct and confluent. The irregular measles however is not so well defined a form of disease as the confluent small-pox, and the division may be more justly compared to that of small-pox into regular and anomalous.

1. Of the Symptoms of Regular Measles.

In laying before the reader the symptoms of regular measles, I shall pursue nearly the same order which was followed in detailing the symptoms of small-pox; in the first place, pointing out the symptoms which precede the eruption; secondly, describing the eruption; thirdly, enumerating the other symptoms which appear while the eruption is present.

It is a more distinct plan to describe the different appearances of the eruption; and having done so, recur to the period of its commencement, and mention the symptoms which accompany it, than constantly to interrupt the account of the eruption, in order to notice these symptoms. The former method is less subject to confusion, and better assists the memory.

Having enumerated the symptoms of the eruptive fever, the circumstances necessary to be known respecting the eruption itself, and the symptoms which accompany it, we shall still find a set of symptoms remaining which demand particular attention. In the fourth place, therefore, I shall enumerate the symptoms which supervene after the eruption has disappeared.

We cannot distinguish the first attack of measles from that of other fevers. The patient, for the whole of the first day, generally complains of alternate heats and chills. On the second day, though sometimes not till the third, the fever is completely formed, and certain symptoms make their appearance by which this fever may generally be distinguished from others. The symptoms of the eruptive fever, therefore, may be divided into those which it has in common with other fevers, and those which characterise it.

Along with other symptoms common to febrile diseases the patient generally complains of much thirst, is often troubled with nausea, sometimes with vomiting. The tongue is generally white and moist. In the more alarming cases subsultus tendinum, spasms of the limbs, delirium, or, what more frequently happens, coma supervene.

The last symptom indeed so frequently attends the eruptive fever of measles, that by some it is regarded as one of its diagnostic symptoms. This symptom indeed is not to be overlooked in forming the diagnosis of any eruptive fever; in all of which it is more apt to supervene than in fevers properly so called.

Adults in particular generally complain of much head-ach; and children, it has been observed, appear unusually morose. Pains of the back and loins also often attend this period; the face is flushed, the pulse frequent and hard, the respiration hurried,

frequent, and sometimes interrupted with sighs. These symptoms generally suffer some remission in the morning, returning
in the evening with increased severity.

On the third day, the nausea and vomiting increasing or appearing now for the first time, the skin becomes hotter and more
parched. If the patient has hitherto escaped delirium, it frequently shews itself on the evening of this day, or increases if it
had supervened at an earlier period. When there is no coma the
inquietude is considerable, and the sleep, if there be any, disturbed. The inquietude and distress of mind, Rhazes observes, is
greater in the measles than in the small-pox.

The matter rejected by vomiting is generally bilious, and when
a diarrhœa supervenes, which is also a frequent symptom, the
stools are frequently of the same kind ; and in children for the
most part of a green colour; " Quo fluxu," Burserius observes,
" ubi supervenit, vomitus et vomituritio fere sedantur." The diarrhœa, he adds, does not impede the appearance of the eruption.
In other cases however the bowels are costive, and sometimes, as
in small-pox, there is a tendency to sweating. Adults, Frank*
says, have been observed to sweat, but not so frequently or pro-
fusely as in small-pox. These sweats, he remarks, often prove
beneficial.

Such are the symptoms which the eruptive fever of measles
has in common with many other febrile diseases. As far as the
prognosis depends on them, it is collected in the same way as in
fevers properly so called. The more parched the skin, the harder
and more rapid the pulse, the more hurried and difficult the
breathing, the more the countenance is flushed, and the greater
the coma or delirium, the less favourable is the prognosis.

A considerable affection of the breathing with an unusually hard
pulse, is particularly to be dreaded, on account of the tendency to
pneumonic inflammation in the measles.

The following may be regarded as the diagnostic symptoms of
the eruptive fever of measles. It is not meant that these symptoms are never met with but in the eruptive fever of measles;
they are the symptoms of common catarrh ; but there they are
not accompanied with the symptoms just enumerated, the fever
for the most part is moderate, and always, we shall find, propor-
-tioned to the affection of the head, fauces, or breast.

On the second day of measles, if not earlier, the patient is attacked with a dry cough and hoarseness, with a sense of heaviness
in the head and eyes. The cough is often severe and obstinate,
Morton* calls it, " Tussis admodum molesta, frequens, pertinax
" et forina, quæ opii ipsius vires soporiferas plane superat." And

* Epitome de Cur. Hom. Morb.
† See Morton de Morbillis in his work De Febribus Inflammatoriis.

although he adds, a cough often precedes the eruption of the small-pox and scarlatina, yet it is seldom so violent as that which attends the eruptive fever of measles.

The cough is sometimes the first symptom of the complaint. Sometimes, Hoffman observes, it troubles the patient for a fortnight before the fever comes on. Other writers make the same observation. Of an epidemic at London in 1753 Dr. Heberden remarks, the cough often preceded the measles for seven or eight days. In such cases the cough is sometimes accompanied with pains of the throat, head, and back.

About the time that the cough generally supervenes, the throat becomes inflamed, impeding deglutition, and increasing the secretion of saliva. And in some cases, Frank observes, a profuse ptyalism supervenes. There is generally a sense of oppression and uneasy tightness about the breast, occasioning a degree of dyspnœa.

The appearance of the eyes however may be regarded as the best diagnostic symptom. They are red, swelled, itchy, very sensible to light, and watery, the tears sometimes falling over the cheeks.

The membrane of the nose is also inflamed, a copious thin secretion often running from it, and occasioning frequent sneezing. " Nec rarum est," Burserius remarks, speaking of the increased secretion from the nose, " sanguinem inde etiam abunde manare, " quo caput, oculi et fauces plerumque sublevantur." The hemorrhagy from the nose however has sometimes been so profuse as to threaten danger. The various hemorrhagies which occur in synocha occasionally appear in the eruptive fever of measles.

The eruption of measles is much less apt to be preceded by epileptic fits, than that of small-pox. In children they now and then occur. Like the eruption of small-pox too, that of the measles is sometimes preceded by severe pain of the back, which is an unfavourable symptom.

These symptoms in various degrees generally continue to increase till the eruption appears.

Such is the eruptive fever of measles ; and it has been observed of this complaint, as of small-pox, that the violence of the succeeding disease is generally proportioned to that of the eruptive fever.

With respect to the prognosis at this period, it may, upon the whole, be observed, that it is derived less from the state of the catarrhal, than that of the febrile symptoms, unless the former threaten suffocation, which sometimes happens, particularly in children, or we have reason to dread an inflammatory affection of the lungs.

It appears from what has been said, that the circumstances which distinguish the eruptive fever of measles from catarrh are, 1. The one complaint arising from contagion, the other from cold . 2. The greater violence of the febrile symptoms compared with the catarrhal in the measles. 3. The state of the eyes; for however mild the other catarrhal symptoms are, the affection of the eyes, which in common catarrh are less generally affected than the nose and throat, is always considerable in the measles. Lastly, certain symptoms' which frequently accompany the eruptive fever of measles, and are seldom observed in catarrh, particularly coma.

When the eruption makes its appearance, it places the nature of the complaint beyond a doubt. The eruption generally, shews itself towards the end of the third, or beginning of the fourth, day; although in some cases it is delayed to the fifth. It comes out on the forehead, in small points, like the bites of fleas, which at first are generally distinct, but here and there increasing in number and size, are soon formed into small clusters of different shapes; so that the face seems marked with red stains of various size and figure. In these clusters the individual pustules are seen with difficulty, but are always readily felt, rendering the parts they occupy rough to the touch. While the eruption is coming out, some degree of moisture is frequently observed on the skin; which is a favourable appearance.

From the face, the eruption gradually spreads to the neck, breast, trunk, and extremities. The eruption generally appears on the extremities, the day after it shews itself on the face, seldom either later or earlier. It sometimes, though rarely, happens that the eruption does not appear on the extremities at all.[*] Frank observes, that the morbillous like variolous eruption, sometimes appears in the mouth affecting the tongue.

On the trunk and extremities the small pustules are often more numerous; but they are generally less prominent, than on the face, so that on the former the red stains are often broader, though seldom so rough, as on the latter; although in all places where there is redness the inequality of the cuticle may be perceived. These stains vary in different cases, being broader and redder in some than in others.

Those in the face continue red or rather increase in redness for two days. On the third they assume a brownish colour. In the course of the fifth or at most of the sixth day of the eruption, that is, about the eighth or ninth day of the disease, the redness on the face disappears, although traces of the eruption often remain for four or five days longer. The cuticle is now broken

* Dr. Heberden.

and raised in the places which the eruption occupied, so that the face appears covered with a light whitish powder.

It is observed by Frank and others, that when the eruption is not very favourable, it sometimes leaves pits in the skin like those which follow the small-pox.

When the redness has almost left the face it is at its height in the extremities, where about a day or two later it runs the same course. The eruption continuing red longer than usual, is an unfavourable symptom. The more early and free the desquamation, which occasions the whitish appearance just mentioned, the more favourable is the prognosis. The eruption sometimes becomes livid and has even been observed to assume almost a black colour. These appearances indicate much danger. Sydenham and others observe, that they are not uncommon when the hot regimen and stimulating medicines have been employed, and are only to be removed by discontinuing the mode of treatment.

During the eruption, the face is turgid, but not swelled as in small-pox, and subsides as the eruption goes off. The eye-lids are sometimes so much swelled as to close the eyes.

It sometimes happens, as in mild cases of small-pox, that on the appearance of the eruption the fever entirely ceases; more frequently however it brings only partial relief. Sydenham observes that he never saw the vomiting recur after the eruption was out. Burserius makes the same observation, adding that the increase of temperature is generally lessened, and the pains of the loins, the delirium, and spasms mitigated. But the cough and difficulty of breathing are often increased at this period, even when the other symptoms suffer a considerable remission. The affection of the eyes and coma also often remain undiminished. More rarely even the febrile symptoms suffer no remission, and in some cases they even become more severe, after the cruption; and continue so till it terminates in desquamation. At the latter period a flow of sweat or of urine, a diarrhœa or other spontaneous evacuation, sometimes supervenes, followed by a remission of all the symptoms.*

Although the fever very generally disappears at the period of desquamation, if not before it, yet this is not universally the case; it sometimes continues and even becomes more alarming than at any former period. The coma in particular, Dr. Heberden remarks, sometimes returns after the eruption, and has even proved fatal at this period.

There is generally a considerable tendency to inflammation

* Dr. Heberden mentions an instance in which the cough was relieved by a copious salivation, which seemed to render the other symptoms milder

throughout the whole course of the measles, and those parts are most subject to it, 'which are most apt to be inflamed in common catarrh, the eyes, nose, fauces, and lungs. The inflammation of the eyes, nose, and fauces, is usually of little consequence ; it seldom becomes very troublesome, and declines with the other symptoms of the complaint. The inflammation of the lungs is more to be feared. It may supervene at any period of the complaint, but is most frequent after the eruption. If the fever continues at this period of the disease, the cough seldom fails to do so likewise, and this cough and fever often become a real pneumonia, or in scrophulous habits degenerate into phthisis pulmonalis.

· Such indeed is the tendency to inflammation in measles, that blood taken 'at any period almost always shews the buffy coat. There can be no doubt however that this tendency has been increased by the treatment formerly pursued in this as well as in other fevers. Those, says Sydenham, who had been treated with the hot regimen and stimulating medicines were most subject to inflammation of the lungs.

When neither the habit nor mode of treatment are bad, such consequences of the measles are far from being frequent, and then in most cases the febrile symptoms are moderate and the danger inconsiderable. Sydenham, from very extensive experience, has pronounced the measles a safe disease. It can only be regarded as such, when the fever abates on the appearance of the eruption, and ceases altogether at the period of desquamation, leaving the patient free from cough and dyspnœa.

The diarrhœa, which is generally salutary towards the termination of the disease, sometimes becomes profuse and troublesome or even dangerous. The same is true of other evacuations. Frank says, a profuse hemorrhagy from the nose has sometimes proved fatal after the eruption had disappeared.

Such is the course of the regular measles. It sometimes happens that it varies, yet in circumstances so trifling, that the disease still deserves the name of regular. Thus it sometimes happens that the eruption makes it first appearance on the neck or shoulders, instead of the face. It sometimes appears sooner, and sometimes later, than the usual time. There is sometimes no desquamation on the disappearance of the eruption. This happened in the measles of 1674 described by Sydenham, and Frank also observes, that he has sometimes seen the measles disappear without any desquamation.

Although these slight varieties do not warrant the name of irregular, yet they seem to indicate a variety, in general more dangerous, and more liable to be attended with inflammation of the lungs, than the more regular forms of the disease. Thus Sydenham observes of the measles of 1674, that more died of this measles than of that formerly epidemic ; for the fever and dyspnœa, which are common in the decline of the disease, were more severe and bore a greater resemblance to true pneumonia. Quarin* indeed remarks, that the eruption of the measles sometimes goes off without desquamation, the state of the patient notwithstanding being quite favourable. These slight variations from the common course, may be regarded as the connecting link between the regular and irregular forms of the disease.

ob 2. Of the Symptoms of Irregular Measles.

The irregular measles is a very dangerous, but fortunately, not a very common disease. Sydenham says nothing of this form of measles, for that of 1674 certainly does not deserve the name of irregular. This is surprising, as the irregular measles raged in London during his practice. He describes the measles of 1670 and 1674, and passes over in silence the regular measles which raged in 1672, as we are informed by the celebrated Morton, who says that this epidemic destroyed nearly 300† weekly.

This epidemic appeared in the autumnal season, whereas the regular measles, like other inflammatory complaints, generally makes its appearance about January, continues to increase to the vernal equinox, and then gradually declines, till it altogether disappears, about the summer solstice. This distinction however is not always observed; the irregular, like the regular, measles most frequently appears in the vernal months.

Since the time of Morton, the irregular measles has been described by a variety of authors, Huxham,‡ Matthiew,|| Burserius,§ Vogel,** &c. In the 4th vol. of the Medical Observations, the reader will find an account of this form of the disease by Dr. Watson, as it appeared in the Foundling Hospital in the springs of 1763 and 1768. Most of the later writers on the measles notice this form of the complaint.

* De Frebibus.

† Dr. Dickson accuses Morton of having greatly exaggerated the fatality of this epidemic. We have reason to believe that Morton was deceived with respect to its fatality. See Dr. Dickson's paper in the 4th vol. of the Medical Observations and Inquiries.

‡ See Huxham de Aere et Morbis Epidemicis, where he gives a short account of the epidemic measles which raged in the autumn of 1742.

|| See a paper by Matthiew in Baldinger's Sylloge Opus. Select. in which he gives a copious account of the irregular measles which raged in Alsace in 1766 and 1767. In this treatise the reader will find references to other writers who treat of this form of the complaint.

§ Institut. Med. Pract. The irregular measles described by Burserius differs considerably from that described by other writers, and resembles more the measles of 1674 described by Sydenham, which Burserius regards as an irregular form of the disease.

** De Cog. et Cur. Morb.

In the eruptive fever of the irregular measles, there are not many circumstances to distinguish it from that of the regular. The symptoms in general are more violent and the fever is sooner formed. The affection of the eyes, cough, and fever, being often considerable from the very commencement of the complaint. On the first night the patient is very restless, and on the next day the fever generally rises high, the cough and inflammation of the eyes increasing.

The eye-lids are sometimes so much swelled that they cannot be separated, and the eye-ball itself is often swelled and prominent; and in some cases there is much pain and inflammation of the meatus auditorius.

The pulse is now often more frequent, but less hard than in the regular measles. For the most part there is some degree of dyspnœa, and little or no expectoration attends the cough. When an expectoration of mucus attends the cough, Matthiew observes, it generally relieves both the febrile and local symptoms.

The restlessness increases, with a parched skin, much thirst, and sense of tightness and oppression about the præcordia. If coma does not supervene, the patient generally complains of an acute pain, often accompanied with a sense of heaviness in the head, or he becomes delirious.

The fauces are of a deep red colour, and sometimes, Vogel observes, assume the same appearance as in the cynanche maligna. Dr. Cameron, in the 21st vol. of the Gentleman's Magazine, mentions several cases in which it had this appearance, so that he regarded the complaint as a combination of the measles and cynanche maligna. The tongue is generally very foul, and the stools often unusually fetid.*

The eruption frequently makes its appearance on the second or third day, it is sometimes delayed to the fourth, fifth, or even a later period. In the epidemic described by Dr. Watson, the eruption generally appeared on the second day; whereas Burserius observes that in the irregular measles, it frequently does not take place till the third, fourth, fifth, sixth, seventh, or even eighth, day. In one of Dr. Cameron's patients the eruption appeared on the sixth day.

When the eruption, Burserius observes, is delayed to the fourth or fifth day, or longer, the excitement is less than in the regular measles. Debility often supervenes at an early period, the fever assuming the form of typhus. This change always indicates much danger, and if the patient escapes, his recovery is generally very slow.

The eruption does not always appear first on the face, as in the

* Matthiew.

more benign forms of the disease, but sometimes on the shoulders, the neck, or breast.

The duration of the eruption in irregular measles, is as various as that of the eruptive fever, though generally proportioned to it. When the eruption appears on the second day, it generally disappears on the fourth, or at most the fifth, or sixth day. When it does not appear till the fifth day, or later, it is often protracted to the twelfth, fourteenth, or seventeenth, or even twentieth day, at different times assuming various appearances; at one time red, at another pale or livid; and in some cases it assumes a black appearance.

Whether the complaint runs rapidly or not, the febrile symptoms generally suffer a considerable remission, and are sometimes for a short time wholly removed, after the disappearance of the eruption. In neither case however, is there any remission of the fever on its first coming out. But on the contrary the symptoms just enumerated are generally increased at this period. If nausea and vomiting have not appeared earlier, they very frequently supervene after the appearance of the eruption, and rise to a greater height than in the regular measles. The affection of the throat increases; the same may be said of the delirium and coma, when these symptoms have appeared at an early period; where they have not, either the one or the other generally makes its appearance now. The pulse becomes more frequent and less full, and when the disease has been protracted, small, feeble, and often irregular; the cough is rendered more violent, the hoarseness increases, the breathing corresponding to the state of the pulse becomes frequent and anxious, the dyspnœa sometimes threatening suffocation. Symptoms denoting the last stage of debility succeed, namely, dropsical swellings, petechiæ, hemorrhagies, tremors, subsultus tendinum, and convulsions which are often the forerunners of death.

In general, however, the fatal termination is delayed to a later period. In the irregular, as well as the regular measles, the symptoms which take place after the eruption has disappeared, are often most to be dreaded. Although the fever at this period generally abates, many of the symptoms become worse. The inflammation of the eyes sometimes degenerates into sores, which, if the patient survives, often continue to barrass him for a long time. The cough, dyspnœa, and oppression frequently remain and are often increased, with a frequent, feeble, and sometimes irregular pulse, and other symptoms of debility.

In this state diarrhœa sometimes supervenes, and generally serves only to increase the debility. When the delirium returns at this period, it is generally a fatal symptom.

When on the contrary the skin becomes moist, the restlessness is diminished, the cough and dyspnœa abate, and the strength begins to return, the pulse becoming fuller and less frequent, the prognosis is good.

. Inflammation of the lungs is more frequent at all periods of the irregular than regular measles. Suppurations of the brain, internal ear, and other parts also, frequently occur in this form of the disease, and sometimes prove fatal. Swellings now and then appear about the neck, on or about the fifth day, and are a very unfavourable symptom. If the patient survives, they often form abscesses and give much trouble.*

From what has been said it appears, that the regular and irregular measles differ chiefly in the four following circumstances.

1. All the symptoms, whether febrile or catarrhal, are generally more violent in the irregular, than in the regular, measles.

2. The fever in the former always shews a tendency to typhus.

3. In the regular measles, the affection of the fauces always resembles that produced by cold ; in the irregular, the fauces are frequently livid, and often assume completely the appearance of the cynanche maligna.

4. The duration of the different stages of the irregular measles is more uncertain. The eruptive fever, as well as the eruption, in regular measles continue for a certain length of time, at least never much exceed, or fall short of, it. In the irregular measles, the course both of the one and the other is sometimes very rapid, at other times very lingering.

The irregular measles might therefore be divided into two varieties, that in which the symptoms run high and are soon terminated, and that in which they are less violent and longer protracted ; and there is the more room for such a division, as the one of these varieties has been epidemic without the other making its appearance. The same epidemic however often assumes both forms.

Besides the regular and irregular forms of the disease, there are certain varieties as in small-pox, which now and then occur in all epidemics. The fever with all its usual symptoms, Quarin observes, has sometimes appeared without the eruption. Others make the same observation, the accuracy of which is called in question by Frank, but not (it appears from a variety of observations) on sufficient grounds. " During this measly season," (it is remarked in the fifth vol. of the Medical Essays) " several people who never had had the measles, had all the preceding symptoms of measles, which went off in a few days without any eruption, which they underwent months or years afterwards." The

---

* Matthiew.

reader will also find a case of the same kind related in Morton's work, " De Febribus Inflammatoriis Universalibus." .The case is entitled, " Febris morbillosa, absque ulla efflorescentia vel co-
" mitante vel subsequente, sanata."

It even appears from the following observation, that the contagion of measles may produce some of the symptoms peculiar to the measles, without either fever or eruption. Dr Home, in his account of the manner of communicating the measles by inoculation, which I shall presently have occasion to describe, observes, " March 27, inoculated a child of eight years old, with the same " blood which had been kept ten days loosely in my pocket-book ; " I was afraid when I used it that it was too weak. The sixth " day this child sneezed much, but never was hot or struck out. " This child took the measles in the natural way about two months " afterwards."

It also sometimes happens that, a few days after every symptom of the complaint is gone, the fever again returns, and is again attended with the eruption of measles. " But it often hap-
" pens," an author in the 2d. vol. of the Medical Museum observes, " after the measles are gone, the patient purged' and re-
" turned to his usual diet, that in the space of ten days he is sei-
" zed with grievous oppression at the breast, and great anxiety, a " fever, thirst, some spots on the skin of a deeper red than the " former. Faint sweats and short breathing conclude the scene, " whereof many have died the last summer. And this fever " seems sometimes induced by cold, and overloading the stomach." The second appearance of the measles is most frequent in the irregular form of the disease. Matthiew observes of that of Alsace that soon after the eruption had disappeared, a new fever came on, followed by a second eruption.

The following are the principal consequences to be dreaded from the measles, all of which are most apt to follow the irregular form of the disease.

There is no complaint more apt than the measles to call into action, if I may use the expression, any scrophulous tendency. Hence the most frequent consequences of the measles are scrophula in its various forms ; glandular tumors, marasmus from obstruction in the mesenteric glands, obstinate sores* often affecting the bones, the most fatal of all forms of scrophula, phthysis pulmonalis.

Even where there is no tendency to phthysis, inflammatory affections of the lungs are frequent after the measles.

---

* See the observations of Dr. Watson in the 4th vol. of the Medical Observations, and Dr. Huxham's Account of the Malignant Measles which raged at Plymouth in 1745.

The bowels are often left in a very weak state, a chronic diarr- hœa remaining, which has sometimes proved fatal.

If we except the lungs, no part suffers so frequently as the eyes, which (as appears from what has been said) are much affec- ted throughout the whole complaint.

. The ophthalmia often remains after the other symptoms, and becomes obstinate ; and in some cases the sight has been 'lost from ulceration of the cornea, in others from an affection of the nerve, a true amaurosis supervening.*

. When the measles has been tedious and severe, it sometimes terminates in dropsy, which, like the marasmus, seems frequent- ly to depend on glandular obstruction.

SECT. II.

Appearances on Dissection.

. . ON this part of the subject, there is little to be observed. If the patient dies under the eruption, the trachea and larger bran- ches of the bronchiæ, as in the small-pox, are often found cov- ered with it ; which may account for the increase of the cough after the appearance of the eruption. .

· When the patient dies with a swelled belly and hectic fever, the glands of the mesentery are found indurated ; when of ph- thysis, indurated tumors of various size, some of them containing pus, are observed in the lungs. · Such appearances however are not connected with the measles, but with other complaints, with which it is complicated. They will afterwards be considered more particularly.

. It was observed above, that inflammation of the viscera is more frequent in the irregular than in the regular measles ; in the for- mer also it is more liable to run to gangrene. Hence, in the ac- counts of the dissection of those who died of irregular measles, we find gangrene of some of the viscera an usual appearance. Dr Watson observes of the putrid measles, " Of those who di- " ed, some sunk under laborious respiration, more from dysen- " terio purging, the disease having attacked the bowels, and of " these one died of a mortification in the rectum. Besides this, " six others died sphacelated in some one, or more parts of the " body. The girls who died, most commonly became mortified " in the pudendum." He also mentions ulcers, which some- times became sphacelated on the cheeks, gums, and jaws.

" Several were opened," Dr. Watson continues, " under dif- " ferent circumstances attending this disease. In some who died

* Vogel.

" of laborious respiration, after the feverish heat and eruption were
" passed, the bronchial system was found very little loaded with mu-
" cus, but the substance of the lungs was tender, and the blood ves-
" sels were very much obstructed and distended. In some who
" died of laborious respiration and extreme debility, many strong
" adhesions were found between the lungs and plevra. The lungs
" were distended with blood, and part of them had begun to
" sphacelate. Part of the jejunum was sometimes inflamed and
" contained several worms." In some who died suddenly, it was
found that the sphacelus of the lungs had occasioned a fatal hemorrhagy. " Collections of purulent matter," Dr. Watson adds,
" were observed in none ; on the contrary, in this putrid disease,
" every morbid appearance indicated a sphacelus."

SECT. III.

Of the Causes of Measles.

THE measles, like the small-pox, seem to have been unknown
to the ancients, although on this indeed there are some disputes.*
The Arabians certainly first accurately described the disease. It
is from them we have the name morbilli. Rhazes, in particular,
gives us both its symptoms and the mode of treatment practised
in Arabia, which as well as the treatment of the small-pox was
more judicious than it had been with us till early in the present
century.

From what we know of the history of measles, and what we
every day see, we cannot doubt that it arises from a specific contagion.

So much was said of contagion in general, that there is little
to be added here. The measles, like other contagious diseases,
is not immediately produced when the cause is applied, but after
the contagion has remained in the body for a certain length of
time. The measles appear earlier after infection than the small-
pox, and the time of their appearance is rather more uniform,
being generally about the sixth and seldom later than the eighth
day. Dr. Heberden observes however, that he has known the
appearance of measles delayed even to the 14th or 15th day after infection.

The habits of body in which the measles are most apt to prove
benign or otherwise, are far from being well ascertained; almost
all we know on this subject is, that they are particularly unfavourable in plethoric, and often still more so in scrophulous, habits.
The measles appear to be less dangerous in pregnant women than
the small-pox. Dr. Heberden says, he never knew any harm

* See the observations of Matthie w and others.

done by this complaint in pregnancy. It sometimes happens however, as in the case of small-pox, that the fœtus in utero receives the measles from the mother.

The measles seldom attack the same person a second time, of which nevertheless there are a few well authenticated instances. " Nunquam enim," Morton observes, " in tota mea praxi novi " quemquam, præter unum puerum, secunda vice hoc morbo cor- " reptum." In the Medical Institutes of Burserius, the reader will find that the measles have not only appeared a second but even a third time in the same person. " Quod secundo et tertio " eundem hominem in eos incidisse ex fidis observatis constet;" and in the fifth volume of the Edinburgh Medical Essays, it is observed of the measles of 1735 and 1736, that many who had formerly had the complaint were seized with all its symptoms, not excepting the eruption, which, it is said, resembled that caused by the stinging of nettles.

The great success which attended inoculation for the small-pox, induced many to believe that similar advantage might be expected from it in the measles. The very prevalent opinion of its being received in the natural way by the lungs, and the lungs being the chief seat of danger in this disease seemed farther to strengthen the opinion. Dr. Home of Edinburgh, however, was the first who actually made the experiment.

He met with some difficulty from the measles not forming matter, and his not being able to collect a sufficient quantity of broken cuticle at the time of desquamation, to produce the disease. " I then applied," he observes, " directly to the magazine of all " epidemic diseases, the blood." He chose the blood when the eruption began to decline in patients who had a considerable degree of fever. He also ordered it to be taken from the most superficial cutaneous veins where the eruption was thickest.

While the blood came slowly from a slight incision it was received upon cotton, and an incision being made on each arm of the person to be inoculated, the cotton, as soon as possible after it had received the blood, was applied over these incisions, and kept upon them, with a considerable degree of pressure. He also used the precaution of allowing the incisions of those to be inoculated, to bleed for some time before the cotton was applied, that the fresh blood might not wash or too much dilute the morbillous matter. The cotton was permitted to remain on the part for three days. How far all these precautions are necessary to the success of the operation has not been determined.

Dr. Home inoculated ten or twelve patients in this way, in whom the operation succeeded equal to his hopes. The eruptive fever generally commenced six days after inoculation, and the symptoms of the complaint were milder than they generally are in the casual measles. The fever was less severe, the cough' either milder or wholly absent, the inflammation of the eyes was trifling; they watered however as much, and the sneezing was as frequent, as in the casual measles; nor did bad consequences follow any case of inoculated measles. No affection of the breast remaining after it.

The chief difference between the casual and inoculated measles seemed to be, the absence of any pulmonic affection at all periods of the latter.

Dr. Home now regarded it as ascertained that the natural measles are received by the lungs, and that on this circumstance depends the danger of the disease. He wished however to ascertain the symptoms of the complaint when evidently received by the lungs. He therefore put a piece of cotton which had remained in the nose of a patient under measles, into that of a healthy child, making him breathe through the infected cotton. The experiment although repeated did not succeed in inducing the disease. Nor, it is evident, if successful, would this experiment have decided the question whether or not the casual measles are received by the lungs. Dr. Home's experiments have not met with the attention they deserve. In scrophulous habits particularly, it would certainly be worth while to try his mode of inoculation. If a more extensive experience prove it capable of producing the effects ascribed to it by Dr. Home, it will certainly be an improvement of considerable importance.

The remains of the measles, to use the language of medical writers, seem to lurk in the body, that is, a morbid tendency remains for some time after this complaint, even where the patient appears to have regained his usual health.

It was observed above, that when the small-pox supervenes on the measles, the former is often of an unfavourable kind. This has been particularly remarked of the small-pox supervening on the putrid measles.

SECT. IV.

Of the Treatment of Measles.

AS the treatment in small-pox is divided into that of the distinct and that of the confluent form of the disease, so we may divide the treatment of measles into that of regular and that of irregular measles.

It has often been observed that the treatment of small-pox and measles, like their symptoms, is similar. It will be found however that almost all which either in the symptoms or mode of treatment of these complaints is similar, is only what is common to them and all other idiopathic fevers in which the synocha prevails.

It is true indeed that catarrhal symptoms often attend the small-pox, but these are not essential to the complaint; and are at most so slight as to demand little attention. In the measles, they not only form an essential but the most alarming part of the complaint.

As inoculation is not practised in the measles, we seldom have the advantage of certainly knowing under what complaint the patient labours as soon as he is attacked. If however we find that he never has had this complaint, that about six days before the appearance of the fever he had been exposed to the contagion of measles, and that the fever is accompanied with the diagnostic symptoms pointed out, there can be little doubt of the nature of the disease. The information required however cannot always be procured, and the diagnostic symptoms are often not alone sufficiently decisive at an early period to mark the disease with certainty, so that in many cases we cannot positively determine the disease to be measles, till the eruption appears. But this is not a matter of much consequence, since the train of symptoms present require very nearly the same mode of treatment, whether the complaint be measles, common synocha, or catarrh; the chief difference being that the same remedies are employed more assiduously in measles.

The treatment of the eruptive fever of measles differs little from that of the eruptive fever of small-pox. The diet should be the same as in the more severe forms of the distinct small-pox. We seldom see the measles so mild a disease as the most favourable inoculated small-pox, for even in the least dangerous forms, inflammatory complaints are to be dreaded. On this account, we find practitioners insisting much on a diluent and antiphlogistic diet, one of the best means we possess of preventing the appearance of inflammatory complaints. " Acarnibus quibuscunque " arcebam," Sydenham observes, of the diet in measles, " juscula " avenacea, hordeacea et similia, nonnumquam et pomum coctum " concedebam." " Dietam vero diluentem," Huxham[*] remarks, " mollem, omni carni vacuam instituere oportet." Morton, Mead, Burserius, and many others, might be quoted to the same purpose ; the last of these even dissuades from the use of milk. M. De Lassone however, having experienced the good effects of milk in the small-pox, made trial of it in measles, and thinks it of great service, particularly when a bilious diarrhœa supervenes and becomes profuse. Dr. Mead recommends asses' milk instead of that of cows.

But in managing the antiphlogistic diet we must always recol-

* De Aere et Morbis Epidemicis.

lect its tendency to produce debility, and in weak habits be careful not to push it too far. When the habit is very weak, Quarin justly observes, we must abstain from too much dilution.

With regard to exercise, if the patient find himself inclined, from the commencement of the febrile symptoms, to remain in bed, he should not be prevented; at the same time there is no occasion to confine him to bed against his inclination. In all cases, towards the period of the eruption, he feels fatigued and averse to motion.

Whether the patient be in bed or not, extremes of heat and cold are equally to be avoided. By the former we always increase the febrile symptoms, by the latter we run a risk of increasing the catarrhal.

After the benefit derived from the application of cold in the small-pox was perceived, many recommended it with equal freedom in the measles, and this practice is still defended by some, particularly the followers of Dr. Brown. Sydenham, who contributed more than any other practitioner of this country, to introduce the cool regimen, when he cautions against keeping the patient too warm in measles, says nothing of the application of cold. " Neque autem, vel stragulis vel igni, quibus sani adsueverant ", quidquam adjici patiebar." In other places he makes similar observations. Morton, the contemporary and almost the rival of Sydenham, adopted the same practice in this respect, and their example has been followed by the best practitioners since their time. This much at least is certain, that if experience has not proved the harm done by a free application of cold in the measles, the practice has not hitherto been sufficiently general to ascertain its safety, ;* at present therefore we may say of the degree of temperature, as of the exercise in this complaint, that it should in a great measure be regulated by the patient's feelings. It is particularly to be observed, that the partial or sudden application of cold, or exposing the patient to a current of air, is dangerous in the measles.

-, In most cases it is necessary to have recourse to other means for diminishing excitement. It is needless to repeat what has been said of nitre, saline draughts, &c. these are useful in all cases of excessive excitement. Acids, Quarin observes, are to be avoided, as they increase the cough.

Gentle cathartics are indispensible in all cases. They are not only useful by removing irritating matter and diminishing excitement, but also by obviating the tendency to inflammation in the head. Neutral salts are here perhaps the best cathartics ; analogy is much in favour of calomel.

* See the 650th paragraph of Dr. Cullen's First Lines.

Emetics have not been much employed in this complaint, except for the removal of certain symptoms, the treatment of which does not come under the general plan of cure.

The remedy which principally demands attention in measles, is blood-letting. Though the utility of blood-letting when the symptoms run high is generally admitted, there has been some difference of opinion respecting the period of the disease at which it should be employed. For the most part Sydenham did not recommend it till towards the end of the disease ; for which he has been criticised by many, particularly by Dr. Mead.*

Had Sydenham however taken the trouble to defend his practice in this instance, he might have found many solid arguments in support of it. Unless the inflammatory symptoms run unusually high, the danger at the commencement of the complaint is inconsiderable ; this period is succeeded by a greater or less remission, which is often followed by a more dangerous train of symptoms than any which preceded them. Why should we unnecessarily reduce the patient's strength in the two former stages, when in the last, should the inflammatory symptoms run high, more strength than can remain after such a disease is requisite to bear without injury the only means which can relieve them ?

" As this fever,'' Dr. Cullen remarks, " is sometimes violent " before the eruption though a sufficiently mild disease be to fol- " low, so bleeding is seldom very necessary during the eruptive " fever, and may often be reserved for the periods of great- " er danger which are perhaps to ensue." The reader will find a paper, in the 4th vol. of the Medical Observations and Inquiries, by Dr. Dickson, in which Sydenham's practice with respect to blood letting in measles is defended, and Dr. Mead censured for his observations on it.†

In some cases however, even unattended by visceral inflammation, the excitement is sufficient to warrant blood-letting at an early period, and we are here to determine as in common synocha. When the excitement is such as threatens immediate danger or much subsequent debility, we must have recourse to venesection.‡

---

* " Sanguis itaque, incipiente morbo, pro ætatis ac virium ratione de- " trahendus est." See Dr. Mead's Monita et Præcepta Med. In this observation we perceive the remains of the hypothesis which led to an indiscriminate use of blood-letting in fevers

† Dr. Dickson's defence of Sydenham rests on the latter not having met with cases in which the excitement was considerable in an early stage. But even when considerable, blood-letting should if possible be avoided at this period.

‡ The presence of the menstrual discharge, Dr. Heberden justly remarks, is no objection, as some have supposed, to the employment of blood-letting in the measles.

With regard to the employment of blood-letting at a late period of measles, it cannot be fully understood till the reader is made acquainted with its employment in inflammatory affections of the chest, which will afterwards be considered.

It is remarkable that blood-letting sometimes removes certain symptoms remaining after measles, for the removal of which under other circumstances very little, is to be expected from it. Thus it has removed cough, although unaccompanied by fever or the other symptoms denoting inflammation. It has even been found a successful remedy in the diarrhœa which remains after measles. " Quin et diarrhœa," Sydenham observes " quam mor-" billos excipere diximus, venæsectione pariter sanatur."

Concerning the use of blisters, so generally recommended in this complaint, it is only necessary to repeat an observation already made. If our view in using them be to remove fever, we shall very constantly be disappointed ; if to relieve local inflammation, we shall find them a powerful remedy. I shall presently have occasion to make observations on the symptoms for which they are employed.

So long a course of antiphlogistic measures, as is sometimes requisite in the measles, often leaves the patient in a state of much debility ; it is therefore necessary as soon as the inflammatory symptoms disappear, to use means for restoring the strength. In most cases a nourishing diet and a moderate use of wine will be sufficient, and the addition of the bark is proper if there is no reason to dread a return of the inflammatory symptoms.

Concerning the treatment of irregular measles, it will not be necessary to say a great deal. Like that of the confluent small-pox, it may be divided into the treatment of irregular measles when accompanied with synocha, and that necessary when the fever is typhus.

In the former the treatment differs only in degree from that of the regular measles. Cooling laxatives and blood-letting are necessary, and must be employed in sufficient extent to reduce the symptoms of excitement, whatever be the period of the disease. In measles, as in small-pox, a prejudice has prevailed against letting blood before the appearance of the eruption ; which demands as little attention in the one case as in the other. When the excitement threatens immediate danger or much subsequent debility, we must in the eruptive fever of measles, as in all other idiopathic fevers, have recourse to venesection. Nitre and kermes mineral are particularly recommended at this period by Matthiew.

The chief difference in the treatment of irregular measles accompanied with synocha, and the regular form of the disease, arises from the fever in the former being apt to assume the form of typhus. There is perhaps no febrile disease of this country more perplexing than a severe case of irregular measles, the excitement often indicating the most vigorous antiphlogistic means, while the succeeding debility frequently supervenes so suddenly as to render the use of these means even in the earliest stage precarious.

What appears to be the best plan in such cases has more than once been pointed out. It consists chiefly, in avoiding blood-letting if the excitement can be diminished by safer means ; if not, employing it only to that extent which the urgency of the symptoms absolutely requires. If the excitement is prevented from rising too high during the first days, the nature of the disease will soon sufficiently overcome it, and then every ounce of blood which has injudiciously been taken, adds to the danger. The tepid bath has been recommended when the excitment runs high; like other debilitating means it is to be employed with caution.*

When the fever has changed to typhus, at whatever period this happens, the opposite plan of treatment becomes necessary.—Evacuations and even refrigerants are then hurtful. Refrigerants, Quarin observes, are particularly hurtful when the patient is weak ; and Hoffman relates the cases of three children under measles, who fell a sacrifice to the use of nitre. There are no observations, as in the case of small-pox, which establish the utility of purging after the typhus appears.

Wine, bark, opiates, and as nourishing a diet as the stomach can receive, are then the remedies to be depended on.

There is nothing to be observed in addition to what has already been said of the use of these remedies. Some have been afraid of the bark in every form of measles ; this fear however appears to be wholly groundless. Among other writers on putrid measles, the reader may consult for the use of the bark in this complaint the observations of Dr. Cameron in the 1st vol. of the Medical Museum, and the 21st vol. of the Gentleman's Magazine.

It only remains to point out the means to be employed when certain symptoms supervene, the treatment of which does not come under the general plan of cure. On this part of the subject there is little to be said here in addition to what was observed respecting the treatment of the corresponding symptoms in small-pox.

The symptom which generally demands most attention is the cough. The medicines which relieve it have been termed pectoral, and are either mucilaginous or oily. A little gum-arabic, syrup, and water, answer as well as any. Hoffman observes,

* See the observations on this remedy in continued fever.

that he has found nothing more effectual for abating the cough than fresh drawn oil of almonds mixed with syrup, and given frequently to the quantity of half a spoonful in water gruel.

Diluting the mixture however renders it less effectual, since it seems to act, as Dr. Cullen remarks, merely by besmearing the fauces, thus allaying irritation at the glottis which is often the exciting cause of the cough. The less diluted it is therefore, provided it does not occasion disgust, the better it is calculated to answer the intention.

But Hoffman and the other physicians of his time believed, that the advantage of pectorals depended on their being received into the mass of blood, and poured out on the lungs. They therefore gave them in large quantity. A quantity of diluting liquors by allaying excitement will often diminish the cough, but they should not be combined with the pectoral mixture, by which the good effects of the latter are almost lost. It should be given in the quantity of about a dram immediately after the patient drinks, that it may remain in and besmear the fauces, repeating it every time he drinks, or when the inclination to cough is frequent. The quantity given at once should be small, as nothing loads the stomach more than mucilaginous and oily medicines. Of the two, the former appear to be preferable; they oppress the stomach less, and are more liable to adhere to the fauces.

When the cough is very troublesome, Quarin observes, inspiring the steam of warm water is often serviceable.

The most powerful however of all the medicines we possess for allaying the cough is opium, but its exhibition requires caution in a complaint where the inflammatory diathesis is so prevalent. Morton regarded opiates as inadmissible previous to the appearance of the eruption. " Utut delirium, tussis vigiliæ, &c. ea " postulare videantur, apprimé, atque religiose abstinendum est."

When the cough remains after the measles, Vogel recommends small doses of the sulphur auratum antimonii, occasionally combined with opium.

A hoarseness sometimes remains after the measles, and when accompanied neither with fever nor dyspnœa is sometimes removed by the bark.*

Difficulty of breathing may often be relieved by inhaling the vapour of warm water. The volatile alkali, or a gentle cathartic, often relieve this symptom. These failing, we must have recourse to venesection if the pulse admits of it; if not, blisters are the best remedy.

* See a paper by Dr. Whytt in the third volume of Essays and Observations Physical and Literary. Testaceous powders are said to be often serviceable in this hoarseness. See a paper in the second volume of the Medical Museum.

When dyspnœa remains after the measles, a perpetual blister on the sternum or a seton in the side are the best remedies, except where this symptom is urgent and attended with fever, in which case, blood-letting is generally necessary; and then the issue will be found the best means to prevent its return. It is proper to use some precautions to prevent the inflammation of the eyes from becoming troublesome; exposure to light should be avoided, and they may be washed occasionally with a little rose or plantain water.

A spontaneous diarrhœa should be kept moderate, but not stopped, particularly by the use of astringents and opiates. When it remains after the disease, Hoffman recommends the cascarilla. If it does not disappear soon after the febrile symptoms, it is to be treated like a case of simple diarrhœa, but still with caution, on account of the tendency to inflammatory complaints, which remains after the measles. For the same reason it is necessary for some time cautiously to avoid exposure to cold, and the other causes of such complaints.

CHAP. IV.

Of the Scarlet Fever.

THE Scarlet Fever, or, as it is termed by medical writers, Scarlatina, is defined by Dr. Cullen,

" Synocha contagiosa. Quarto morbi die facies aliquantum
" tumens; simul in cute passim rubor floridus, maculis amplis
" tandem coalescentibus, post tres dies in squamulas furfuraceas
" abiens, superveniente dein sæpe anasarca."

He divides the Scarlatina into two varieties, the Scarlatina Simplex, and the Scarlatina Cynanchica.

The former is defined, " Scarlatina nulla comitante cynanche."

Dr. Cullen observes, that although in the space of forty years he had seen the scarlet fever epidemic six or seven times, it had always assumed the appearance of the scarlatina cynanchica, and was, for the most part, attended with ulceration of the fauces. It appears however from the observation of Sydenham and others, that the simple scarlatina has sometimes been epidemic, without the other form of the complaint showing itself. It generally happens, that in the same epidemic some have the scarlet fever with, and others without, the affection of the throat; while others have the affection of the throat without any eruption.*

* " During the prevalence of this epidemic," Dr. Clark observes, " some patients had erysipelatous inflammation of the throat without ul-

It has long been disputed whether the scarlet fever and malignant sore throat ought to be esteemed different diseases, or only varieties of the same disease. This dispute is only of consequence from its having made some noise. I shall delay any observations on it till the symptoms of both complaints have been laid before the reader.

The second variety of scarlatina, Dr. Cullen defines, " Scarla-" tina cum cynanche ulcerosa." This is the most common form of the disease. Some think it should be regarded as a different complaint from that attended singly with the eruption or affection of the throat.* This question will be considered with the former ; it is enough at present to observe, that they are both of little consequence, since neither, take it which way we will, affects the mode of practice.

In considering the symptoms of scarlet fever, I shall follow the same mode of arrangement as in the foregoing exanthemata. In the first place, enumerating the symptoms which precede the eruption ; secondly, describing the eruption ; thirdly, enumerating the symptoms which accompany it ; and lastly, those which follow it.

It may seem proper, in laying down the symptoms of scarlatina, to keep in view the division of this disease into the two varieties just mentioned ; and this division might aptly be compared to that of the small-pox into distinct and confluent, or that of the measles into regular and anomalous.

For several reasons however it is unnecessary to insist much on the symptoms of scarlet fever unaccompanied by cynanche ; it is not often met with ; it may be readily known from what will be said of the scarlatina cynanchica ; and it does not require any particular mode of treatment. It is so mild a disease indeed that the assistance of the physician is seldom necessary. The following is Sydenham's description of this form of the complaint. The patient, as in other fevers, is seized with chills and rigors, but does not complain of much sickness ; soon after this the whole skin is covered with small red stains, more numerous, broader, redder, but not so uniform as those in measles ; these stains remain for two or three days and disappear with a desquamation of the cuticle, which appears in small scales that fall off and appear again two or three times in succession.†

ceration, others had ulceration of the tonsils without any rash, and some " had the scarlet eruption and fever without any affection of the throat." See Dr. Clark's Treatise on Fevers.

* See Dr. Cullen's Synopsis Nosologiæ Methodicæ. p. 138.

† See the 2d chapter of the 6th section of Sydenham's work, Circa Morborum Acutorum Historiam et Curationem.

SECT. I.

Of the Symptoms of Scarlet Fever.

AT the commencement, this fever differs little from others. It comes on with confusion of thought, lassitude, languor, dejection, chills, and shivering, often alternating with fits of heat. The thirst is generally considerable, and the patient is often troubled with anxiety, nausea, and vomiting. But the anxiety and vomiting are rather symptoms of the cynanche maligna, than of the scarlatina, and have been ranked among the diagnostic symptoms of the former.

, Soon after the appearance of these symptoms the patient feels some degree of pain about the throat, increased on swallowing. This is to be regarded as a favourable symptom; in cynanche maligna there is little pain in swallowing, and it is only as it approaches to this disease that the scarlatina is dangerous.

The uneasiness of the throat is sometimes among the first symptoms, and in some cases, Aaskow* observes, it appears before any other. The sore throat is not often attended with cough or other catarrhal symptoms, but frequently with a sense of stiffness in the muscles of the neck. These circumstances distinguish the eruptive fever of scarlatina from that of measles, the sore throat which seldom attends the latter assisting the diagnosis.

In some cases of scarlet fever however, as in the measles, the eyes are inflamed, watery, and incapable of bearing the light, the eye-lids are swelled, and the patient is troubled with sneezing†. More frequently cough has attended the eruptive fever of scarlatina, cases of which the reader will find in the works of Morton, one of the earliest writers on the complaint, and in Dr. Cotton's letter to Dr. Mead on a particular form of scarlatina prevalent at St. Alban's in 1748. Dr. Sims also observes of an epidemic scarlatina, that a short cough was a very frequent symptom, which was most severe when the throat was least affected.

On examining the internal fauces they are found very red and more or less swelled. A florid appearance and a considerable degree of swelling are favourable symptoms.

On the tonsils, velum pendulum palati, and uvula, the parts chiefly affected with inflammation, there generally, not always, appears a number of small, whitish, or greyish specks or sloughs. The darker their colour the less favourable is the prognosis.

The skin is now very hot, the pulse frequent, sometimes full

* Acta Societ. Hafniensis.
† See Frank's Epitome De Cur. Hom. Morb.

and strong which is a favourable symptom, at other times, particularly where the throat is of a purplish hue, and the specks of a dark colour, it is small and weak, though at the same time often hard, a state of the pulse which always indicates danger. The breathing is hurried, difficult, and sometimes rattling. The fever generally suffers an exacerbation towards night, and delirium sometimes supervenes; or the patient becomes comatose; either of which symptoms indicates considerable danger.

What first seemed greyish specks often now appear small ulcers. The internal fauces and mouth are loaded with viscid mucus, and the swelling of the fauces increasing, the swallowing becomes more difficult and painful.

In milder cases the sloughs continue till the fever is passed, and then falling off, an ulcer appears on one or both tonsils, which for the most part is well conditioned, and heals readily.

If hemorrhagy from the nose occurs at an early period, it often considerably relieves the fauces. A thin discharge from the nose, especially if fetid and if it excoriate the lips and nostrils, is a bad symptom. The same may be said of the diarrhœa which sometimes supervenes, and seems often to proceed from the morbid secretion of the fauces being swallowed.

But the purple colour and ulceration of the fauces, the coryza at least when the matter discharged is acrid, and the diarrhœa, are rather to be regarded as symptoms of the cynanche maligna than of the scarlatina.

Nausea and vomiting are more frequent in the progress than at the accession of the eruptive fever; and the vomiting, Frank observes, as in the eruptive fever of small-pox, is sometimes attended with pain at the stomach.

If the swelling of the throat at any period of the disease subside, a swelling sometimes appears in a neighbouring part. In an epidemic mentioned by Dr. Rush, a swelling behind the ear often followed that of the throat. Such a translation of the swelling generally denotes an unfavourable form of the disease. That mentioned by Dr. Rush approached to the nature of the cynanche maligna.

In less favourable cases, a little before the eruption appears, the face is sometimes flushed and somewhat swelled, and the eyes blood-shot and watery. It sometimes happens, though very rarely, that in children the eruption is preceded by an epileptic fit.*

The period of the eruption is more uncertain than in the other exanthemata. When the symptoms are moderate, it is general-

---

* See Sydenham's work on Acute Diseases, sect. 6th, chap. 2d, and a paper by Bang in the 2d vol. of the Acta Scc. Med. Hafniensis.

ly delayed to the third or fourth day; in more severe cases, it often appears on the second or even on the first day. Bang often saw it on the first day, Dr. Clark met with it within twelve hours from the commencement of the disease, and Dr. Cotton mentions cases in which the eruption appeared as soon as the fever.

The eruption first appears on the face, most frequently, Eikel observes, about the nose and mouth. like a red stain or blotch, which disappears on pressure.* Itsoon spreads over the neck, breast, trunk, and at length over every part of the body which often appears uniformly red. When this is the case the prognosis is better than when the redness appears here and there in blotches, which is sometimes the case on the trunk, while at the same time the redness is uniform on the extremities. The degree of redness also varies much; it is sometimes so pale, (in certain cases, for example, mentioned by Dr. Cotton) as not to be very remarkable; in other instances, as in some mentioned by Dr. Withering† and De Meza,‡ the whole body is so red that it has been compared to a boiled lobster.

When the eruption is nearly inspected, it appears to consist of innumerable little pimples running together. Upon the extremities and in the interstices of the blotches on the trunk, small points are often observed more prominent than those forming the stains, which is generally an unfavourable appearance.

The eruption seems much connected with the state of the throat, so that the former is seldom completely and uniformly diffused if the latter is alarming; and on the contrary if the affection of the throat be slight, the redness is more general.

Exceptions to this are mentioned by some writers. De Meza observes, that the sore-throat sometimes occurs without the eruption, and it often happens, he remarks, that in this case the sore throat is milder than it usually is when attended with the eruption. It is probable however, that the cases of sore throat alluded to by De Meza were of a different nature from that which attends the scarlatina. Dr. Rush, Frank, and others observe, that while the scarlatina anginosa prevails, other kinds of sore-throat are generally frequent.

A degree of swelling sometimes attends the eruption, appearing first on the face, especially on the eye-lids, afterwards on the neck, hands, and feet; in the majority of cases however this symptom is hardly perceptible.

The duration of the eruption is as uncertain as the time of its appearance. It frequently remains for three or four days, some-

* It sometimes makes its first appearance on the neck. See the observations of Eikel in the Act. Soc. Med. Haf, &c.
† See Withering on the Scarlatina Anginosa.
‡ See the observations of De Meza in the Act. Soc. Med. Haf.

times disappears within twenty-four hours. In general, however, the red colour begins to change into a brown in the space of two or three days; soon after this the skin becomes rough, and the cuticle begins to peel off, sometimes in small scales at other times in large pieces, which process now and then continues as late as the twenty-eighth or thirtieth day. In most instances it is finished much sooner.

The nails have now and then been cast off with the cuticle; sometimes the cuticle of the tongue peels off at the same time.* In other cases the tongue only becomes clean. The tongue, Eickel observes, becomes clean while the desquamation goes on, which is a favourable appearance.

When the desquamation begins, a gentle sweat very generally appears, while all the symptoms abate and are soon wholly removed.

Such is the general course of the eruption in scarlatina; considerable variations have been occasionally observed. " Die au-
" tem morbi quarto, quinto, vel sexto, singuli scarlatinam efflo-
" rescentiam per cuticulam ubique sparsam perpetiebantur, eam-
" que per septem, octo vel decem dies protensam."† Varieties of this kind however are rarely observed. The most remarkable variety in the eruption of scarlatina is analogous to the variety of measles, termed Rubeola Variolides. " In some," Dr. Rush observes, " an eruption like the chicken-pox attended the sore-throat." This variety is called by Sauvages Scarlatina Variolosa.

The symptoms which accompany the eruption differ little from those which precede it. The febrile symptoms are seldom relieved by its appearance. The inflammation and swelling of the internal fauces in some cases abate; in others, they are increased; and the viscid mucus, which is now often secreted in considerable quantity, renders the deglutition more difficult. The swelling however is seldom so considerable as it frequently is in other kinds of sore-throat. When the maxillary and parotid glands partake of the swelling, it is sometimes so considerable as to affect the breathing.

The viscid mucus frequently assumes the appearance of a crust covering the tonsils and neighbouring parts. When by the use of gargles this mucus is washed off, which may readily be done, the surface sometimes appears inflamed but sound, at other times covered with small ulcers. In the worst cases, small masses resembling coagulated blood are frequently spit up, and the acrid secretion from the nares is increased or supervenes if it did not appear before the eruption, excoriating the lips and nostrils. The eyes assume a dull and heavy appearance, and the face appears bloated, and affected with œdematous swelling; the hands

* See the Observations of Bang and others.
† Morton De Feb. Scarlat.

and fingers, are often affected in the same way, and painful on
pressure ; or severe pains of the extremities without swelling,
much restlessness, delirium or coma supervene. But such cases
rather deserve the name of cynanche maligna than scarlatina.

In the most favourable cases the symptoms upon the whole become milder after the appearance of the eruption. The febrile
symptoms indeed are seldom much relieved, but the inflammation
and swelling of the fauces begin to abate, and by the time the
eruption is over, if there be a free desquamation with moisture
on the skin, have wholly disappeared, at most leaving only superficial ulcers of the tonsils which soon heal.

The fever now abates, and for the most part in a short time
wholly disappears ; more or less of an œdematous swelling appearing on the legs and sometimes over the whole body, which
in two or three days goes off without the assistance of medicine,
some degree of debility remaining, which as the appetite is generally keen, is soon removed by a nourishing diet. In less favourable cases, though more rarely, the febrile as well as other
symptoms continue to harrass the patient after the eruption has
disappeared.

It sometimes happens that although the patient is free of complaint for some days after the eruption disappears, yet in a short
time, particularly if the skin has remained dry during the desquamation, symptoms of fever again shew themselves, and as
sometimes happens in the other exanthemata, are now and then
followed by a second eruption. If the skin remains dry, Eickel
observes, after the beginning of the desquamation, the disease will
either be dangerous or protracted, the affection of the fauces and
fever become worse, and in some cases a new eruption appears
on the face and neck ; which unfavourable symptoms, he adds,
generally disappear as soon as the skin becomes moist.

The same author remarks, that a similar train of symptoms
often supervenes both in the measles and erysipelas, when the
skin remains dry at the time of desquamation.

If there be no moisture on the skin at the time of desquamation, a running from the ear, sometimes very copious and fetid,
now and then supervenes, and the hearing has sometimes been
impaired or wholly lost. It sometimes happens that a swelling
of the parotid glands comes on at this period, which is now and
then relieved by a spontaneous salivation. The swelling of the
parotid glands is unfavourable, the running from the ear more so,
and the prognosis is still worse if both symptoms attend, especially, Eickel observes, if the parotids shew a tendency to suppuration, from which, he says, he never observed any benefit.

The swelling of the parotids is generally relieved when the
running from the ears is considerable, and again increases when

this is lessened. Eickel remarks that while the running from the ear and the swelling of the parotids remain, the best diaphoretics cannot produce a general moisture on the skin. The swelling of the parotid glands, Dr. Sims observes, occurs at various periods of the disease, and seems when it is late of appearing to protract all the symptoms of the complaint, or even to renew them after they had ceased, the eruption itself not excepted.*

Sometimes the symptoms which succeed the eruption take a different turn, the patient falls into obstinate anasarcous swellings, or is attacked with dropsy of some of the cavities. At other times the swelling of the glands about the neck suppurate, obstinate sores forming in the nose and ears and even affecting the bones. The mouth, lips, and palate, and the parts in the neighbourhood of the anus, also occasionally suffer from ulceration.

The inflammation sometimes spreads to the trachea and lungs, occasioning hoarseness, violent coughing, and wheezing or rattling breathing; † or as in cases mentioned by Drs. Rush, Home, and others, a squeaking voice similar to that which attends the croup. ‡

Symptoms of debility often attended with scanty, sometimes with bloody, urine, have now and then appeared after the patient has remained well for some days or even weeks. This train of symptoms is mentioned by Plenciz, Quarin, and De Haen in the continuation of the 1st vol. of his Rat. Med.|| Dr. Sims and Dr. Withering mention a similar train of symptoms, after the complaint seemed almost removed : there often supervened, the former remarks, an extreme degree of languor, which appeared to the patient the fore-runner of death, but which was not attended with much if any danger, and generally went off without the assistance of medicine. It was otherwise in the cases which Dr. Withering saw. In ten or fifteen days from the termination of the fever, he observes, and when a complete recovery might have been expected, another train of symptoms often appeared, and frequently proved fatal. The patient complained of an unaccountable languor and debility, and a stiffness in the limbs, the pulse became frequent,§ the sleep was disturbed, and the appetite lost, the urine

<hr/>

* See a paper by Dr. Sims in the 1st vol of the Memoirs of the London Medical Society. Plenciz in his Tractatus de Scarlatina, Quarin in his work De Febribus, and others, make similar observations.

† See the observations of Dr. Clark.

‡ In the case of Dr. Morton's daughter, related by him, the scarlatina terminated in an intermitting fever, which was removed by the bark.

|| These symptoms indicate a tendency to dropsy, as farther appears from the treatment found most successful in them. Diuretics and cathartics, De Haen observes, were sometimes serviceable, diaphoretics very rarely. The medicine chiefly recommended by Plenciz and De Haen, has for its principal ingredients calomel and squills. The cases mentioned by Dr. Withering often terminated in confirmed dropsy.

§ Some of the other authors just mentioned remark that the danger was greatest when fever supervened.

was scanty, and the patient soon after fell into dropsy, which sometimes appeared in the form of ascites, sometimes in that of anasarca, and resisted all the usual means.

The train of symptoms mentioned by these writers seems to
be only a greater degree of that condition of body which in almost
all cases remains after the scarlatina, and gives rise to the more
trivial dropsical affection which follows this disease.

Although the swelling of the parotids has not previously appeared, it sometimes supervenes with the anasarca, and even goes
on to suppuration. The reader will find cases of this kind mentioned by Bang, who observes that epileptic fits sometimes both
precede and follow the dropsical swellings. De Meza also says,
that during these swellings he has seen both children and adults
seized with epilepsy, which did not however prove dangerous, and
seemed generally owing to exposure to cold, or some error in
diet.

Death seldom happens at a very early period of the scarlatina.
Where the symptoms run high and the eruption appears on the
first or second day, the patient is sometimes carried off on the
fourth or fifth, in other cases seldom sooner than the eighth or
ninth day, and often later. " The length of the disease," Dr.
Clark observes, " was uncertain ; there was seldom any sensible
" crisis, some soon recovered, others had no favourable signs till
" the twelfth or sixteenth day. Five only that I attended died
" before the eighth, four on the ninth, and in all, the other cases
" that proved fatal the patients protracted their miserable exist-
" ence to the thirteenth, fifteenth, sixteenth, seventeenth, and
" sometimes to the nineteenth day of the disease."

It may be observed upon the whole, that the true scarlet fever
is a very mild disease. It is only in proportion as it partakes of
the nature of the cynanche maligna that it becomes dangerous.
In collecting the prognosis, therefore, the symptoms shewing a
tendency to the cynanche maligna particularly demand attention.
These I shall recapitulate, contrasting them with the corresponding symptoms of the mild scarlatina. They are not only of consequence in determining the prognosis, but of the first importance
in regulating the treatment of the disease.

If the scarlatina makes its attack with only a degree of lassitude,
languor, dejection of spirits, and shivering, the disease promises
to be less dangerous, and to approach less to the nature of cynanche
maligna, than when, along with these symptoms, the patient is
troubled with anxiety, nausea, and vomiting.

If the internal fauces are of a florid colour, and considerably
swelled, with difficult and painful deglutition, the prognosis is better, than when they appear of a dark red or purple colour, without swelling, the deglutition being easy and attended with little
or no pain.

If the specks, which appear about the tonsils, velum pendulum, and uvula, be of a whitish colour and are not soon changed into ulcers, the disease is more favourable, than when they are of an ash or brown colour, and become ulcerous at an early period.

When there is no running from the nose, or such as produces no excoriation, the prognosis is better, than when a thin acrid and fetid secretion runs from it.

It is also a sign of the mildness of the disease to be unattended with purging, and of great danger when the purging excoriates the anus.

When the pulse is strong and full the complaint is less dangerous, than when it shows a tendency to become weak and irregular.

When the patient bears the complaint well, and without much loss of strength, his situation is more favourable than when he is restless and debilitated.

When the mental functions remain unaffected, the prognosis is better than when delirium or coma supervene.

If the eruption is delayed till the third or fourth day, the disease is safer than when it appears on the second. When it appears on the first day the prognosis is generally bad.

When it is universal, every part of the body becoming uniformly red, the prognosis is better than when it comes out here and there in stains or blotches, or in small points.

When its appearance is followed by a remission of the symptoms in the throat, the prognosis is more favourable than when the affection of the throat increases. A tendency to swelling in the neck, hands, and feet, and the eruption being less considerable on the trunk than extremities, add to the unfavourable prognosis.

The same may be said of the eruption appearing unsteady, and the fever not remitting at the period of desquamation.

Glandular swellings also are unfavourable symptoms.

When the dyspnœa is considerable, without much swelling about the throat, there is reason to apprehend that the inflammation has spread to the trachea, which is always an alarming accident. The inflammation also sometimes extends along the œsophagus to the stomach, or along the eustachian tube, occasioning acute ear-ach.*

Hemorrhagies in general are unfavourable, unless at an early

* See Withering on the Scarlatina.

period and when the excitement is considerable. Bloody "saliva" in particular denotes an unfavourable state of the fauces.

All anomalous consequences of the scarlatina are to be dreaded:

SECT. II.

Of the Causes of the Scarlet Fever.

THERE is no mention of the scarlet fever in the works of Hippocrates; nor do we find it mentioned as a distinct disease by any other of the Greek or Roman writers. Some of them have taken notice of a scarlet rash as an accidental occurrence in fever, but not as marking a distinct genus.

Prosper Martianus, an Italian physician, is among the earliest writers on this complaint. He gave an account of the scarlatina as it appeared at Rome about the middle of the seventeenth century. It soon after made its appearance in London, and was described both by Sydenham and Morton, who term it Febris Scarlatina. They met with it however, under different forms. Sydenham describes it in its mildest state. Morton met with many instances, in which alarming symptoms appeared, and which, as was hinted above, varied in some respects from the ordinary course of the disease; but he did not always distinguish very accurately between measles and scarlatina. The disease described by Prosper Martianus resembles that described by Sydenham.†

Since the days of these writers the complaint has been described by a variety of authors. This disease, De Haen observes, was hardly known in the sixteenth and seventeenth centuries, but has appeared very frequently in the present.

The cynanche maligna, so much connected with the scarlatina,* is said to have made its first appearance about the year 1610 in Spain, where it is called Garrotillo. From Spain it soon spread to other countries of Europe. It appeared in Naples in 1618, where it raged for twenty years, destroying great numbers. If we compare the accounts of these epidemics with what Sydenham and Prosper Martianus say of the scarlatina, we shall be inclined to believe that this fever and the cynanche maligna, on their first appearance were more distinct diseases than we now find them to be.

It appears from the history of the scarlatina, that its exciting

* See Plenciz' Tractatus de Scarlatina.

† The scarlet fever which Morton describes prevailed in the same year in which Sydenham died, which is the reason we do not find it mentioned by the latter.

cause is a specific contagion. Concerning its predisposing causes little has been determined. It has only been ascertained that
children are more subject to it than adults, and those of a lax habit of body than the more robust. Females have generally been
supposed to be more liable to the scarlatina than males. Many
more of the female than of the male sex, Dr. Sims observes,
were seized with the scarlatina anginosa. It seemed particularly fatal to girls from two to eight years of age. He saw but one
child at the breast who had the complaint, and that but slightly.
Dr. Fothergill also observes, that women are more subject to it
than men. This however is contradicted by the observations of
Dr. Clark.* And some have even doubted whether young peo-
people are more subject to the scarlatina than adults. Bang asserts that all under thirty are equally subject to it. But whatever
may have happened in the particular epidemics which he saw, it
has been well ascertained, that those under puberty are most liable to this disease.

The scarlet fever, Sydenham observes, may appear at any season of the year, but it most frequently shews itself about the end
of summer. Fothergill and others make the same observation.
It is sometimes checked by a severe winter. Dr. Sims remarks
that he has seen it wholly at a stand during some days of sharp
frost, after which however it seemed to recover new vigour. It
generally disappears in the spring, but has been known to continue for several years, and consequently has withstood the different seasons.

Physicians have endeavored to ascertain the circumstances
which determine the severity of this disease. " The remote
" and external causes," Dr. Clark observes, " which had the most
" obvious influence in rendering the epidemic malignant, may
" be reduced to the three following, namely the heat and moist-
" ure of the air, and effluvia arising from many persons being
" crowded together in the same house, or often in the same
" room."

The constitution of the patient has a considerable effect in
rendering the disease mild or otherwise. I have seen it at the
same time assume all its various appearances in different individ-
uals of the same family. But what circumstances in the constitution render the disease mild or otherwise, have not been ascertained. We have reason to believe that it is most severe in the
debilitated and the plethoric. In the latter I have known it assume its worst form, while in others similarly circumstanced it
proved very mild.

* See Dr. Clark's Table of Patients labouring under Scarlatina received into the Newcastle Dispensary.

Respecting the means of prevention, there is nothing to be added to what was said when speaking of contagion in general.*

It has been asserted by some, that the scarlatina never attacks the same person a second time. Bang and others declare they never knew this happen. More extensive observation has contradicted this opinion. It appears however that the scarlatina properly so called, namely, that in which the eruption is complete, is less apt to attack the same person a second time, than that in which the eruption is imperfect and the affection of the throat considerable. The recurrence of the true cynanche maligna in the same person has not been questioned; although there is reason to believe that this complaint also is less apt to attack those who have formerly laboured under it. It is observed in the Edinburgh Medical Essays, that such as formerly had had scarlet fever without sore-throat, were now attacked with the sore-throat without the eruption; those who had formerly had the sore-throat, now had the fever and eruption without any affection of the throat. All the others had both the eruption and sore-throat. There are even instances in the same epidemic of the same person having the disease first in the one form, and then in the other.

SECT. III.

Of the Treatment of the Scarlet Fever.

AS the treatment of small-pox was divided into that of the distinct and that of the confluent form, and as the treatment in measles was divided into that of regular and that of irregular measles, so the treatment of scarlatina may be divided into that of simple scarlatina, and that of the scarlatina cynanchica.

It is unnecessary to enter particularly into the treatment of the former; it differs little from that of a mild synocha, and consequently little from that of the distinct small-pox or regular measles. The particular nature of the complaints, however, points out some difference in the treatment of even the mildest cases of small-pox, measles, and scarlatina, which is not to be overlooked.

In the small-pox, the application of cold can hardly be too free; in the scarlatina, from the greater tendency to inflammatory affections, it requires more caution. Any sudden or partial appli-

---

* Dr. Sims says, he found Rhubarb given in small doses, so as to support a moderate catharsis, a good preventive, while the scarlatina anginosa raged. He also thought it was useful in moderating the ensuing disease, when given between the period of infection and the commencement of the complaint.

cation of cold in measles is still more precarious, the catarrhal symptoms always demanding particular attention, which is not the case either in the distinct small-pox or simple scarlatina.

As the fever in distinct small-pox ceases when the eruption is completed, and as the application of cold is very free, other antiphlogistic measures are less necessary than in the measles and scarlatina, where even in mild cases the fever usually does not cease while the eruption is out, and an equally free application of cold is inadmissible. Besides, the greater tendency to inflammation in the measles and scarlatina, enforces the necessity of an attention to the antiphlogistic plan ; and as the measles are most apt to be accompanied with or followed by visceral inflammation, in this complaint a strict attention to the antiphlogistic regimen is least dispensable ; yet on this very account the more powerful antiphlogistic means, blood-letting or much purging are to be employed with greater caution at an early period, than in either small-pox or scarlatina, because visceral inflammations supervening when the strength has been reduced, very frequently prove fatal.

With regard to the treatment of the scarlatina cynanchica, as this form of the disease may be regarded as a combination of the simple scarlatina and cynanche maligna, its treatment cannot be understood without being acquainted with the treatment of the latter complaint. For the treatment of the scarlatina cynanchica therefore, I must refer to what will be said of the treatment of cynanche maligna in the next volume.

CHAP. V.

Of the Plague.

THE Plague is defined by Dr. Cullen,

"" Typhus maxime contagiosa. Incerto morbi die eruptio bu-
" bonum vel anthracum."

Although few British physicians have occasion to practise in the plague, the propriety of being acquainted with a disease, which has demanded so much attention, and bears so strong an analogy to complaints which every day fall under their care, is too apparent to require any comment. Besides, we cannot foresee in what circumstances we may be placed; and for a physician to betray ignorance of the plague would be unpardonable.

There are few diseases so remarkably varied, and there are few, perhaps none, of which it is more difficult to give an account, which shall be at the same time sufficiently full and distinct.¹ The reader will find the best writers, who have had an opportunity of seeing the disease, complaining of this difficulty.

As much as possible to prevent confusion, they have divided the plague into different classes ; nor is it possible without this to give a just view of the complaint, since no two diseases are more opposite than the different forms of the plague. In one we shall find it the most dreadful of all fevers, destroying without exception all whom it attacks ; in another we shall find it consisting chiefly of an eruption unattended by danger. Why, it may be said, are diseases so different, regarded only as varieties of the same ? However different these extremes, they are not only produced by the same specific contagion, but almost insensibly run into each other ; from which we may form some idea of the variety which the plague presents It will not then appear surprising that the difficulty of arranging its symptoms, so as on the one hand to avoid confusion, and on the other to give a comprehensive view of the complaint, be very great. In fact there is no author, although most of those who have written on the plague speak from their own observation, who has overcome this difficulty. In all we find the account either short, and consequently more or less imperfect, or of considerable length and more or less confused. So varied are the symptoms of the plague, that if the common varieties are given, the account must be tedious, and then it is impossible perhaps to prevents it being in some degree perplexed.

I shall not spend time by laying before the reader the modes of division adopted by different writers, or by pointing out the objections which might be made to them. The objections consist chiefly, in many of the divisions not being marked with sufficient precision, so that it is often impossible to say what are the corresponding divisions in the different accounts of the disease ; as the reader will perceive if, for example, he compare together the different accounts of the plague in the Traité de la Peste, or any of these with the division adopted by Dr. Russell in his Treatise on the disease.

In dividing a disease into varieties, each variety must be marked by some symptom which constantly attends it. This symptom must not be accidental or unconnected with the state of the symptoms in general, which would render the division useless ; but must mark a variety, in which the symptoms on the whole, and, what renders the division of more importance, the prognosis, differ from those of other forms of the complaint.

I shall not defer a particular account of the eruptions, namely, the buboes, carbuncles, &c. till after the different forms of the disease have been considered, as has usually been done ; by which we are forced to use terms before they have been defined ; nor on the other hand, is it proper, where the variety is so great, to interrupt the account of the general course of the disease, in order to describe the different eruptions. It therefore appears necessary to depart from the order which has been pursued in laying down the symptoms of the other exanthemata, and to regard bubo, carbuncle, &c. as terms which must be defined, before proceeding to give the symptoms of the plague.

SECT. I.

Of Pestilential Eruptions.

1. OF Pestilential Buboes.

A pestilential bubo at its commencement is a small, hard, round tumour, readily perceptible to the touch, about the size and shape of a pea, it is moveable under the skin, the appearance of which is not altered at an early period, the bubo lying at a greater or less depth, and the swelling not appearing externally.

As the tumified gland enlarges, it changes from a round to an oval shape, becoming at the same time less moveable. The integuments now begin to thicken and the swelling to appear externally.

The appearance of the bubo is often preceded by a sense of tightness and pain sometimes lancinating, or itchiness, in the part where it is about to appear, now and then by shivering. In many cases however, the small swelling just described comes on without being preceded by any peculiar symptoms.

Some buboes are indolent and insensible, others very sensible and rapid in their progress. The tumour advancing quickly to suppuration, is generally regarded as favourable. When the buboes suppurate properly, De Mertens observes,* and there is a separation of eschars from the carbuncles, with a remission of the febrile symptoms, the prognosis is good. No general rule however can be laid down. Cases where early suppuration takes place often prove fatal; and there are many histories of cases terminating favourably where the buboes were extremely indolent and terminated in resolution.

It is difficult to foresee in what way a bubo will terminate. The fluctuation is often scarce perceptible where suppuration has taken place, and buboes are sometimes resolved after fluctuation has been very evident. Their progress indeed is almost always more or less irregular, especially after the first week. At one time they seem advancing to suppuration, at another show a tendency to resolution. " But these variations," Dr. Russell re-

* See his Account of the Plague of Russia.

marks, " chiefly respected the integuments ; for the gland itself
" when carefully explored was seldom found to alter, and where
" the tumour actually dispersed, it was not suddenly, but by slow
" degrees. , Thus from the alteration in the teguments alone, the
" whole tumour, on a superficial view, seemed to lessen or in=
" crease, though the gland remained the same ; and I am inclined
" to think that this deception was often the cause of the bubo be-
" ing said to fluctuate, or to vanish in appearance entirely, and
" again return." He adds however, " At the same time I am far
" from thinking that this fluctuation was never real," And Chenot* observes, " Vidimus quoque abruptam suppurationem in his
" resuscitari ac demum per effusionem puris absolvi."

The bubo as it increases in size becomes somewhat flat ; and
generally about the second week, the skin over it grows tense and
painful, and begins to be inflamed. In some eases the inflammation is moderate, in others considerable ; but it seldom terminates in gangrene, although the skin now and then assumes a
bluish colour.

It sometimes happens however, that the bubo runs to suppuration without any degree of inflammation appearing on the skin,
and then, as it is generally harder than a suppurated venereal bubo, it is often difficult to determine whether suppuration has taken
place or not. When buboes break spontaneously, it generally
happens in the third week, sometimes at a later period.

The buboes most frequently appear in the groins or a little lower, among the lowest cluster of the inguinal glands ; they also
frequently appear among the axillary glands ; sometimes, though
more rarely, they have their seat in the parotid, and the disease
is then by many reckoned more dangerous than when the buboes
appear in the groins or armpits. Still more rarely they appear
in the maxillary or cervical glands.

" The latter two," namely the maxillary and cervical glands,
Dr. Russell remarks, " were seldom observed to swell without
" either the parotid swelling at the same time or soon after, or a
" carbuncle protruding near them ; they never were the sole
" pestilential eruptions, and I recollect few instances of their com-
" ing to maturation." It has been remarked by others, that the
parotid bubo seldom appears unaccompanied by one or more in
the axillæ or groin.

It may upon the whole be observed, that the axillary buboes
suppurate more frequently than those situated about the fauces,
and the inguinal more frequently than the axillary.

Buboes often make their appearance on the first day of the
complaint ; sometimes indeed they are among the first symptoms.

* See his Treatise on the Plague.

It has been observed, that when they appear later than the third
or fourth day, they are generally preceded by an exacerbation of
the febrile symptoms. Those which come out at so late a period,
however, are not, for the most part, the first which appear in the
course of the complaint; for a succession of buboes sometimes
takes place, till three or four have made their appearance. In
this case several hours usually intervene between the appearance
of any two of them.

" It sometimes happens that no buboes appear, and these cases
are upon the whole the most fatal. This is a circumstance which
particularly demands attention, as the cases unattended by buboes
and other pestilential eruptions generally make their appearance
at the commencement of the epidemic, and have often, in consequence of the absence of the eruptions, been mistaken for other
complaints. In other cases, particularly towards the decline of
the epidemic, the buboes and other eruptions often form the principal part of the complaint, which is then unattended by danger;
from which it would appear, that the eruptions in the plague are
to be regarded as favourable symptoms; but of this I shall presently have occasion to speak more particularly.

Where the inflamed gland advances to suppuration more rapidly than the integuments troublesome fistulous ulcers are sometimes formed, if an artificial opening has not been made in the
skin. This accident however is rare; in general the buboes, left
to themselves, do not prove troublesome.

When they do not suppurate, and the patient recovers, they
gradually disperse, generally in the space of a few weeks. In
some cases they are succeeded by an induration of the gland,
which remains for many months. Even where suppuration has
taken place, if the cure proves tedious, either in consequence of
the matter having been discharged by too small an opening, or
the opening having repeatedly closed in the progress of the
cure, a similar induration sometimes succeeds, which in like
manner sooner or later disappears, these indurations never terminating in cancer.

Such are the circumstances to be learned from attending to the
external appearances of the buboes; some further circumstances,
of less moment however, have been ascertained by dissection.

It has been the practice of many, particularly the French surgeons, to extirpate the buboes; which gave them an opportunity
of observing the internal changes which take place in them.
From the appearances on dissection they have been divided into
several different species. It is unnecessary to detain the reader
with an account of this hitherto useless division; he will find it at
length in the Traité de la Peste from the 428th to the 434th page.
One observation deserves attention; it has just been remarked,
that the skin covering the buboes never runs to gangrene; dis-

section shows that it is otherwise with respect to the gland itself.
" Je cou_{pai} par le milieu celle (h. e. the bubo) qui etoit sur les
" vaisseaux, que je trouvai tout noire." " Le lendemain j'ouvris
" le bubon, j'y trouvai le corps glanduleux, comme un rein de
" mouton, tout noir."*

ı. ı. Besides the true bubo, another pestilential eruption has also
received the name of bubo. This eruption is so rare that some
who mention it have been accused of misrepresentation. This
accusation we are now assured is groundless†.

The principal circumstance in which the spurious, differs from
the true, bubo, is in the former appearing indiscriminately on
almost every part of the body, while the true bubo is confined to
the groin, axilla, and parts about the fauces. " Spurious buboes
" were observed," says Dr. Russell, " on the head, the forehead,
" the throat, the shoulder, above the clavicle, the neck, on or above
" the scapulæ, the back, the side under the breast, the belly, the
" hip, hind part of the thigh near the ham, the leg, the scrotum,
" the arm near the usual places of issues, inside of the arm near
" the elbow, outside of the forearm and near the wrist."

Some of these buboes, if they are not lanced at a proper time,
grow to a great size, particularly those on the scapulæ or back,
in other parts however they seldom much exceed the size of a
common hen's egg. They generally make their appearance about
the second or third day, and for the most part after the protrusion
of true buboes or carbuncles. They generally suppurate, though
less rapidly than the true buboes.‡

2. Of Carbuncles.

Next to buboes, carbuncles are the most remarkable of the pestilential eruptions.

The reader will find carbuncles divided by different writers into several varieties. One makes three, another four, a third five
different kinds.

Dr. Russell divides the carbuncles he met with, into five varieties.

The first appeared in the form of a small pustule about the size
of half a pea, on its upper surface of a dusky or yellow colour,
and a little wrinkled. The skin which immediately surrounded
this pustule was hard and inflamed. The pustule itself soon became very painful and continued to increase till it became a tumour of the size of a nutmeg, and sometimes that of a walnut;

* See Traité de la Peste, p. 447, 448.
† See Dr. Russell's Treatise on the Plague, p. 119.
‡ See Traité de la Peste, part 1st, p. 435.

and a yellowish matter was secreted under the cuticle, which was sometimes moist, at other times dry and crusty ; the rest of the tumour assumed a dark reddish colour, the circle which surrounded it appearing at different times of various hues.

On the third, fourth, or fifth day of the carbuncle, a gangrenous crust appeared on the middle of it, which soon occupied the whole surface of the tumor, exactly resembling the black eschar formed by caustic.

This crust, when the termination was favourable, was thrown off by suppuration, leaving an ulcer of various depth, which for some time continued to discharge matter. When the case terminated fatally, the crust remained dry and often spread to the inflamed circle, surrounding the carbuncle, so as to form a gangrene of considerable extent.

The second kind of carbuncle appeared in the form of a small angry pustule, not rising so high as the former, more disposed to spread, and becoming gangrenous on the second day. In this state it was not easily distinguished from the other, but was generally surrounded with a more highly inflamed ring. It chiefly attacked tendinous parts, particularly the joints of the fingers and toes.

In the third variety, the cuticle was at once raised into a blister of the size of a horse-bean, filled with a dusky yellow or blackish fluid, and the skin which surrounded this variety of the carbuncle, was less tense and of a paler red, than that surrounding either of the foregoing. When the blister broke, the cuticle fell upon the flat surface, which was of a dark colour and soon became black. At this period, that is about the third or fourth day of the carbuncle, it resembled the preceding varieties, except that it was flatter. The circle surrounding the eschar gradually assumed a very dark red, but never became gangrenous. The eschar was about the size of a six-pence. This carbuncle was very painful, and five or six times appeared on the same patient.

The fourth variety was a small red spot raised only to the touch, which gradually rose higher and spread, till in 24 hours it was a flattish dusky pustule, surrounded by a light rose-coloured margin. This carbuncle was very painful, and when it appeared on the face occasioned swelling but without inflammation of the skin. It often became black beyond the rose-coloured margin on the second day, and the mortification spread to the neighbouring parts. This species of carbuncle always accompanied other eruptions, and was usually pretty numerous.

The fifth and last variety appeared at first a pustule, which, on the second day, resembled that of the small-pox ; it rose in the form of a cone to twice the size of a large distinct pock with a blunt yellowish point, which, instead of advancing to suppuration, became black to the size of a large field pea. The gangrene in this case however did not spread farther. The margin became of a dusky red, but appeared brighter as the suppuration which threw off the eschar advanced. After the second day, this differed from the third and fourth varieties only in the gangrenous part being of less extent and the pustule more raised.

In other writers we find an account of carbuncles in some respects differing from the foregoing. Samoilowitz, in his Account of the Plague of 1771 in Russia, observes, that the petechiæ or maculæ are very large and confluent, and often turn to carbuncles a short time before death, which happens in the following manner: two, three, or four large petechiæ run rogether and form a large pustule; sometimes a similar pustule arises on each petechiæ; in either case, on opening the pustules a true carbunele appears beneath. In the Traité de la Peste, it is observed of a plague which raged in the eastern parts of Europe, that purple spots appeared on various parts of the body, in the middle of which arose small gangrenous tubercles.

In the same publication Geoffry takes notice of a carbuncle, no part of which assumed a black appearance. Dr. Russell, however, thinks that Geoffry describes its appearance at one period only.

Dr. Gotwald describes a carbuncle, which on its first appearance was a small swelling, on the surface of which there soon arose a number of little vesicles in clusters, which in a short time were formed into an eschar. These carbuncles were generally situated in membranous and tendinous parts, about the knee, behind the ears, upon the toes, &c. A streak proceeding from carbuncles on the fingers has sometimes been observed and compared to a tail.

Dr. Hodges mentions an eruption of vesicles, which in one case he found covering the whole body. When the inflammation was considerable, they sometimes became gangrenous, and were changed into carbuncles; they then resembled Dr. Russell's third variety.

There are certain eruptions which now and then appear in the plague in some respects differing considerably from any one of the carbuncles just described; in others resembling them. Such is the eruption which has been termed papulæ ardentes, or fire bladders. Gotwald, (says Goodwin in his Historical Account) observed the papulæ ardentes or fire bladders in two patients only, both of whom recovered. They were as broad as a shilling, of an irregular shape, and the skin seemed as if it were shrivelled by fire; at length they emitted a small quantity of moisture, and vanished in a few days. They appeared on the belly, thighs, and legs.

But it would be tedious to enumerate all the various eruptions of this kind which have been observed in different epidemics. The true pestilential carbuncle may be defined, a pustular or vesicular eruption, sooner or later running to gangrene.

The eruption called anthrax, is nothing more than a carbuncle after it has become sphacelated.

Carbuncles, to whatever variety they may belong, for the most part do not exceed the size of a walnut ; they have sometimes been observed considerably larger. The time of their appearance is uncertain ; they sometimes shew themselves on the first day of the complaint, but more commonly not till a later period ; and when several appear on the same person, they generally succeed each other rapidly. They have been known to come out as late as the eighteenth or twentieth day.

Respecting the number which appears on the same patient, Dr. Russell observes, " Of those of the first and second species " seldom more than one or two were observed in the same subject, " in general one only. The other varieties occurred in greater " number, and including those of the fifth, I have sometimes " counted between twenty and thirty, but this happens very " rarely."

This eruption is always attended with considerable pain, which in some cases is very violent. No external part of the body is exempted from carbuncles. " I have observed them every where," the author just quoted remarks, " the penis and scrotum not ex- " cepted, but never observed them on the tongue, the tonsils, and " internal parts of the mouth, (there have been instances however " of their appearing on the tongue) though in carbuncles on the " cheek, near the corner of the mouth, the gangrene spreads in- " wards, and in one instance of a carbuncle on the eye-brow, the " gangrene spreading upon the globe of the eye had destroyed " part of it."

The carbuncle is a less favourable eruption than the bubo. Carbuncles were regarded by the Russian physicians, Dr. Guthrie informs us, as a sign of greater malignity than buboes; but of this presently. They thought the carbuncle indicated less danger when red than when livid; when it suppurated than when it did not. When the hands and feet were the seat of carbuncles, Dr. Guthrie observes, the patient seldom or never recovered. Carbuncles on the spine were also regarded as particularly unfavourable.

It is remarked, in the Traité de la Peste, that in those cases in which little or no eruption appeared, and in which the patients died on the fourth or fifth day, some of the viscera were generally found much affected, the intestines, chiefly the small intestines, the mesentery, the liver, the internal parts of the stomach or the lungs, being eroded, or having large pustules or gangrenous spots formed on them.

Carbuncles and buboes often appear separately; they are also frequently combined, and when this happens it has been remarked, that the carbuncles most frequently appear on the same side of the body with the buboes. This however is far from being universally the case. The carbuncle sometimes comes out very near the bubo. but rarely upon it. Dr. Guthrie observes that carbuncles sometimes appear on the buboes.

Carbuncles now and then give rise to buboes, for it frequently happens that when the former appear on the arm, the glands of the axilla swell; these have been observed to be less painful than primary buboes, and they disperse when the carbuncles come to a favourable suppuration; which is not the case with primary buboes. These lymphatic buboes, as they have been termed, are also observed, but much more rarely, in the groin when the carbuncles appear on the thighs, legs, or feet.

Such are the eruptions which chiefly distinguish the plague. There are some others however which occasionally attend this disease.

3. Of the other Pestilential Eruptions.

Common boils or furuncles, as they have been called, appear more rarely than buboes or carbuncles. They are protruded suddenly, and are very much like the pustule which precedes some kinds of carbuncles, but considerably larger. They soon rise to a point, suppurate, and discharge good matter.

From what has been said of petechiæ the reader will not be surprised to find this eruption in so well marked a typhus as we shall find the plague usually is. They are not however a constant attendant. In some epidemics they have been rarely observed, in others more frequently. It is chiefly this eruption which has been called tokens; by some, God's tokens; but these names have not been used in a very definite sense.

The appearance of petechiæ in the plague adds to the unfavourable prognosis. By the Russian physicians they were regarded as a very fatal symptom.

I need not say much of the different classes into which, from their different appearances, they have been divided. At one time they appear red, afterwards becoming brown, or even black; in other cases they are brown from the first, and become black sooner. In some cases they are few in number, and confined to

the superior parts of the body, in others they are more numerous and appear on every part. They are sometimes small circular spots, at other times larger and of a more irregular shape.
As in other fevers, the darker their colour the more danger they
indicate.

Eruptions very different from petechiæ are mentioned under
this name by writers on the plague. Thus Gotwald's fourth species of petechiæ is described in Goodwin's Historical Account as
not unlike the eruption of measles. " In two or three days, it is
" observed they seem to rise to a head in little blisters, but con-
" tain no matter; on the fifth day they are dry, and then the pa-
" tient's death is not far off.

As in other malignant fevers, petechiæ often run together,
forming blotches of various size and figure. Sometimes blotches
appear without petechiæ properly so called, the skin being varie-
gated with stains of different colours, so that it has been compared to the clouds and stains in marble. In different places it
is blue, yellow, red, brown, black, of various shades and bright-
ness. " The skin," Dr. Russell observes, " in various places was
" sometimes deformed by narrow streaks of a reddish, purple,
" or livid colour. When such took possession of the face they
" gave a frightful appearance to the countenance, and frequently
" produced such an alteration of features and so completely dis-
" guised the patient as to render him hardly known by his ac-
" quaintance. A streak nearly of the same kind was sometimes
" observed darting from the edges of the buboes and carbuncles."

Very often the stains or blotches do not appear till af er death,
and then, particularly on the fleshy parts, the body seems as if
it had been bruised. " Sometimes," Dr. Russell continues, " the
" whole skin of the thighs, back, and shoulders, turned livid
" while the corpse was yet warm."

These appearances, he remarks, are not often observed at the
commencement of the epidemic ; which is to be regretted, as
it is then that a characteristic mark of the plague is most wanted.

Such are the pestilential eruptions. In Dr. Russell's Treatise,
the reader will find tables, giving the proportional frequency of
the different kinds of buboes and carbuncles. The following are
the results.

Of 2700, 1841 had inguinal buboes, 569 axillary, 231 parotid,
74 spurious buboes, 490 carbuncles. From these tables it appears that buboes in the right groin were more frequent, than
in the left, 729 had the former, 589 the latter. In another instance, 161 the former, 130 the latter. Buboes were also rather
more frequent in the right axilla, than in the left though not in
so great a proportion ; 184 had buboes in the right, 165 in the

left, axilla. In another table the numbers of those who had
them in the right and left axilla differed only by one, and that was
in favour of the left.   Not above one in 10 or 12 had buboes in
both groins or both axillæ.

The fourth table shews the number of cases in which buboes
in the parotids, carbuncles, or spurious buboes, were the sole
eruptions, compared with that in which they were combined
with inguinal or axillary buboes.

Buboes in the parotids in 130 were unattended, in 110 were
attended, by inguinal or axillary buboes.

Carbuncles were the only eruption in 85 cases; they were combined with axillary or inguinal buboes in 405.

Spurious buboes appeared alone in 37 cases; they were combined with axillary or inguinal buboes in the same number.

In 143, inguinal and axillary buboes were variously combined.
In 602 there was a complication of various eruptions.

It is to be remembered however that these proportions are
drawn only from one or two epidemics, and will not perhaps apply with much accuracy to others ; as the result of extensive experience however, they may serve upon the whole to give some
idea of the comparative frequency of these eruptions.

SECT. II.

Of the other Symptoms of the Plague.

That I may abridge the following account of the symptoms of
the plague, and consequently render it more distinct, it is proper
to observe, that all the symptoms both of synocha and typhus
occasionally attend this fever.   It is unnecessary again to detail
all of these, for which I refer the reader to the first volume ; and
shall here consider at length, those which characterize the plague,
or appear in this disease under peculiar modifications.

It has already been remarked, that in the several divisions of
the plague adopted by writers, many of the varieties are ill defined.
They seem to be marked by accidental symptoms, and some of
them by no particular symptom, but by the general mildness or
severity of the disease.   In the former case the division can be of
no use ; in the latter it can admit of no precision.   Besides, most
writers on the plague, speaking from their own observation alone,
describe the complaint as it appeared in one or two epidemics,
and in almost all epidemics there are peculiarities.   It is only by

comparing many, that we can form an account of the disease generally applicable. . . . .

On comparing different epidemics we shall find, that whatever be true of other eruptions, buboes are salutary. They almost always mark a form of the disease less generally fatal, than that unattended by this eruption. "Those perished," Dr. Russell remarks, "sometimes within the twenty-four hours, sometimes on "the second or third day; they had neither buboes nor carbun- "cles, and it was very rare to find suspicious marks of infection "on the dead bodies." In another place he observes, "The to- "tal absence of buboes in those who died suddenly I have no "doubt of." He also remarks, "That the plague, under a form "of all others the most destructive, exists without its characteristic "eruptions or other external marks reckoned pestilential, can ad- "mit of no doubt." The Russian physicians, Dr. Guthrie informs us, found the cases attended with buboes less fatal than those attended with carbuncles. Carbuncles and petechiæ, De Mertens, in his Account of the Plague of Moscow, observes, are not critical eruptions, they only denote a putrid condition of the humors, whence it follows that in proportion as buboes are more common, and petechiæ and carbuncles more rare, the milder is the plague. Orrœus, in his Treatise on the same Plague, observes indeed, that buboes often attended the most accute form of the disease; yet in another place he informs us, that there were no buboes in the worst form, their germs only being sometimes observed after death; and Samoilowitz,* in his account of this epidemic, in describing the worst form of the disease, notices petechiæ and carbuncles as frequent symptoms, but makes no mention of buboes.

Upon the whole then, the plague unattended by buboes, runs its course more rapidly and is more generally fatal, than when accompanied by this eruption. The plague may therefore be divided into that which is, and that which is not, attended with buboes.†

The first of these includes many varieties, from that in which the prognosis is almost uniformly good to a form of the disease little less fatal than that unattended by buboes. The appearance

---

* Mémoire sur la Peste qui en 1771 ravagea l'Empire de Russie, surtout Móscow, par M. Samoilowitz.

† Some writers have divided the plague into three species; that attentended with buboes, that attended with carbuncles, and that attended with petechiæ. It will appear, I think, from a very cursory view of the disease, that there is no room for such a division.

In some of the older writers we find plagues mentioned, in no case of which, it is said, any eruption appeared. This is said of a plague which raged in Europe in the 15th century. We have every reason however to believe, that these epidemics were not the true plague. That of the 15th century appears to have been of the same nature with the Sudor Anglicus.

of the buboes also affords the means of, subdivision, for it will be found, on comparing the accounts of different epidemics, that upon the whole the earlier the buboes appear, the milder is the disease ; thus, for example, in the first class of Dr. Russell's division, which was the most fatal, buboes were very rare ; in the second, which was also very fatal, though less uniformly so, buboes appeared on the third day or later ; in the third class, which was less fatal, they appeared earlier ; in the fourth, which was still milder, buboes generally appeared on the first day ; in the fifth, which never proved fatal, they were among the first symptoms of the complaint.

To the two foregoing forms of the disease a third might be added, since the pestilential eruptions towards the end of the epidemic sometimes appear unattended by fever. This form, however, which is merely a local affection unattended by danger, demands little attention.

The most fatal form of the plague makes its attack in various ways, sometimes merely with depression of strength, a sense of weight in the head, confusion of thought, giddiness, dejection, and oppression about the præcordia, often accompanied with a bitter taste in the mouth:* The patient is inclined to be silent, shews much anxiety in his countenance, but makes few complaints ; the febrile symptoms are very moderate. The attendants suppose the patient a little indisposed, but suspect nothing alarming ; yet such patients often die within the first twenty-four hours, sometimes on the second day.†

In general however this form of the plague makes its attack less deceitfully. In an epidemic described by Chenot,‡ that of Marseilles,‖ and many others, the symptoms from the first were alarming, the complaint often appearing with violent and irregular shaking.

Delirium is sometimes the first symptom observed. At other times, a remarkable state of the pulse, which very suddenly becomes so weak that it can hardly be felt, frequent, and intermitting, with much debility and languor, introduces the disease. The prostration of strength is sometimes so sudden and complete, that Mr. Smith, Dr. Guthrie§ informs us, saw men in apparent

* The bitter taste in the mouth the reader will find mentioned by different writers as characteristic of the plague. It is observed by some that a favourable change seldom happened while this symptom continued.

† See Russell's Treatise on the Plague, and Orræus on the Plague of Moscow.

‡ See Chenot de Peste.

‖ See the Traité de la Peste.

§ See Dr. Guthrie's Observations on the Plague of Russia.

good health, on being infected by the plague, suddenly drop down as if shot by a musket ball. Sometimes, instead of mere debility and lassitude, the patient is affected with extreme horror and despair, and his spirits so low that nothing can recall them.

At other times, the disease attacks with very slight chills, soon followed by a burning heat, which remains during the disease; as soon as the heat commences, the patient complains of insufferable head-ach and excessive thirst. Sometimes, as in the plague of Russia described by Orrœus, the patient is suddenly seized with violent shivering succeeded by a hot fit, the shivering and hot fit alternating several times.

The first symptom of the plague is sometimes a violent beating of the temporal arteries, while the pulse at the wrist is small and feeble. In this case the heat is generally moderate, but the head-ach intolerable. In the plague which raged at Lyons in 1628, a burning heat in some of the viscera, and a dull pain or rather great heaviness of the head, announced its approach. I

The plague sometimes comes on with violent palpitation, and strong convulsive tremblings. The plague which raged in London in 1665 often made its attack in this way.

As the complaint advances, it assumes more of the appearance of the fevers we have been considering. The inflammatory symptoms generally run high for the first day or two; but for the most part the plague assumes the form of typhus at an early period; and the patient soon becomes delirious or comatose.

The delirium is sometimes of the furious kind, particularly, Orrœus observes, in those of a robust and full habit, and in whom a full meal appeared to be the immediate exciting cause. In general however, the delirium is of that species which characterizes typhus, the patient appearing rather stupid than outrageous, and complaining of a pain at the heart, a symptom frequently observed in the plague. When coma comes on early, it has been looked upon as affording a worse prognosis than delirium, particularly if it suffers no evident remissions during the day time. Both delirium and coma indeed are almost always most considerable during the night. The remission in the day time is generally more evident when the patient is delirious than when he is comatose.

Whether he becomes comatose or not, there is always present a very remarkable muddy appearance of the eyes, which is sometimes observable at the very commencement, and is one of the most characteristic symptoms of the disease. This appearance of the eyes in some degree resembles that in the last stage of malignant fevers. It is not however described as altogether such, for with the muddiness there is blended a degree of lustre. It is an appearance in short very remarkable to those who have seen it, but not easily conveyed in words.

Chicoyneau observes of this appearance of the eyes, " Les
" yeux etoient ternis, le regard fixé et egaré annoncoit la terreur
" et le désespoir."*

Chenot calls it, " Oculorum languor et mæstitia ;" in another
place, " occuli tristes scintillantes," which last may almost be
looked upon as a translation of Dr. Russell's account of the eyes.
The eyes, Orrœus observes, are unusually prominent and preternaturally red, watery, and of a sparkling fierceness, but in the
advanced stage of the disease, they sink, the redness goes off, and
a little before death, they appear dull and as if covered with a
film. This change may be observed to a greater or less degree,
during each remission, for it is in the exacerbations that the peculiar appearance of the eyes is most remarkable.

Almost all writers on the plague take notice of a peculiar cast
of countenance, which to those who are conversant with the disease, is one of its best diagnostics. It was the state of the eyes,
Dr. Russell remarks, which contributed chiefly to occasion that
confusion of countenance which he does not attempt to describe,
but from which, after repeatedly observing it, he could with some
certainty pronounce whether the disease was the plague or not.

The danger is very generally proportioned to the degree of this
symptom. When the eyes resume the natural appearance, particularly when this happens after sweats, the prognosis is favourable. But in the form of the plague we are considering, this
hardly ever happens. In the comatose the muddiness of the
eyes is most remarkable. Their fierceness is most striking in
those who labour under delirium, particularly. the furious delirium ; and it sometimes happens, that the coma and delirium, with
the peculiar casts of countenance which accompany them, alternate with each other. In the delirious, however, there is still an
appearance of muddiness, and the eyes retain some lustre in the
comatose. These appearances of the eyes are less remarkable
in children than in adults. Such is the best account I have been
able to collect from the observations of those who were conversant
with the disease, of that peculiar appearance of the eyes which all
who have seen the plague agree, so remarkably characterizes it.

The changes which take place in the eye are not always confined to its appearance only ; the retina is sometimes much affected. The patients complain of seeing sparks, flashes of fire,
and various colours passing before the eyes ; this is only a greater degree of the symptoms termed muscæ volitantes. Deceptions of sight, however, are not frequent symptoms in the plague.
Deceptions of hearing are still more rare. Deafness, as in other
fevers, is generally a favourable symptom, but it seldom attends
the plague. With respect to the other senses, nothing particular is to be observed. The depravation of the taste, which is in

* Traité de la Peste.

some measure characteristic of the plague, I have already had occasion to notice.

The anxiety in many cases is extreme, the patient constantly changing his posture, and soon finding the present as uneasy as the last, so that he is sometimes perpetually in motion. When this symptom is considerable, it affords a very unfavourable prognosis. The appearance it assumes when at its height, which generally indicates the approach of death, is described by authors, who have termed it a mortal inquietude in very strong terms. The patient incessantly twists his body as if in agony, but is incapable of giving any account of his feelings, so that it is difficult to determine whether it is occasioned by a great degree of anxiety or severe pain.

. The temperature, in the progress of the disease, is various. While the chills continue to recur, its increase is not considerable, and in the cases where it is most considerable, it seldom equals that which we often meet with in common synocha.

-The state of the pulse is also various. In most cases after the first days of the disease, in many after the first hours, and in some from the commencement, it is feeble and frequent. Sometimes it is remarkably hard and small but regular, at other times it is irregular or intermitting, and at length fluttering.

During the exacerbations, it often becomes full, open, and strong, as Dr. Russell expresses it; after which it again sinks; but in a more advanced stage, a different change is observed during the exacerbations, the pulse becoming so feeble that it can with difficulty be felt.

It has been observed of the pulse in the plague, that though to a slight touch it is strong and full, it is often easily compressed; a state of the pulse not readily accounted for, which is mentioned however by more than one author from their own observation.[*] The most striking fact relating to the state of the pulse in the plague is, that it has often been observed nearly natural while the other symptoms indicated much danger.

As the disease advances the increase of debility is generally indicated by a considerable affection of the speech; in some cases amounting only to a degree of confusion and faltering, or a change of tone; in others the voice is greatly impaired or wholly lost. The affection of the voice appears the earlier, the greater the debility. When this is excessive from the beginning, when, as Chenot observes, " Ægri erecti stare aut sedere impotes, proprio

* In the Traité de la Peste the reader will find this state of the pulse mentioned both by Chicoyneau and Conzier. " Il etoit ouvert et animé." The former observes, " Il disparoisoit cependant si on pressoit l'artere " avec le doigt."

" pondere labebantur," a considerable affection of the speech is generally observed on the first night, or the second at farthest. When the debility is less considerable, it is delayed to the third day or later.

The state of the tongue, as in other fevers, is various. It often retains the natural appearance throughout the greater part of the disease. Sometimes it is moist, and covered with thick mucus, at other times dry. " Sometimes," Dr. Russell observes, " it be- " came parched with a yellow streak on each side, and reddish " in the middle, but it never was observed to form so thick a fur " or become of so dark a colour as in the advanced stages of some " other fevers. The dryness or moistness of the tongue," he adds, " rarely corresponded with the febrile symptoms, for the " tongue was often moist where the external heat was intense " and the pulse indicated high fever; and on the contrary, parched " where the fever in appearance was very inconsiderable."

Vomiting, though more frequently observed in less violent forms of the plague, sometimes attends this variety. The pain at the heart, so frequently complained of, Dr Russell thinks situ- ated about the orifice of the stomach. As it often accompanies vomiting, he was at first led to believe that it arose from bile or other irritating matter in the stomach. He found however that it was not relieved by the discharge. It seems more than proba- ble, from the nature of the symptoms, that this pain proceeds from an inflammatory affection of the stomach. The matter evacuated by vomiting is generally bilious. It is sometimes of a dark co- lour and mixed with blood; and it is not uncommon in the plague for worms to be thrown out by vomiting. Whatever be the ap- pearance of the matter rejected, when vomiting occurs at an early period and returns at intervals, the prognosis is bad.

Nausea without vomiting is a frequent symptom. It does not seem to proceed from irritating matter in the stomach, as repeat- ed vomiting is not found to relieve it. There are few means more effectual for allaying nausea and vomiting than those which pro- mote the perspiration. It has been observed of the plague, that if the repeated reaching occasions a moisture on the skin, the nausea abates.

A diarrhœa is apt to supervene, sometimes during the first days, more frequently at a later period. This is invariably a dan- gerous symptom. The matter passed by stool is similar to that rejected by vomiting, often bilious, frequently with an evident admixture of blood; sometimes blood only is passed. Chenot of- ten met with dysenteric purging in the plague.

As there are few fevers in which purging is so unfavourable, so there are none in which constipation appears to be less injurious.

" A number of the sick," Dr. Russell observes, " were disposed
" to be costive throughout the disease, and some had no stool for
" several days, the popular dread of provoking a diarrhœa proving
" a bar to laxatives and even to simple clysters, which are readily
" admitted at other times. The consequences of this sluggish-
" ness of the bowels were by no means what might have been ex-
" pected; for on comparing a number of cases in which the body
" had been all along regular, with others in which there had been
" no stool, the former did not appear to have been particularly
" exempt from those symptoms which might plausibly have been
" imputed to costiveness in others."

The urine is often observed in no respect different from that of
a person in health ; at other times it is found pale, high coloured,
clear, turbid, without sediment, or with a great deal, and sometimes
more or less tinged with blood ; in short, it assumes in different
patients, or sometimes in the same at different times, all the various appearances observed in other fevers.

There is no excretion of such consequence in the plague as
that by the skin. When the skin remains parched, or when only
slight, clammy, partial sweats appear, the prognosis is bad ;
when on the other hand a thin, general, and copious sweat takes
place, it often proves more or less critical.

Dr. Russell observes, that the breath and perspiration were seldom or never fetid. Other writers however have observed that
they are often fetid to a great degree.

As in many, perhaps in all the other exanthemata, epileptic
fits now and then occur. They are a rare symptom in the
plague. When they appear, they generally precede an eruption.

Slight convulsive motions of the limbs and subsultus tendinum
are frequent ; with respect to other convulsive motions, hiccup,
rarely, and sneezing almost never, attends the plague.

Hemorrhagies are a common symptom, and unless very moderate, generally indicate much danger. They are frequent, as
appears from what has been said, from the stomach, intestines,
and kidneys.... They are more common however from the nose,
and in women from the uterus, than from other parts. These,
particularly the hemorrhagy from the nose, when they occur early in the disease, and the patient is young and plethoric, sometimes bring relief. At a later period, hemorrhagies are always
unfavourable, and when they become profuse, the patient seldom
recovers. It has been remarked, as might have been inferred a
priori, that the blood which flows in these hemorrhagies is thinner
in proportion as the disease is further advanced.

Such are the symptoms of the worst form of the plague. The
strength gradually sinks, till the pulse impresses the finger with
only a weak undulating, or tremulous motion, with frequent in-

termissions. The surface, particularly .on the extremities, be-comes cold and covered with clammy moisture, the pulse cannot be felt, and the patient calmly expires, or, as frequently happens in all idiopathic fevers, is carried off by convulsions. ...

The second and more common form of the plague, that accom-panied with buboes, includes endless varieties. What I am about to say of this form, may be divided into two parts ; the circum-stances in which it differs from the preceding form, and those in which its principal varieties differ from each other. In the first place, of the circumstances in which this form differs from the preceding.

In the second form of the plague, according to the division I have adopted, buboes always make their appearance on the first, second, or third day, or later. If we except the appearance of buboes, we shall find no symptom constantly attending the one, and never present in the other, form. There are certain symp-toms however more frequent in the one than the other.

Both vomiting and diarrhœa are most frequent in cases where buboes are about to appear. They sometimes attend from the commencement ; at other times supervene at a later period. When the vomiting and purging commence early, they often continue to harrass the patient through a great part of the com-plaint.

Although the delirium and coma are sometimes as uniform in this, as in the preceding form of the disease, it is not generally the case. In most instances indeed, some degree of these affec-tions comes on in the evening, and continues through the night, but in the majority of cases. unless the disease is far advanced, the patient during the day is nearly and sometimes altogether free from them. The sudden depression of strength also is upon the whole less remarkable, and the pulse for the most part contin-ues longer full, and is less apt to become irregular.

The duration of the complaint upon the whole is longer, pe-techiæ and vibices are more common, and the body more fre-quently becomes livid and black after death. In short, the differ-ence between the general course of the symptoms in the first and second forms of the plague, is, that in the latter they are upon the whole less alarming and more protracted, the patient often labour-ing under various symptoms for some days before the fever is formed.* In the danger and rapidity of the second form how-ever there is great variety ; it varies from a degree of severity nearly equal to that of the first form, to a degree of benignity ap-proaching to that of the last, in which the eruptions are unaccom-panied by fever.

* See what Orrœus calls the period of infection, in his Account of the Plague of Russia.

Although the varieties of the second form are in reality endless, there are only three which can be distinctly marked, for (notwithstanding the numerous divisions of authors) I can discover no symptom which characterizes different gradations included under any one of these varieties; and varieties ill characterized, instead of rendering the subject clearer, increase its perplexity, by holding forth distinctions which the reader soon perceives, nature has not made. Surely vomiting occurring more or less frequently, or coma supervening at an earlier or later period, afford no sufficient marks for characterizing different varieties of the plague, unless it can be shown that the general course of the disease is materially influenced by the absence or delayed appearance of such symptoms, which on perusing the account of different epidemics we do not find to be the case.

The first variety of the second form, according to the division I have adopted, is characterized by the buboes not appearing till the second or third day.

In this case the symptoms are generally more violent, and the prognosis worse, than when they appear on the first day of the complaint, which characterizes the second variety of this form; in the third, the eruption of buboes is among the first symptoms in which case the febrile symptoms are for the most part still milder.

Many cases of the first of these varieties so much resemble some of the first form, that the difference consists almost solely in the appearance of buboes in the former; thus the first and second forms of the plague imperceptibly run into each other; but the symptoms of the first variety of the second form are in general less severe.

The pulse generally continues pretty full and tolerably strong till the second day, during which, for the most part, it becomes weak, and sometimes intermitting. The peculiar dejection of countenance, with the muddiness of the eyes, which come on more early in the very worst cases, frequently supervene at this time. Irregular flushing, a sense of internal heat, pain about the præcordia, and incessant inquietude, at this period afford a very fatal prognosis; as in the first form, these symptoms often precede that diminution of temperature and cold dampness of the surface, which announce the patient's death to be inevitable, which is often however, after the appearance of these symptoms, at the distance of a day or two. After this however, although the heat of the body returns, the symptoms upon the whole gradually become worse. When the strength has not been greatly reduced by the vomiting and purging, a remission is often observed on the third day, but if the foregoing train of symptoms has previously occurred this remission is always fallacious, the disease returns with redoubled violence, while the powers of resisting it are enfeebled. The patient often survives to the fifth or sixth day or later, the remissions constantly becoming slighter, and the exacerbations more severe.

On the second or third day, sometimes later, buboes make their appearance, in general without bringing relief; carbuncles also frequently supervene with no better effect. This however is not uniformly the case; Chenot observes, that the eruption of buboes and carbuncles was often attended with an evident remission of the symptoms. In some epidemics, Waldshmidt* remarks, when the symptoms were most alarming, the appearance of buboes often saved the patient, but in others they were not followed by any remission.

In this variety the body is frequently covered with petechiæ or vibices, and the corpse often becomes black.

The malignant train of symptoms just mentioned as appearing on the second day, sometimes do not supervene till a later period. At whatever time they occur, however, they almost always afford a fatal prognosis. In some favourable instances, especially where the vomiting and purging do not occur or at least not in such a degree as greatly to reduce the strength, the foregoing train of symptoms does not appear at all, and the patient escapes. In such cases the delirium or coma seldom comes on before the second night, and the remissions which take place in the morning are more considerable. These flattering appearances however often prove deceitful, and even a salutary sweat on the morning of the third day is sometimes succeeded by a fatal train of symptoms.

These sometimes do not appear till the fourth day, and the patient after their appearance frequently experiences a remission in the mornings; the exerbations however gradually become more severe, and death is only delayed.

In this variety, death for the most part happens on the fifth day, sometimes not till the sixth, seventh, or eighth, and then the symptoms are generally milder, and the buboes appear early on the second day. Few recover from this variety.

In the second variety of the second form of the plague, according to the division I have adopted, buboes appear on the first day. Here the symptoms are wonderfully varied. Many cases are equally fatal with those which have been considered, but this variety upon the whole is less so.

Dr. Russell observes of his fourth class, which corresponds to this variety, " The fourth class was the most numerous of all, " comprehending those forms of the disease, which from the " various and sudden changes in their course so often though not

* See Haller's Disput. ad Hist. et Cur. Morb. Pert. vol. v.

" constantly met with, cannot easily be represented in concise
" and connected description ; I therefore enter on the attempt
" with diffidence, and as a supplement for defects, must refer to
" the cases themselves noted below. The distinctive marks of
" this class are, the continuance of the inflammatory and febrile
" symptoms with less interruption than in the former ; a pulse
" more constantly sustained or soon recovering itself when sunk
" and hurried in the excerbations ; the length and rigour of the
" excerbations decreasing in the advance of the disease ; and a-
" bove all, the prevalent tendency to a favourable crisis by the
" skin, with the critical sweats on the third, fifth, or subsequent
" days."

Vomiting is not so frequent a symptom in this variety as in the
former, but upon the whole the first symptoms of these varieties
are not very different.[1] Some hours after the commencement,
a bubo begins to shew itself, and now and then more than one.—
Notwithstanding this, the symptoms are sometimes as severe as
in the foregoing variety ; for the most part however they are
milder.

. The fever is more moderate ; delirium or coma still more rarely
appear on the first night, during which the patient is less restless
and anxious. But from the state of the symptoms at the commencement, we cannot judge with certainty respecting the event,
those often escaping in whom the first symptoms are severe ;—
whilst others, in whom the febrile symptoms are milder at an early period, are carried off after lingering for many days.

The remission on the second morning is generally considerable
in this variety, and during the second day the symptoms often
undergo many different changes ; at one time the febrile symptoms running high, now and then even accompanied with a degree
of coma, soon afterwards a very evident remission taking place,
which in many cases is only a prelude to a new exacerbation.

These exacerbations are often followed by a sweat more or
less general, and which is found in proportion as it is general to
bring relief. The most general sweats commonly occur in the
morning, and consequently the most evident remissions. At other times the sweats for the most part are partial, and the patient
during the remissions, anxious and oppressed. The morning
sweat of the third day often proves completely critical, or brings
such relief that the patient remains free from danger.

These may be regarded as the most favourable cases of this
variety ; they seem to be the same which M. Chicoyneau describes in the following manner. If all those of the former class
die, he observes, others might indulge more hope. The latter
were seized at first with the same symptoms as the former, but
they disappeared on the second or third day. Nature and art, he
remarks, seemed equally to conduce to this happy effect; the for-

mer collected the poison which had been every where diffused through the system into the buboes and carbuncles, which suppurating, spreading, and throwing out the matter they contained, formed a kind outlet through which the pestilential virus flowed,[*] while art aided this evacuation, which always proved salutary when it was not neglected.[†]

But many cases of this variety are less favourable. The remission on the third day is but imperfect, and the exacerbation soon returns. If during this there be an evident change in the state of the pulse, if from having been pretty full and strong it become weak and fluttering, the prognosis is bad. After this, the pulse varies in frequency, but seldom recovers its strength.

When the change in the pulse is less remarkable, however, the sweat which returns on the morning of the fourth day often brings more relief, and if the exacerbation on this day be less considerable, the sweating is more profuse and brings more relief on the fifth, and a third profuse sweat on the morning of the seventh day often completes or nearly completes the recovery. It has been remarked, that the sweats in this class of patients are more profuse and bring more relief on the morning of the odd, than on those of the even days.

All the patients who escape however do not recover in this way, but often very slowly, and without any sweat or with very little, the complaint gradually abates.

In the last variety of the second form of the plague, namely, where the eruption of buboes is among the first symptoms, many cases are attended with a considerable degree of fever, sometimes protracted for six or eight days ; but comparatively few are attended with much danger.

Chenot gives the following short account of his first division of the plague, which nearly corresponds with this variety. " Su- " binde vix ulla bubonis ortum præcedit stipatve ægritudo. Ipse " carbunculus nonnunquam prodit. prævia tantum miti commo- " tione febrili, manifestior tamen plerumque est quam in bubone."

In this variety the patient is sometimes not even confined to the house, and very often not to bed. In short, the mildest cases of this variety almost resemble the last form of the plague, namely, that in which the eruptions are the only symptoms.

Such are the symptoms of the plague, and such the gradations, by which the first form runs imperceptibly into the last, a disease, as different from it as can be imagined.

* It is almost unnecessary to warn the reader of the groundless nature of this hypothesis.

† See the observations of M. Chicoyneau, in the Traité de la Peste.

Before leaving this part of the subject it is necessary to observe, that although most cases of the plague will be found referable to some of the foregoing heads, yet there are many anomalous cases which cannot be arranged under any one description, as they differ from each other, as well as from all other cases. The only way of describing these is to give the cases themselves; this the reader will perceive would be endless.

Dr. Russell forms a separate class for such anomalous cases, without however attempting any general account of them; all he observes is, " This class being reserved for such cases as were " dubious, anomalous, or extraordinary, varying more or less in " some material circumstances from any of the foregoing classes, " admits of course of no general description. The particular " cases, to which have sometimes been subjoined occasional re- " marks, may be consulted agreeably to the references made be- " low to the journals."

An account of such cases would not only be tedious but of little use, since the anomalous cases of one epidemic are not always found to resemble those of another. All that can be done, is to warn the practitioner that anomalous appearances are to be looked for, which do not however seem materially to influence the mode of treatment.

SECT. III.

Of the Causes of the Plague.

THE history of the plague is involved in much obscurity, so that it is impossible to say from what source, or where, it originated. The earliest plagues of which we have any account raged in Egypt and other parts of Africa.*

We are sufficiently acquainted with its history however to be assured, that like the other exanthemata it arises from a peculiar contagion. Professor Stoll of Vienna indeed, and some others, have combated this opinion, but it would be mispending time to trouble the reader either with the arguments of these writers, or any refutation of them, as they have scarcely now a single advocate.†

It will be unnecessary here to make many observations on contagion, as this subject has already been considered at length. It is needless to repeat what has been said of the means of preventing the generation and checking the progress of contagious dis-

---

* See Waldshmidt's Treatise on the Plague, in the fifth volume of Haller's Disput. ad Morb. Hist. et Curat. Pert.

† See the Traité de la Peste, and Dr. Russell's work on the Plague.

eases ;* and it would be tedious here to describe lazarettos and the various' precautions employed to prevent the introduction of the plague from foreign countries ; for these I shall refer the reader to the works of Mr. Howard and Dr. Russell.

Some facts would lead us to suppose that peculiar states of the air are favourable to the production of the plague ; it has some-times appeared in many parts of a country at the same time.† More generally however it appears at first in one place, and spreads gradually to others.

Like other contagious fevers, warm weather is generally fav-ourable, and cold weather unfavourable, to its progress. The plague was greatly weakened, De Mertens informs us, while the thermometer stood between sixteen and twenty degrees below frost. It often happens however, that its violence is not checked by the winter, and there are many instances of the plague ceasing in the warmest seasons of the year. In all the plagues with which Aleppo has been visited during this century, the Rev. Mr. Dawes observes, it is said to have regularly and constantly ceased in August or September, the hottest months of the year.

Like other contagions, that of the plague is active only for a very short distance around the patient. The physicians, De Mertens observes, often went within a foot of the patients, with-out being infected.

The young and robust, the same author observes, were more liable to infection than the old and infirm. It has often been re-marked of the plague, as of most other contagious fevers, that infants are less liable to it than adults. Waldhsmidt saw several infants who sucked nurses ill of the plague, and yet escaped in-fection. He even observes, that one infant sucked two nurses ill of the plague, both of whom died, yet the child did not receive the disease. A woman who suckled her child five months old, was seized with the plague and died after a week's illness, but the child who sucked her and lay in the same bed with her, escaped the distemper.‡ De Mertens and others make the same obser-vation.

It is remarkable, however, that the fœtus in utero sometimes re-ceives the disease, and that even where the mother escapes.

* De Mertens recommends, as a good preventive, wearing a cloak of oiled cloth over the cloathes, while in the rooms of the sick. It has also been recommended to anoint the body with oil. De Mertens thinks is-sues not to be depended on. The reader will find, in his Treatise on the Plague of Moscow, formulæ for what have been termed antipestilential powders; they are similar to the fumigating powders mentioned in the first volume when speaking of the purification of fomites; the manner of using them also, is there pointed out.

† See a Letter by the Rev. Mr. Dawes from Aleppo, in the third vo-lume of the Medical Museum.

‡ Mr. Dawes's letter.

" Last year as well as this, says Mr. Dawes, there has been more
" than one instance of a woman's being delivered of an infected
" child with the plague sores on its body, though the mother her-
" self has been entirely free from the distemper."*

It was observed of some of the other exanthemata, that certain constitutions are incapable of undergoing them; the same
seems to be true of the plague. Waldshmidt knew a woman
who was servant in a family where seven people died of the
plague, and afterwards in another all of whom died of it, and yet
remained uninfected. A Greek lad, Mr. Dawes observes, made
it his business for many months to wait on the sick, and to wash,
dress, and bury the dead, yet escaped the disease.

Those who have once had the plague are less subject to it than
others. This circumstance, together with the success which had
attended inoculation for the small-pox, induced some to recommend inoculating for the plague, which has actually been done.
In Dr. Guthrie's Letter to Dr. Duncan there is an account of a
surgeon, Mathias Degio, who inoculated himself for the plague.
He inserted, with a lancet, under the cuticle of the arm, a little of
the matter from a pestilential abscess. On the fourth day after
inoculation the fever appeared; he treated himself in all respects
in the same way as if he had been inoculated for the small-pox,
paying particular attention to the cool regimen. His only medicines were cold water and vinegar, with a little wine. The complaint proved so mild that he was never confined to bed, but was
generally in the open air. It was not a more severe complaint
than the common inoculated small-pox.

This surgeon afterwards regularly attended an hospital allotted
for the reception of patients under the plague, without feeling
any symptom of the disorder; while most of the other surgeons
fell a sacrifice to it. From one case however nothing conclusive
can be drawn; besides, it is far from being uncommon for the
plague to attack the same person a second or third time.

It appears from the foregoing case, that the contagion of
plague produces the disease about four days after infection. De
Mertens also observes, that the attendants on the sick generally
fell ill about the fourth or fifth day, and Dr. Guthrie relates a case
in which the patient sickened on the fourth day. Sometimes however its effects are much more sudden. Waldshmidt mentions
the case of a person, who while he was drying some wet clothes
which had been worn by a patient under the plague, was immediately seized with nausea and head-ach, and died on the sixth day;
a bubo and other pestilential symptoms having made their appearance.

Brutes are incapable of receiving this disease, although, like

* In pregnant women the plague generally produces abortion.

other things which have been in contact with or near the sick, they are often the means of conveying the contagion from one person to another. It appears however from an instance alluded to in the Introduction, and some similar ones mentioned by Waldshmidt, that the contagion of the plague, if received into the stomach, often produces violent effects on brutes ; a circumstance which affords a strong argument against contagion, in casual infection, making its first attack on the stomach.

The contagion of the plague, like that of typhus, seems sometimes to act merely as a predisposing cause. When speaking of the latter, it was observed that the observations of Dr. Lind have proved the contagion of typhus may sometimes lurk in the body and remain inactive for a considerable length of time, if the patient is not exposed to other causes of the disease, which seem to subject the system to its action. De Mertens makes a similar observation with respect to the plague ; many, he observes, were suddenly seized after a hearty meal, a fit of anger, or violent exercise.

It is of great importance to determine how long the contagion of plague will lurk in the human body, or in fomites while freely exposed to the air, and retain its activity, as this circumstance determines the duration of quarantine. Dr. Cullen thinks forty days longer than necessary for the quarantine of people ; and with regard to that of goods, he is of opinion that were they properly unpacked and aired, the term of their quarantine might also be shortened.

" I suggested," Dr. Guthrie observes in his Letter to Dr. Duncan, " to Baron Ash, physician general to the Russian army, a " doubt of the possibility that the very active contagion of the " plague could remain so long latent in the body, as the quar- " antine of persons seems to imply, and that it appeared to me " to be founded on an imperfect knowledge of the disease drawn " from a period of ignorance or of general consternation and " terror. His answer was, that he did not think that the conta- " gious nature of this violent disease could remain longer in the " body than fourteen days without declaring itself on, or before, " that period, but that from his own observation and experience " he could not take it upon him to say that it could be con- " cealed so long. Such were likewise the answers I received " from the other medical gentlemen whom I consulted on the " subject. Some gave a little more latitude, and some less, as it " can only be a matter of opinion, but none exceeded fourteen " days."

It appears from different facts, above alluded to, that the plague generally appears as early as the fourth or fifth day after infection ; but we do not know how long a person who has laboured under the disease is capable of infecting others, nor how long the con-

tagion may lurk in an unfavourable habit without producing the
disease, and may yet be communicated and excite the disease in
habits more susceptible of the infection. Upon the whole we
have reason to believe, that a quarantine of forty days is considerably longer than necessary for persons, and probably for goods also. Experience however has not yet determined how much of
this term may be abated.

It appears from what was said above, that the plague at the
commencement of the epidemic is very frequently uncharac-
terized by the proper pestilential symptoms; it has also been observed that at this period it is less contagious than at the height of
the epidemic; a circumstance which further contributes towards
a deception respecting its real nature.

But the most unaccountable circumstance respecting the contagion of the plague, and which has also been observed more or
less strikingly of the contagion of other fevers, is, that it often
suddenly and without any apparent cause ceases to produce the
disease. The plague, says De Mertens, ceased at one time over the
whole Russian empire, after having prevailed at Moscow and other places for a year and an half. "But a greater difficulty," Dr.
" Russell observes, than that of all persons not being susceptible
" of infection, arises from the cessation of the plague at a pe-
" riod when the supposed contagious effluvia preserved in appa-
" rel, furniture, and other fomites, at the end of a pestilential
" season, must be allowed not only to exist in a much greater
" quantity than can be supposed to be at once accidentally impor-
" ted by commerce, but in a state also of universal dispersion
" over the city. The fact, however unaccountable, is unques-
" tionably certain, the disease seems to be extinguished by some
" cause or causes equally unknown as those which concurred to
" render it more or less epidemical in its advance and at its
" height. In Europe something may be ascribed to the means
" employed for the cleansing of houses and goods supposed lia-
" ble to retain the latent seeds of infection. But at Aleppo,
" where the distemper is left to take its natural course, and few or
" no means of purification are employed, it pursues nearly the
" same progress in different years. It declines and revives in
" certain seasons, and at length, without the interference of human
" aid, ceases entirely." "Ubi pestis nondum penitus extinc-
" ta fuit," says Waldshmidt, " hæ sua sponte præter omnium
" expectationem ita cessavit, ut ne vestigium quidem ejus pos-
" tea appuruerit." Nor was any one infected by another, he
adds, although the latter still had the pestilential buboes about
him, while articles which had been in contact with the sick entirely lost the power of communicating the disease.

The plague is generally most fatal at the beginning of the
epidemic.

It is remarkable that the convalescents from the plague have the venereal appetite unusually strong, a circumstance which often counteracts the endeavours of the magistrate, and tends to spread the distemper. The same thing has been observed respecting other malignant fevers. It is particularly remarked by Dr. Rush of the late dreadful fever of North America.

SECT. IV.

Of the Treatment of the Plague.

" In the cure of the plague," Dr Cullen justly remarks, " the " indications are the same as those of fever in general." I therefore refer the reader to what was said of the treatment of continued fever, and shall now only make a few additional remarks particularly applicable to the plague.

In the first place, of blood-letting in this complaint. It is a remark of Sydenham, that blood should be let if the physician see the patient before any appearance of a bubo. This maxim, although very different from that which seems warranted by experience, is, notwithstanding, the result of observation ; for it is in those cases where buboes do not appear or are delayed to a late period, that the inflammatory symptoms most frequently run high.

Many, particularly the Asiatics, make it a rule to let blood in all cases of the plague, if they see the patient at an early period ; and some recommend it as late as the fourth, fifth, sixth, or seventh day, and even some European practitioners have gone nearly as far. Dr. Alexander Russell in his Natural History of Aleppo observes, " It seemed to me that very plentiful bleeding at the " first appearance of the disease was of great service." Others run to the opposite, but safer extreme, and declare that blood-letting is hurtful in all cases of the plague. The proper mode of practice seems to lie between these extremes.

The reader will find many declaring that, in the cases of plague which fell under their observation, they could not perceive that a small blood-letting at the commencement did harm. But although this were true, is it sufficient to recommend a remedy, that it does no harm ? The truth seems to be, that the general prejudice has always been in favour of blood-letting, and no physician's experience has been sufficiently extensive to ascertain its hurtful tendency, unless in cases where the injury done by it is very apparent, and almost constantly follows its employment.

But if there are other cases in which blood-letting has never been attended with any sensible advantage, and which nearly resemble the fevers in which it has been found hurtful, we surely have every reason in such cases to believe it improper.

It is in vain to ask what advantage is expected from blood-letting in these cases ; authors seem to have assumed it as an axiom, that if blood-letting is not evidently hurtful, it must be beneficial in this complaint ; and all that they seem anxious about is to adduce cases and arguments in support of its innocence.

Nor can there be any thing more fallacious than the arguments employed to prove the innocence of this practice. This the reader will readily perceive, if he ask himself, what are the consequences of blood-letting to be dreaded in the plague ? what are its consequences when it evidently does harm ? They are, the symptoms indicating a general loss of tone, the pulse sinks, instead of the febrile heat a cold damp spreads over the body, which is often the forerunner of death. But these are the unfavourable train of symptoms to be expected in all the more alarming forms of the plague, and in different cases they supervene at different periods. How extensive then must that experience be, which has ascertained that in any one case blood-letting has not hurried on these symptoms, nay has not occasioned them, where they would not otherwise have appeared. Is it from reviewing the result in eight or ten cases, in half of which blood-letting was, and in the other half was not employed, and observing the course of all nearly the same, that the safety of so important a step is to be determined ?

Besides, if such observations prove any thing, they prove that blood-letting in the plague does neither good nor harm, and ought therefore to be laid aside as an useless remedy ; a conclusion very different indeed from the result of our experience in similar cases, and not to be admitted except of blood-lettings so trifling that neither good nor harm could be expected from them, and which do not therefore deserve the name. Many of the Turks indeed employ local instead of general blood-letting, and in the latter they generally draw much less blood than we are accustomed to do ; a circumstance which has probably contributed much to establish the safety of blood-letting in the plague.

" Upon finding the pulse sink so suddenly after bleeding," an author I have frequently had occasion to mention observes, " I " was at first inclined to attribute it to that evacuation, and to sus- " pect in less plethoric habits bleeding must prove still more pre- " judicial ; but I afterwards found the low state inseparable " from certain forms of the disease, and often could observe no " material difference in its progress in cases where blood-letting " had or had not been omitted." The author in this quotation confesses that the symptoms of debility were those which he dreaded, and also those to be feared from the remedy he employ- ed, without informing us of any advantage to be expected from it, to counterbalance the risk.

The more we study the observations of the original writers, the more reason we shall find for believing, that the employment of blood-letting in the plague is to be regulated by the same maxims as in other idiopathic fevers. " The measures," says Dr. Cullen, " for moderating the violence of reaction, which op-" crate by diminishing the action of the heart and arteries, have " seldom any place here, except so far as the antiphlogistic regi-" men is generally proper. Some physicians indeed have re-" commended bleeding, and there may occur cases in which " bleeding may be useful ; but for the most part it is unnecessary, " and in many cases hurtful."

An opinion has prevailed, as respecting the other exanthemata, that blood-letting is apt to repel the eruption, which it is feared might be attended with bad consequences. Dr. Russell thought that in one case blood-letting had this effect. Direct experience is not sufficiently extensive and accurate to decide the question, whether blood-letting, if otherwise indicated, should be delayed when an eruption is expected ; if we admit of inference from analogy, it is easily answered.

We are led from analogy to believe that emetics may often be useful at the commencement of the plague, and they have sometimes been employed with advantage. " Vomiting," Dr. Alexander Russell,[*] observes, " was also of the utmost conse-" quence at the beginning." " The mode of treatment," says Dr. Guthrie, ."which the Russian physicians found the most " successful in the plague was, beginning with a vomit on the " appearance of the first symptoms, and working it off with acid " drinks. If the nausea and bitter taste in the mouth were not " relieved by the first, they gave a second and sometimes a third " and fourth ; nay if the symptoms were very urgent, they gave " two or three in the space of twelve hours, as there is no time " to be lost in this disease; for they did not find this evacuation " subject to the same objections as brisk purges, which a man " in the plague is unable to support." Dr. Patrick Russell also approves of emetics at the commencement, although the preju-dice of the Asiatics against them, prevented his employing them at an early period.

We have reason to believe, that in the progress of the disease they will seldom be of much service, unless when necessary for evacuating offending matter ; and by their debilitating effects they may do much harm. When retching occurs without vomit-ing, an emetic is often serviceable. When it fails to allay this symptom, opiates generally succeed.

There can be no doubt of the propriety of opiates for the pur-pose of allaying restlessness and procuring sleep in all cases

· * See his Natural History of Aleppo.

where the excitement is not considerable. Dr. Patrick Russell says he never saw them produce coma.

From what we observe in similar fevers, we should a priori believe, that much purging would prove pernicious in the plague ; but that gentle laxatives or clysters, sufficient to keep the body regular, would be found indispensible ; and a great part of this inference has been confirmed by experience.

Almost all physicians who have practised in the plague agree, that much purging is hurtful ; but I have already had occasion to observe, that costiveness appears to be less pernicious than we should have expected. A spontaneous diarrhœa in the plague is always a dangerous symptom ; on this account, in those places where the disease is frequent, there is the utmost dread of any means which tend to induce this symptom ; and this often proves an obstacle to the exhibition of any laxative or clyster however mild.

Suppositories are much used in Eastern countries, but even these are avoided in the plague, so that the patient often remains costive for a long time, and it is said without suffering from it.

We may say of this, as of blood-letting, that in a complaint the symptoms of which are so varied, it requires much experience to determine the effects of any mode of practice. But we have a double reason for drawing our conclusion cautiously, when the measures which appear safe have in similar cases been found per_nicious. Besides, although the common inconveniences of cos_tiveness be less felt in this complaint than in many others, it seems often to occasion an accumulation of irritating matter in the intestines, which sometimes induces the very symptom which we are endeavouring to prevent. Clysters or suppositories, as they are less apt to occasion diarrhœa, are preferable to cathartics taken by the mouth.

When diarrhœa does occur, whether spontaneously or from the use of cathartics. it is for the most part readily checked by opiates at the commencement of the disease ; but in the advanced stages, opiates, astringents. and every other means we can em-ploy, often fail to relieve this symptom, and then the prognosis is fatal.

" From some principles with respect to fever in general," Dr. Cullen observes, " and with respect to the plague in particular, I " am of opinion, that after the exhibition of the first vomit, the " body should be disposed to sweat, which ought to be raised to a " moderate degree only, but continued at least twenty-four hours " or longer, if the patient bears it easily."

We found in enumerating the symptoms of the plague, that spontaneous sweating is often attended with the best effects, and sometimes proves completely critical. There is however in most fevers a wide difference between the effects of spontaneous sweating and that produced by art, and we have reason to believe that the observations made on this subject, when speaking of continued fever, are applicable to the plague.

It has not been determined whether antimonial diaphoretics are useful in the plague. Dr. Russell thinks that, combined with opium, they promise to be serviceable.

Little is to be expected from valerian, contrayerva, bezoar, and other similar articles, regarded as diaphoretics, which have been celebrated in this complaint. Nor is much to be expected from camphire, which has also been particularly recommended.

A method of promoting sweat, however, very different from those employed in ordinary cases of fever, has lately been attended, it is said, with very great success. It was proposed by Mr. Baldwin, the British agent and consul general at Alexandria, in Egypt, and has been made known to the public by a small Treatise in the Italian language by Count Bertchtold; the following extract from which has been translated into different languages and circulated throughout Europe.

" The directions are simply these : immediately after a person
" is perceived to be infected with the plague he must be taken
" into a close room, and over a brazier of hot coals, with a clean
" sponge dipped in warm olive oil, his body must be very briskly
" rubbed all over, for the purpose of producing a profuse sweat.
" During the friction, sugar and juniper berries must be burnt in
" the fire, which raise a dense and hot smoke that contributes to
" the effect.

" The friction ought not to be continued more than four minutes,
" and a pint of oil is enough to be used at each time.

" In general, the first rubbing is followed by a very copious
" perspiration ; but should it fail of this effect, the operation may
" be repeated, first wiping the body with a warm dry cloth ; and
" in order still farther to promote perspiration, the patient may
" take any warm sudorific drink, such as elder-flower tea, &c.
" It is not necessary to touch the eyes; and other tender parts
" of the body may be rubbed more gently.

" Every possible precaution must be made use of to prevent
" the patient taking cold, such as keeping covered those parts of
" the body not directly under the operation ; nor must the linen
" be changed till the perspiration has entirely subsided.

" The operation should be repeated once a day, until evident
" symptoms of recovery begin to appear. If there are already
" tumours on the body, they should be gently and more frequently
" rubbed, till they appear to be in a state of suppuration, when
" they may be dressed with the usual plaisters.

" The operation ought to be begun on the first appearance of
" the symptoms of the disease; if neglected till the nerves and
" the mass of blood are affected, or a diarrhœa has commenced,
" little hopes can be entertained of cure; but still the patient
" should not be despaired of, as, by an assiduous application of
" the means proposed, some few have recovered even after diar-
" rhœa had commenced.

" During the first four or five days the patient must observe
" a very abstemious diet; the author allows only a small quan-
" tity of vermicelli, simply boiled in water. Nor must any thing
" be taken for the space of 30 or 40 days, except very light food;
" as, he says, an indigestion in any stage of the disorder might be
" extremely dangerous. He does not allow the use of wine till
" the expiration of forty days.

" There is no instance of the person rubbing a patient having
" taken the infection. He should previously anoint himself all
" over with oil, and must avoid receiving the breath of the infect-
" ed person into his mouth and nostrils. The prevention to be
" used, in all circumstances, is that of carefully anointing the
" body, and living upon light and easily digestible food."

Mr. Baldwin observes, that among upwards of a million of
people who died of the plague in Upper and Lower Egypt, during the space of four years, he could not discover a single oil-
man or dealer in oil.

With respect to diet there is nothing to be added to what
was said when speaking of continued fever. While the synocha
lasts it must be light and diluent, being rendered more stimulant
and nourishing in proportion as the fever assumes the form of
typhus. At all periods of the complaint acids and acidulous fruits
are serviceable, and while the synocha lasts, other refrigerants
should be employed. Nitre in particular has been much recommended.

I may here also refer to the treatment of continued fever, for
what was said respecting temperature and ventilation, and likewise respecting the use of bark, wine, and the other medicines
termed tonic. Although it has not been customary to employ
the latter medicines very freely in the plague, we have reason to
believe that they should be had recourse to, as early as the degree
of excitement admits of, and, after the typhus has commenced,
employed with the same freedom as in other cases of this fever.

Nor is any thing further to be said of the use of blisters and
rubefacients.

The buboes and carbuncles generally require some treatment,
but this part of the subject belongs to the province of surgery.

CHAP. VI.

Of the Urticaria.

THE Urticaria or Nettle-rash is defined by Dr. Cullen,

" Febris amphimerina.* Die secundo rubores maculosi urti-
" carum puncturas referentes. interdiu fere evanescentes, vespere
" cum febre redeuntes, et post paucos dies in squamulas minutis-
" simas abeuntes."

SECT. I.

Of the Symptoms of the Urticaria.

DR. Cullen remarks, that he gives the character of the nettle-
rash rather from the accounts of others than from his own observation, as he had seldom seen the disease, and never a single case
of it in which it run the course described in his definition.

Sydenham considers it a species of erysipelas, and describes it
to be a slight fever, soon followed by an eruption of small pustules over the whole body, resembling the appearance produced
by the stinging of nettles Vogel† regards it as characteristic of
this eruption that it comes out when the skin is exposed to cold,
and disappears when it is kept warm.

Small vesicles filled with matter are sometimes formed on the
tops of the pustules, or as Eller‡ observes, without any matter
forming in the pustules the cuticle breaks. which gives a roughness to the parts occupied by the eruption. This eruption is
attended with intolerable itching, and when it disappears, scratching is apt to renew it.

It appears most frequently, Burserius‖ and Vogel observe, on
the face, neck, and arms Before the appearance of the eruption, the former author remarks, an increase of debility and some
anxiety are frequently observed.

The eruption generally appears after the fever has lasted a few
hours, and for the most part relieves it. It is said in the definition,
that the eruption generally disappears in the day time, but accor-

---

* The term amphimerina is generally used to express a fever, which
returns daily and is always finished within the day, so that it is a quotidian intermittent. The term however has not always been employed in
precisely the same sense.

† Vogel's Prælect. Acad. de Cog. &c.

‡ De Cog. et Cur. Morb.

‖ Institut. Med. Pract.

ding to Burserius it sometimes remains out for two or three days.

Such are the symptoms of the urticaria which do not require to be considered at greater length. The complaint is seldom met with,* and is usually so trifling as to require no medical assistance.

Dr. Heberden† describes an eruption similar to that of the urticaria, which was unattended by fever. Burserius regards the essera of authors as a species of urticaria. It only differs from it in the pustules being generally larger and not itchy.

SECT. II.

Of the Causes of the Urticaria.

LITTLE has been determined concerning the causes of this complaint. We have reason to believe it, like many other eruptive fevers, connected with the state of the primæ viæ. Sydenham observes, that it occurs at all seasons of the year, and seems often produced by too free an use of thin wines or other similar liquors. Burserius says, he has seen it arise from irritating matter in the stomach, or from the perspiration being checked ; so that it is doubtful whether it be properly arranged among the exanthemata, from which it also differs in not being contagious. It however, seldom if ever, appears as a symptomatic affection, and in one species of it at least, that described in Dr. Cullen's definition, it is always preceded by fever.

SECT. III.

Of the Treatment of the Urticaria.

WITH regard to the treatment of this complaint, if it arises from impurities of the primæ viæ, these must be cleared. When this is not the case, it generally requires only a gentle laxative to prevent the irritation of retained fæces ; or if any thing else be necessary, the treatment is the same as in synocha. Vogel says of the essera that the retrocession of the eruption is not attended with danger.

* Vogel says it is not uncommon about Gottingen.
† See the first volume of the Medical Transactions.

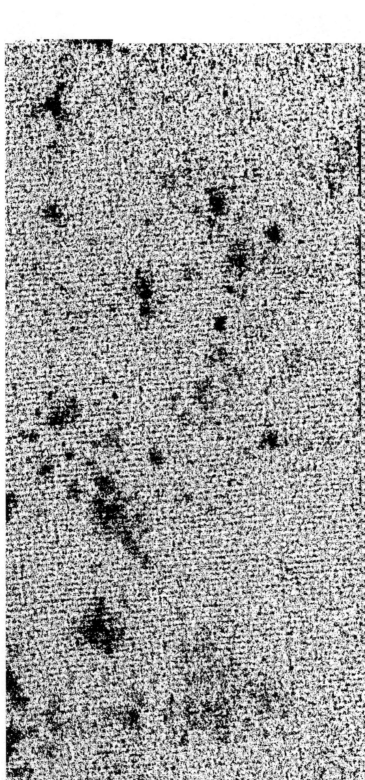

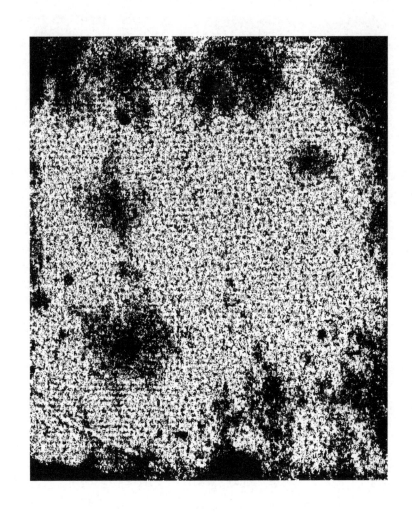

Lightning Source UK Ltd.
Milton Keynes UK
UKHW021925180219
337529UK00011B/978/P

9 780260 233943